EXECUTIVE FUNCTION IN EDUCATION

Executive Function in Education

FROM THEORY TO PRACTICE

Edited by Lynn Meltzer

THE GUILFORD PRESS
New York   London

© 2007 The Guilford Press
A Division of Guilford Publications, Inc.
72 Spring Street, New York, NY 10012
www.guilford.com

Printed in the United States of America

This book is printed on acid-free paper.

Last digit is print number: 9 8 7 6 5 4 3 2 1

Library of Congress Cataloging-in-Publication Data

Executive function in education : from theory to practice / Lynn Meltzer,
editor.
    p. cm.
   Includes bibliographical references and index.
   ISBN-13: 978-1-59385-428-7 (hardcover : alk. paper)
   ISBN-10: 1-59385-428-5 (hardcover : alk. paper)
   1. Educational psychology. 2. Executive ability in children. 3. Learning
disabled children—Education. I. Meltzer, Lynn.
   LB1057.E94 2007
   371.94—dc22

                                                          2006033425

To my parents, Jack and Thelma Segal,
who taught me that all my dreams could become a reality
with focus, determination, and resilience

To my husband, Peter, and my children, Colin and Danny,
for their unwavering support, flexibility, and use of humor
to maintain balance in our lives

About the Editor

Lynn Meltzer, PhD, is cofounder and codirector of the Institutes for Learning and Development (ILD and ResearchILD) in Lexington, Massachusetts. She holds appointments as an Associate in Education at the Harvard Graduate School of Education and as an Adjunct Associate Professor in the Tufts University Department of Child Development. For the past 4 years, she has been President of the International Academy for Research in Learning Disabilities. In her 25 years of clinical work with children, adolescents, and adults, Dr. Meltzer has emphasized the critical importance of the theory-to-practice cycle of knowledge. Her research, publications, and presentations have focused on understanding the complexity of learning and attention problems using a multidimensional model to bridge the gap between theory, research, and practice. Her extensive publications and professional presentations include articles, chapters, and books on the assessment and treatment of learning difficulties, with an emphasis on the importance of metacognition, strategy use, cognitive flexibility, self-concept, and resilience. Dr. Meltzer is the founder and chair of the national Learning Differences Conference, now in its 22nd year at the Harvard Graduate School of Education. She is on the editorial boards of a number of prestigious journals, including the *Journal of Learning Disabilities*. Her recent work, together with her ResearchILD colleagues, includes books for professionals (*Strategies for Success,* Pro-Ed, 2005) and parents (*Parent's Guide to Hassle-Free Homework,* Scholastic, 2007) and two award-winning interactive software products (BrainCogs and Essay Express), all with an emphasis on teaching metacognitive strategies and executive function processes.

Contributors

Mirit Barzillai, MEd, Research Institute for Learning and Development (ResearchILD), Lexington, Massachusetts

Jane Holmes Bernstein, PhD, Department of Psychiatry, Children's Hospital and Harvard Medical School, Boston, Massachusetts

Samantha G. Daley, MA, Harvard Graduate School of Education, Cambridge, Massachusetts

Martha Bridge Denckla, MD, Kennedy Krieger Institute, Baltimore, Maryland

Kurt W. Fischer, PhD, Harvard Graduate School of Education, Cambridge, Massachusetts

Howard Gardner, PhD, Harvard Graduate School of Education, Cambridge, Massachusetts

Irene West Gaskins, EdD, Benchmark School, Media, Pennsylvania

Steve Graham, EdD, Department of Special Education, Vanderbilt University, Nashville, Tennessee

Karen R. Harris, EdD, Department of Special Education, Vanderbilt University, Nashville, Tennessee

Kalyani Krishnan, MA, Research Institute for Learning and Development (ResearchILD), Lexington, Massachusetts

Lynn Meltzer, PhD, Institutes for Learning and Development (ILD and ResearchILD), Lexington, Massachusetts; Harvard Graduate School of Education, Cambridge, Massachusetts; and Department of Child Development, Tufts University, Medford, Massachusetts

Seana Moran, MA, Harvard Graduate School of Education, Cambridge, Massachusetts

Natalie Olinghouse, PhD, Department of Counseling, Educational Psychology, and Special Education, Michigan State University, East Lansing, Michigan

Sally Ozonoff, PhD, Department of Psychiatry and Behavioral Sciences, M.I.N.D. Institute, University of California at Davis, Sacramento, California

Laura Sales Pollica, MA, Research Institute for Learning and Development (ResearchILD), Lexington, Massachusetts

Michael Pressley, PhD (deceased), Department of Teacher Education and Department of Counseling, Educational Psychology, and Special Education, Michigan State University, East Lansing, Michigan

Bethany N. Roditi, PhD, Research Institute for Learning and Development (ResearchILD), Lexington, Massachusetts

David Rose, EdD, Center for Applied Special Technology, Wakefield, Massachusetts; Harvard Graduate School of Education, Cambridge, Massachusetts

Katherine Rose, BA, Yale School of Medicine, New Haven, Connecticut

Eric Satlow, PhD, Benchmark School, Media, Pennsylvania

Patricia L. Schetter, PhD, Autism and Behavior Training Associates, Woodland, California

Judith A. Stein, PhD, Research Institute for Learning and Development (ResearchILD), Lexington, Massachusetts

Joan Steinberg, MEd, Research Institute for Learning and Development (ResearchILD), Lexington, Massachusetts

Deborah P. Waber, PhD, Department of Psychiatry, Children's Hospital and Harvard Medical School, Boston, Massachusetts

Preface

Education should inspire students to turn their full intelligence on a problem, to think creatively, originally, and constructively instead of defensively, and to carry these new ways of thinking into new situations
—HOLT (1964, p. 27)

As we enter the 21st century with greater reliance on technological expertise, life success depends increasingly on the mastery of executive function processes such as goal setting, planning, organizing, prioritizing, memorizing, initiating, shifting, and self-monitoring. Beginning in the elementary grades, teachers now require students to complete lengthy reading and writing assignments, as well as long-term projects, both of which rely heavily on these executive function processes. Students are also expected to become proficient at note taking, studying, and test taking, all tasks that require the simultaneous organization and synthesis of multiple subprocesses. Academic success is thus dependent on students' ability to plan their time, organize and prioritize materials and information, distinguish main idea from details, shift approaches flexibly, monitor their own progress, and reflect on their work. Nevertheless, executive function processes are not taught systematically in schools and are not a focus of the curriculum, which primarily emphasizes competency and proficiency in the three Rs: *reading*, *writing*, and *arithmetic*. Furthermore, classroom instruction generally focuses on the content, or the *what*, rather than the process, or the *how*, of learning and does not systematically address metacognitive strategies that teach students to think about *how* they think and learn. As a result, a large gap separates the skills and strategies taught in school from the executive function processes needed for success there and in the workplace. Both these settings now require individuals to take greater responsibility for their independent learning and to organize and integrate an ever-changing body of information that is available through the Internet and other web-based media.

The rationale for writing this book stems from the current confusion surrounding explanations about the failure of so many students to perform at the level of their potential. In fact, as is emphasized by Denckla (1996, and Chapter 1, this volume), the concept of executive function emanates, in part, from the efforts of clinicians to explain why certain students present as "poor students" despite their strong performance on psychometric measures of intelligence and cognitive processes such as perception, memory, and language. This book brings together experts from a cross-section of disciplines and includes developmental, cognitive, and educational psychologists as well as neuropsychologists, neurologists, and educators. These experts provide a theoretical and conceptual framework for understanding executive function processes as well as methods of addressing these processes in various disorders and in the classroom. The four chapters in the first section of the book discuss the varied understandings of executive function processes and the "fuzzy definitions" that still abound (Lyon & Krasnegor, 1996). The authors focus on the challenges and opportunities that educational professionals face in an era of brain-based approaches to diagnosis and standards-based education. In the second part of the book, experts address the implications of executive function research for the assessment and treatment of students with language-based learning disabilities, nonverbal learning disabilities, and autism spectrum disorder. In the third part of the book, the chapters focus on approaches to teaching at the level of the individual child, the classroom, and the entire school. The authors discuss methods for systematically teaching strategies that address executive function processes, such as planning, organizing, prioritizing, memorizing, shifting, and checking. Specific teaching methods are discussed for enhancing executive function processes in the context of reading, writing, and math. A number of the chapters also focus on the importance of creating strategic classrooms that address executive function processes systematically in the context of a curriculum that provides the sustained support needed by all students.

In summary, the chapters in this volume present a broad range of perspectives that seek to integrate the neurosciences with education. Our hope is that this volume will help to clarify the confusion in the field surrounding the definition and critical role of executive function processes in learning. Our goals are to narrow the lingering gap between research and educational practice and to improve our methods of identifying and teaching students with executive function difficulties. We hope that schools will begin to shift their focus and teach strategies for lifelong learning so that students can perform at the level of their potential and gain an enduring education without sharing the sentiments of Albert Einstein that "education is what remains after one has forgotten everything one learned in school."

REFERENCES

Denckla, M. B. (1996). A theory and model of executive function: A neuropsychological perspective. In G. R. Lyon & N. A. Krasnegor (Eds.), *Attention, memory, and executive function.* Baltimore: Brookes.

Holt, J. (1964). *How children fail.* New York: Pitman.

Lyon, G. R., & Krasnegor, N. A. (Eds.). (1996). *Attention, memory, and executive function.* Baltimore: Brookes.

Acknowledgments

I would like to acknowledge a number of people whose support has been so important for the completion of this book. First, I would like to thank Rochelle Serwator, Editor, at The Guilford Press, for her energy, commitment, and willingness to problem-solve during the long process of creating a book, from the initial concepts and ideas to the final product. I am also grateful to all the staff members at Guilford for their help with the different stages of this project. Special thanks are due to the dedicated staff of the Research Institute for Learning and Development (ResearchILD) for their thoughtful suggestions, creative ideas, and help. Finally, my thanks to the many children and young adults whose struggles with their daily learning challenges have taught me so much about persistence, resilience, and the executive function processes that are the subject matter of this book.

> Explaining metaphysics to the nation
> I wish he would explain his explanation.
> —LORD BYRON, *Don Juan*

Contents

I. Executive Function: Theoretical and Conceptual Frameworks   **1**

1. Executive Function: Binding Together the Definitions   5
of Attention-Deficit/Hyperactivity Disorder
and Learning Disabilities
Martha Bridge Denckla

2. "Hill, Skill, and Will": Executive Function   19
from a Multiple-Intelligences Perspective
Seana Moran and Howard Gardner

3. Executive Capacities from a Developmental Perspective   39
Jane Holmes Bernstein and Deborah P. Waber

4. Connecting Cognitive Science and Neuroscience to Education: 55
Potentials and Pitfalls in Inferring Executive Processes
Kurt W. Fischer and Samantha G. Daley

II. Executive Function Difficulties in Different Diagnostic Groups: **73**
Challenges of Identification and Treatment

5. Executive Function Difficulties and Learning Disabilities: 77
Understandings and Misunderstandings
Lynn Meltzer and Kalyani Krishnan

6. Nonverbal Learning Disabilities and Executive Function: 106
The Challenges of Effective Assessment and Teaching
Judith A. Stein and Kalyani Krishnan

Contents

7. Executive Dysfunction in Autism Spectrum Disorders: 133
From Research to Practice
Sally Ozonoff and Patricia L. Schetter

III. Interventions to Address Executive Function Processes — 161

8. Executive Function in the Classroom: 165
Embedding Strategy Instruction into Daily Teaching Practices
Lynn Meltzer, Laura Sales Pollica, and Mirit Barzillai

9. Executive Control of Reading Comprehension 194
in the Elementary School
Irene West Gaskins, Eric Satlow, and Michael Pressley

10. Addressing Executive Function Problems in Writing: 216
An Example from the Self-Regulated Strategy Development Model
Steve Graham, Karen R. Harris, and Natalie Olinghouse

11. The Strategic Math Classroom: Executive Function Processes 237
and Mathematics Learning
Bethany N. Roditi and Joan Steinberg

12. Teaching Metacognitive Strategies That Address 261
Executive Function Processes within a Schoolwide Curriculum
Irene West Gaskins and Michael Pressley

13. Deficits in Executive Function Processes: 287
A Curriculum-Based Intervention
David Rose and Katherine Rose

Index 309

PART I

Executive Function

Theoretical and Conceptual Frameworks

Executive functions perhaps make possible many of the goals we live for and permit ways to identify and achieve those goals. However, to know where one is going, it is necessary to know where you have been and where you are. In this sense, development and elaboration of executive functions are critically dependent on memory and attention and, when built upon this foundation, can provide a basis for continuing adaptation, adjustment, and achievement throughout the life span.

—ESLINGER (1996, p. 392)

More than a decade after Eslinger's chapter was published in the seminal book *Attention, Memory, and Executive Function* (Lyon & Krasnegor, 1996), fuzzy definitions still abound. Furthermore, different theories and models still compete to explain the development of executive function processes. There is general agreement, however, that executive function is an umbrella term for the complex cognitive processes that serve ongoing, goal-directed behaviors. In this regard, most of the definitions of executive function include many, but not all, of the following elements:

- Goal setting and planning
- Organization of behaviors over time

1

- Flexibility
- Attention and memory systems that guide these processes (e.g., working memory)
- Self-regulatory processes such as self-monitoring

The authors in this section provide somewhat different conceptualizations of executive function processes, based on their theoretical roots in neurology, cognitive psychology, developmental psychology, and neuropsychology. The different chapters provide a microcosm of this emerging field that is still grappling to develop a unitary definition of executive function processes and to describe the relationship among cognition, metacognition, and executive function (Denckla, 1996, 2005; Lyon & Krasnegor, 1996). In the first chapter, Denckla presents a neuropsychological perspective in which she advocates a move away from the hierarchical models of executive function and emphasizes its central importance for cognition. She addresses the ideas that learning disabilities and attention-deficit disorders both influence and are influenced by the executive function domain and that the effects of "executive dysfunction" on students' performance change over time. In the next chapter, Moran and Gardner discuss the developmental trajectory of executive function processes in the context of Gardner's theory of multiple intelligences. They conceptualize executive function as the integration of three important parameters: hill, the establishment of a clear goal; skill, the abilities and techniques needed to attain this goal; and will, the volition to begin and persevere until the goal has been reached. Their paradigm provides a framework for the developmental perspective discussed by Holmes Bernstein and Waber, who emphasize that executive function processes are best understood as relatively domain-general resources that can be influenced by context and specific task demands. They also discuss caveats to the emphasis on the role of the frontal cortex in controlling executive function processes in the developing child. In the final chapter of this section, Fischer and Daley highlight the strengths and limitations of recent research in the cognitive and neurosciences for improving our diagnostic and intervention methods for executive function weaknesses in clinical and educational settings.

REFERENCES

Denckla, M. B. (1996). A theory and model of executive function: A neuropsychological perspective. In G. R. Lyon & N. A. Krasnegor (Eds.), *Attention, memory, and executive function.* Baltimore: Brookes.
Denckla, M. B. (2005). Executive function. In D. Gozal & D. Molfese (Eds.),

Attention deficit hyperactivity disorder: From genes to patients. Totowa, NJ: Humana Press.

Eslinger, P. J. (1996). Conceptualizing, describing, and measuring components of executive function: A summary. In G. R. Lyon & N. A. Krasnegor (Eds.), *Attention, memory, and executive function.* Baltimore: Brookes.

Lyon, G. R., & Krasnegor, N. A. (Eds.). (1996). *Attention, memory, and executive function.* Baltimore: Brookes.

CHAPTER 1

Executive Function

Binding Together the Definitions
of Attention-Deficit/Hyperactivity Disorder
and Learning Disabilities

MARTHA BRIDGE DENCKLA

The purpose of this chapter is to review the historical context in which the term "executive function" rose to a prominent position among descriptors of domains of neurocognitive elements relevant to developing children's adaptive repertoire.

EXECUTIVE FUNCTION DISORDERS: HISTORICAL OVERVIEW

The term "executive function" was familiar to those who were trained in adult-oriented behavioral neurology and kept up with developments in the elaboration of the dementias, especially cortical versus subcortical in origin. Thus it was of particular interest to learn in the late 1980s that no less an authority on a major developmental disability than Russell Barkley was beginning to talk and later write about deficient executive function as central to the meaning of the syndrome of attention-deficit/hyperactivity disorder (ADHD) (Barkley, 1997). Since 1980, the cognitive emphasis on "attention" has taken the lead position in terminology and has inspired theorizing about frontal lobe analog status of ADHD-related behaviors. Nevertheless, it was the more sophisticated cognitive neuroscience implied by the term "executive function" that captured the imaginations of behavioral neurologists and neuropsychologists devoted to disorders of development. The emerging possibilities of magnetic resonance imaging further enhanced the enthusiasm of researchers who wanted to explore both cortical and subcortical candidates for the brain locales most relevant to executive function (EF) and dysfunction (EDF). By 1991, Bruce Pennington had boldly outlined the neuropsychology of the most common non-retardation-associated developmental disabilities in a slender volume; he clearly placed reading and language disorders in a classically posterior (parietotemporal) frame of reference neurologically, while his ADHD/EDF localization pointed frontally (and to frontally interconnected regions) (Pennington, 1991). Most helpfully, in the 1990s, both Pennington and Harvey Levin produced normative developmental papers that began to elucidate the trajectory of executive control maturation (Levin, Culhane, Hartmann, Evankovich, & Mattson, 1991; Pennington, 1997). Levin's studies of children with traumatic brain injuries showed how similar their most common clinical pictures were both to ADHD and to frontal lobe injury, thus closing the theoretical circle implied in the speculations of the 1980s (Levin et al., 1993). Furthermore, as cognitive phenotyping became a popular side effect of the era of genetics and was correlated with magnetic resonance imaging, it emerged that a very common neurogenetic disorder, neurofibromatosis 1 (NF1), frequently presented with ADHD-syndromic characteristics and with demonstrably subcortical abnormalities (Koth, Cutting, & Denckla, 2001). It was ever clearer that there were three levels of description to be connected: (1) ADHD at the surface syndromic level; (2) EDF at the intermediate cognitive analysis level; and (3) not just frontal but striatal and cerebellar localizations at the neurological level. Heterogeneity characterized each level, most clearly at the neurological level, but many subdivisions of the ADHD syndrome are still debated, and certainly the domain of EF is a broad-ranging one (Denckla, 2005).

EF AND EDF: CONNECTING THE MEDICAL AND EDUCATIONAL PERSPECTIVES

Departing from the neuropsychiatric and neuropsychological perspectives (which together might be called "the medical model"), those who are comfortable with EF/EDF terminology can communicate with the important related fields of education and educational psychology by translating or analyzing EF into more familiar words like planning, organization, study skills, and self-monitoring/checking skills. These are all terms of less strange or formidable resonance than is EF and exist in literature concerning learning disabilities (LDs) and special education as far back as 40 years ago. More problematic are how the domains of "attention" and "memory" straddle the concepts as understood between the brain-based and the school-based backgrounds of various professions. Those of us from the brain-based disciplines are notorious "splitters," who are comfortable explaining that some aspects of attention (indeed, executive/selective or "top-down") and some aspects of memory (working memory, not short-term or long-term) are subsumed under the "executive" domain. Rather than being theory-driven, these "splits" or distinctions are grounded in a systems-and-circuits analysis of the brain.

Less helpful to all who wish to communicate about and apply the concepts summarized under the EF/EDF nomenclature is the prefix "meta-" as applied to cognition; thus, even the recently developed Behavior Rating Inventory of Executive Function (Gioia, Isquith, Guy, & Kenworthy, 1996) could be faulted for choosing "*meta*cognitive" as the name for the index under which are grouped Initiation, Working Memory, Planning/Organizing, Organizing Materials, Self-Monitoring (Gioia et al., 1996). The "meta-" prefix gets us into the difficulty exemplified by Seana Moran and Howard Gardner's chapter (see Chapter 2, this volume), or what is essentially a "homunculus" dilemma, in which there is a sort of little meta-person running all of cognition. Since EF develops slowly, starting at about 9 months of postnatal age and continuing into the early part of the fourth decade of life, the "meta-" prefix may be unnecessarily static. In terms of observed behaviors and brain system/circuitry, EF starts as much as infrastructure for other cognitive systems as overseer thereof; EF develops in a constant back-and-forth, up-and-down, interactive, looping fashion involving other cognitive domains. For example, the "baby step" of sensorimotor inhibition, permitting delayed responding, is an EF infrastructure that permits choice responses to sensory discrimination, which in turn provides the substrate for selective attention (Diamond, 2000). Another example of a developmental spiraling loop is that without the building blocks of words one cannot provide the central EF working memory with the ingredients to be worked on; yet, without working memory, one cannot develop receptive language for complex sentences.

Like "higher cortical function" in the medical model or "higher-order thinking skills" in the educational model, "meta-cognition" is a term that disguises the developmental dynamics of EF, leading us to ignore many subcortical contributions in the brain.

Thus, we need to put EF/EDF back on a humbler, more equal footing with other domains of brain–behavior correlative functions, like language, visual–spatial ability, visual object discrimination, verbal and visual memory storage, motor coordination learning, social skill learning, and the other system/circuit-based modular brain functions displayed in a Howard Gardner chart. No "higher" (and sometimes "lower" than any of these well-described ingredients of cognition) are the harder-to-describe action controls (initiate, sustain, shift, inhibit) subsumed under EF. Perhaps, just as the elaborated view of visual (and, more recently, auditory) perceptions is colloquially captured as "where" and "when" functions, we could speak of EF as encompassing "how and when" functions. Even more colloquially, speaking to adolescents and parents, EF can be defined as "getting your act together." (There are also earlier-developing elements of the EF domain, such as inhibition and delayed responding, that are not so conscious or effortful, yet provide the infrastructure for speed and refinement of action and stand at the interface between basic automatic motor and more intentional output efficiencies.) Much is to be gained by avoiding fancy words when laboring to describe and hopefully understand EF/EDF in a developmental context.

EDF: THE BRIDGE BETWEEN ADHD AND LDs

In a practical and applied context, there appeared about 20 years ago to be comorbidity between the diagnostic categories of ADHD and LDs, the source of which turned out to be best described as EDF. Using different summarizing terminology but descriptive assessment data clearly convergent upon EDF, health care and educational professionals began to try to document in research studies what they could observe in clinics and/or classrooms. The results so far have been relatively unimpressive, at least in terms of replicability; the subject heterogeneity within each category (ADHD and LDs) and the sparsely normed or inadequately control-sampled assessment instruments leave plenty of questions. The one subdomain of EDF that has repeatedly emerged as ADHD-related is that of inhibitory control (Barkley, 1997; Denckla, 2005). The other aspect of EDF is more elusive, lacking even a name, and that is "excessive variability." The index of inadequate inhibitory executive control is found in many studies of children with ADHD and in some (largely language-mediated) studies of children with LDs, which usually means reading disability (RD) (Block, 1993; Lovett et al., 1994; Loranger, 1997; Rosenshine & Meister, 1997; Vidal-Abarca & Gilabert, 1995). Further complicating understanding of EDF in either general category

(ADHD or LD) is the rather perfunctory way in which each-comorbid-with-the-other is delineated within most published studies.

For example, many neuropsychologically oriented studies of EF/EDF in populations with ADHD do not explicitly exclude or covary for LD. It has proven difficult in research studies to control for the cognitive demands that constitute the "ingredients" of tasks purported to target EF, since in group studies individual variations in capacity, even when controlled on a group basis, may obscure the EF component; for example, an individual with great verbal gifts may appear unimpaired on a verbal fluency task because the abundant lexicon, the substance or "ingredient" of the task, obviates or compensates for the need to "search the lexicon." (It would be as if for such a person items spill out of an overflowing basket rather than having to be rummaged around for and plucked from the depths of the basket.) What is done more easily on a clinical basis, the intraindividual profiling resulting in conclusions such as, "For a person with superior verbal ability, it is striking that the verbal fluency score is barely average," seems persistently difficult in a study with statistics focused on between-group differences controlling groupwise for broad-brush indices (like IQ scores) of cognitive comparability. Thus far, even in the hands of those who have tried to construct variable-by-variable "ingredient-controlled" EF measures, the traditional studies have failed to reflect the clinical experiences (Denckla, 2005).

Another difficulty in documenting the role of EF, beyond heterogeneity of the cognitive profiles aside from EF, is the breadth of functions and developmental dynamics of what is included under EF. As a clinician who may have the privilege of following individuals from kindergarten through college, one may see that the component of EF glaringly apparent at one age is later replaced by another component. Furthermore, in patients with the diagnosis of ADHD, the developmental dynamics often do not (but sometimes do) parallel the hierarchy of EF components reported in normative studies (although rare is the truly longitudinal, as opposed to the cross-sectional, age-related data). Clinically, across the school-age portion of the lifespan, what is often surprising is that the more advanced or demanding components of the EF domain "leapfrog" the basic or infrastructural elements. One may see, in clinic, college students with ADHD who excel at Tower tasks or Proverb interpretations while failing dismally a search-and-circle task that involves target and nontarget shapes and was originally designed for preliterate kindergartners. While this disparity may reflect underlying brain localization to more basic/infrastructural circuits still impaired but compensated for by later, more adequate cortical development, it is equally possible that the boring nature of the basic/infrastructural tasks cannot trigger the gratifyingly novel and intrinsically interesting higher-order challenges to EF. At each age/stage, therefore, it would be desirable to contrast the basic/infrastructural component with the novel/challenging component of EF and track each longitudinally. Of course, such a design would tax the ingenuity of researchers to come up with multiple novel developmentally appropriate forms of each component assessment.

Dividing the EF domain into these low-level and high-level components might provide behavioral data to correlate with the three levels of the brain (and their reciprocal interconnected circuits) under scrutiny in ADHD: frontal, striatal, and cerebellar. At the crossroads of all, we cannot forget the thalamus—and in traumatic brain injury (Gerring et al., 2000) and NF1 (Wang, Kaufmann, Koth, Denckla, & Barker, 2000) ADHD-like syndromes can be correlated with thalamic pathology. It is possible that once our magnetic resonance imaging techniques have made possible some sorting out of ADHD, not on the basis of clinical subtypes, but on the basis of brain localization, the developmental dynamics of "low-level" and "high-level" EF components may be similarly sorted. We may, however, be in for some surprises. Hierarchically based notions of subcortical being "below" may be turned upside down, especially in regard to the cerebellum. The status of the cerebellum has too long been concretely conceived under the influence of its posterior and inferior geography, forgetting that its name means "little cerebrum."

In short, there is heterogeneity within the most common clinical developmental syndrome associated with EDF (ADHD), within the brains of those with ADHD, and within the EF domain.

IMPLICATIONS FOR THE DIAGNOSIS OF ADHD AND LDs

With all this heterogeneity, is it too confusing to bring EF/EDF into the educational landscape? Does such a preliminarily and tentatively understood aspect of brain development provide improved understanding of the life histories of those with just plain LD or just plain ADHD versus LD-plus-ADHD? The remainder of this volume will answer these two questions in various ways. This chapter comes down on the side of yes; a few examples follow, case composites of how the EF factor plays out in each of the three major categories (LD, ADHD, and LD-plus-ADHD). These examples are drawn from clinical experience and illuminated by a research-derived framework.

Language-based LDs that appear to be complicated by ADHD, what have sometimes been described as "dyslexia-plus," in clinical follow-up often resolve themselves into language-based LDs complicated by performance anxiety (giving rise to restlessness) and/or a kind of overload/exhaustion phenomenon (giving the appearance of inattentiveness). At younger ages, children struggling with school skills often meet criteria for ADHD of one type or another and even seem to do poorly on those challenges to EF that are assessed with words (verbal content), depending upon the "phonological loop" to subserve verbal working memory or word retrieval to subserve speed-based assessments of fluency. Even with recent improvements, there are still many "pseudo-ADHD" and "pseudo-dysexecutive" pronouncements made about elementary-school-age children with language-based LDs; if re-evaluated in middle and high school, such children often show remarkable late blooming of their executive abilities, even strategically on verbal learning tests, but most obviously on more visual–spatially loaded tasks, such as Tower Task or Design Fluency. Working memory for purely verbal instruction, including lectures and unillustrated written text, remains the victim of many a persistently weak phonological loop (Baddeley, 1983). In addition, those students with language-based LDs who have remained in environments that do not reduce their performance anxiety will show the secondary type of EDF that anxiety can produce and/or maintain. As high-stakes testing and overzealous homework assignments have escalated in recent years, the role of anxiety as EDF generator/perpetuator/amplifier has made assessment of tweens and teens remarkably complicated. (It seems of late that clinicians have time-traveled back more than three decades, when referral questions were often phrased, "Is this child's school problem neurodevelopmental or emotional?") Under optimal environmental conditions, the clinician may see the emergence of valuable compensatory executive competence in adolescents whose language issues may even cause more academic underachievement than before (a subject for an entire chapter in itself). The general picture of adaptive development, however, even academically, looks remarkably successful. Optimal conditions include not only direct skills remediation, but also accommodations in curriculum, teacher style, and assessment/feedback; at home and personally, understanding of what a weak language system does and does not imply, for the present and the future, is essential.

As for the child with ADHD and EDF (let us for the moment focus on the one without any LD) there may be an impact on basic reading skills. One little boy of 8 years captured the EDF issue better than most professionals do; he explained that although he could recite the rule of the silent terminal *e* and explain short and long vowels, he found that when he got involved in reading text, he "forgot to look ahead." He could recall the strategy but forgot to be strategic, the very "curious dissociation between knowing and doing" that is at the core of EDF. As this child grew older, the repetitive practice effect obviated strategic approaches, but he did poorly in extracting from texts answers to questions posed by teachers to assess reading comprehension. Written expression, with all its planning, organizing, and formal rules to be applied, became the next academic struggle for a boy with quite excellent "ingredients" of all cognitive domains other than that of EF. In such a way do those with EDF (usually, but not always, attached to an ADHD diagnosis) grow into school-assessed LD, written expression first in prevalence and reading comprehension next (Singer, Schuerholz, & Denckla, 1995).

When assessed clinically, the purely ADHD/EDF profile loses over time the prominence of motor correlates of ADHD such as overflow (a subclass of which is known as mirror movements). ADHD is defined by impairments at the level of cognitive and behavioral control, with deficits in response inhibition contributing to excessive impulsive, hyperactive, and/or inattentive behavior. In contrast, impairments in motor control have been identified as a defining feature of developmental coordination disorder (DCD), which is commonly comorbid with ADHD (Denckla & Rudel, 1978; Diamond, 2000; Schuerholz, Cutting, Mazzoco, Singer, & Denckla, 1997). The clinical overlap between the two disorders likely reflects common abnormalities in parallel frontal-subcortical circuits distinctly involved in cognitive, behavioral, and motor control. Dysfunction within the circuits involved in cognitive and behavioral control may contribute to impairments in effortful response inhibition (as assessed on go/no-go and Stop Signal tasks), whereas dysfunction within the circuits involved with the motor executive may contribute to impaired motor control, including failure to inhibit extraneous overflow movements. Overflow movements, of which children are not even aware, occur at an automatic level. It is therefore unlikely that overflow movements, which are not under effortful control, are a direct consequence of higher-level impairments in response inhibition. The co-occurrence of overflow movements and impaired response inhibition in children with ADHD more likely reflects common dysfunction across parallel circuits. The anomalous motor signs observed in children with ADHD (in particular, impaired inhibition of overflow movements) are therefore viewed as potentially important co-localizing biomarkers for behavioral abnormalities associated with ADHD of inhibitory immaturity/insufficiency. Similarly, slow-for-age movements, skill milestones (like hopping), and slow reaction times on various versions of continuous performance tasks slow completion times (color-naming) are seen in elementary school-age children with ADHD but generally become less prominent at pubertal or postpubertal ages (Denckla, 2005). The inhibitory insufficiency comes out as rule breaking, intrusions, digressions,

and commissions or false positives. On the verbal side, where more practice and less novelty is usual, verbally gifted adolescents with ADHD/
EDF may by virtue of sheer "ingredient" superiority coupled with practice look very good even on a timed task like Word Fluency but
are remarkably challenged by here-and-now online memorization such
as the California Verbal Learning Test for Children (Cutting, Koth,
Mahone, & Denckla, 2003). Research groups have been surprised to
find that very amply verbal youngsters with ADHD are characterized
not only by poor semantic clustering or error excesses, but also by poor
levels of recall and recognition. Thus, there appears to be a very literal
route whereby the non-LD but ADHD/EDF status of a student may wilt
into difficulty in learning all that must be memorized in the curriculum
of the higher grades, even starting with the second half of elementary
school.

EDF IN ADHD AND LDs:
IMPLICATIONS FOR EDUCATIONAL INTERVENTION

From time to time, research studies support clinical observations, not
subjected to statistics yet advantageous in their longitudinal nature, that
suggest that EDF, even when unaccompanied by cognitive weaknesses in
other school-relevant domains, carries a risk of academic early wilting,
whereas the language-based difficulties, no less academically serious,
may with proper handling permit late blooming in subjects or in accom-
modative curricula that permit foreign language exemptions or give latitude to capabilities other than the specifically linguistic (narrower than
"verbal").

The developmental dynamics of interaction between LD and EDF
(usually, but not always, manifest as ADHD) show up in the life histories
of the substantial overlap group, those who are first diagnosed with LD
and ADHD. Behaviorally, meaning at play and in the non-academic
pauses punctuating the early years in school, the troubles of this LD/
ADHD group are predictable from studies concerning self-regulation by
speech (Vygotsky, 1962), and self-regulation by speech also predicts cognitive issues such as affect or stabilization of perception. Most LD is language-based, no matter how subtle. Weaknesses in the language/speech
system and the regulation-of-behavior system make each other worse,
while the normal early development of each facilitates the maturation of
the other. Just as a physiological system like vision requires visual input
to mature properly, in a process recognized as activity-dependent brain
development, so too are there brain-to-brain activity-dependent developmental dynamics; furthermore, these are not unidirectional, although in

the case of language the normal sequence of outward production appears strikingly more obvious than does the self-regulatory executive control. This outward asymmetry may overemphasize unidirectional hierarchy (EF "later and higher") because human beings use language so preferentially in their interpersonal relations that they may not notice the recursive loop whereby delayed responding facilitates the nature and content of the child's communication (verbal and nonverbal). In social negotiations with authority figures and/or peers, these mutually activity-dependent relations between language and executive capacities are probably of even greater importance than in academic success, although more elusive to document or quantify.

Unlike the language-gifted dysexecutive young child, the doubly deficient (LD/ADHD) cannot learn to read by doing what comes naturally. (In terms of selective attention, such a child cannot learn with "half an eye and half an ear.") This is because the cognitive capacity for sound–symbol association must be selectively attended to unless one is blessed with a superabundance of this "ear for language." In terms of working memory, again one is in double trouble if both phonological loop and central executive are weak senders and receivers of each other's processing. The LD/ADHD combination is a more fortunate one than the ADHD-alone profile in terms of probable early recognition of an academic skills deficit and a well-established processing deficit enfranchising an individualized education plan (IEP) into which are incorporated the ADHD-related (albeit not separately specified as such) dysexecutive needs; this is the source and rationale for organizational planning (often called "sequencing" in an LD context) and working memory (often called "short-term memory"), aspects of EF long recognized in special education. In digging these aspects of LD, as it were, out from under the LD coverage in IEPs and recognizing their overlap with the cognitive correlates of ADHD alone, assigning this overlap domain the name EF/EDF, these issues have been articulated only lately; this lateness echoes what happens late in the school careers of children with ADHD. Unfortunate enough to learn early skills with "half an eye and half an ear," linguistically gifted children with ADHD/EDF have also benefited from the greater degree of structure, supervision, and support afforded by elementary school. By middle school (which has been pushed back often to start with sixth grade and sometimes fifth or even fourth grade), the shift to greater expectations of independence, responsibility, planning, organization, and keeping in mind (i.e., in working memory) a complex schedule/agenda of school and other activities will cause a crash even for this early-succeeding child with ADHD/EDF. Since no IEP was seen as needed before middle school, at most there a

504 Plan will be offered. (Ill-conceived for ADHD as we now understand it, since the language of the law that is parent to 504 speaks of "limited alertness," the 504 Plan rarely comes near meeting EDF needs.)

Almost as unlucky by middle school is the mixed LD/ADHD profile. Because the underpinnings of the LD part, the processing deficit, may have been only moderate but amplified by the EDF bundled under the ADHD part of the profile, the elementary school IEP may have sufficed to bring the child with this profile to the door of the middle school with assessed-as-adequate academic skills. This child, too, will be at risk from the escalated demand for EF in middle school and, without continued special education support, will also be in danger of both slipping backward in academic skills and being dysexecutively unable to build on and apply academic skills in the independent and responsible manner expected. Dysexecutive children in middle school are in danger of being emotionally traumatized by being called lazy, unmotivated, irresponsible, and other such words implying moral turpitude instead of neurodevelopmental disability or immaturity. Probably the greatest value in recognizing the neurodevelopmental/neurocognitive domain called EF is to protect a sizable minority of children from being traumatized by what amounts to adult name-calling. Much research needs to focus on the milestones and progression of brain development subserving EF so that for middle school the educational construct of "school readiness" can be given neurodevelopmental rationale. (Sadly, the educational establishment seems to have ignored or perhaps misinterpreted "readiness" at the academic entry level, so middle school will be challenging to address.)

Why has linguistic domain interaction with the executive domain been stressed and other cognitive domains (e.g., visuospatial) ignored in this chapter? This book is about the classroom, and in terms of academic skills the nonlinguistic endowments (strong or weak) of a student ordinarily account for very little of success or failure, although strong endowments may help in compensatory ways to avoid failure. The phrase "compensatory ways," however, implies the use of EF to bring to bear upon academic skills the nonlinguistic strengths that are ordinarily of minimal relevance. The dysexecutive child will need a coach or tutor to become explicitly aware of how to use his or her strengths as compensatory. Sometimes a language-deficient child will arrive at a visualization strategy for a verbal retrieval task on his or her own, but surely that child is not one who suffers from ADHD/EDF. Another example is that of the child with weak visuospatial capacity (expected to influence negatively arithmetical calculation skill acquisition) who uses strong EF strategies to compensate by calling upon strong linguistic and verbal memory capacities. The problem is that often the child with a language-based LD but free of ADHD may lack in academic settings the self-confidence and freedom from anxiety to call upon strong executive strategies; yet that very same child will show EF in athletic, social, musical, and other performing artistic pursuits. The neuropsychological evaluation may be needed to act as a form of cognitive-behavioral therapy by interpreting results and explaining to the child in positive terms the EF strengths that can, with some coaching, be brought to bear on the language-loaded academic challenges.

CONCLUSION

The EF domain as it influences the student in the classroom is not above other cognitive domains, not some reified and exalted higher-order pinnacle of cognition, not meta- but intra- and intercognitive. A homely analogy that seems to get the idea of EF across to youngsters and parents is as follows: to put a cooked meal on the table, the cook needs both the ingredients and recipes for the component dishes. No meal is produced simply by setting out a bunch of ingredients; equally, there is nothing to eat in a book or a recitation of recipes. The "how and when" of EF is meaningless without reciprocal interaction with other cognitive and motor domains.

REFERENCES

Baddeley, A. D. (1983). Working memory. *Philosophical Transactions Royal Society London Biological Sciences, 302*, 311–324.

Barkley, R. A. (1997). *ADHD and the nature of self-control.* New York: Guilford Press.

Block, C. C. (1993). Strategy instruction in a literature-based reading program. Special issue: Strategies instruction. *Elementary School Journal, 94*(2), 139–151.

Cutting, L. E., Koth, C. W., Mahone, E. M., & Denckla, M. B. (2003). Evidence for unexpected weaknesses in learning in children with attention deficit hyperactivity disorder without reading disabilities. *Journal of Learning Disabilities, 36*(3), 259–269.

Delis, D. C., Kaplan, E., & Kramer, J. H. (2001). *The Delis–Kaplan Executive Function System.* San Antonio, TX: Psychological Corporation.

Denckla, M. B. (2005). Executive function. In D. Gozal & D. Molfese (Eds.), *Attention deficit hyperactivity disorder: From genes to patients* (pp. 165–183). Totowa, NJ: Humana Press.

Denckla, M. B., & Rudel, R. G. (1978). Anomalies of motor development in hyperactive boys without learning disabilities. *Annals of Neurology, 3,* 231–233.

Diamond, A. (2000). Close interrelation of motor development and cognitive development and of the cerebellum and prefrontal cortex. *Child Development, 71,* 44–56.

Gerring, J., Brady, K., Chen, A., Quinn, C., Herskovits, E., Bandeen-Roche, K., et al. (2000). Neuroimaging variables related to development of secondary attention deficit hyperactivity disorder after closed head injury in children and adolescents. *Brain Injury, 14*(3), 205–218.

Gioia, G. A., Isquith, P. K., Guy, S. C., & Kenworthy, L. (1996). *Behavior Rating Inventory of Executive Function.* Odessa, FL: Psychology Assessment Resources, Inc.

Koth, C. W., Cutting, L. E., & Denckla, M. B. (2001). The association of neurofibromatosis type 1 and attention deficit hyperactivity disorder. *Child Neuropsychology, 6*(3), 185–194.

Levin, H. S., Culhane, K. A., Hartmann, J., Evankovich, K., & Mattson, A. J. (1991). Developmental changes in performance on tests of purported frontal lobe functioning. *Developmental Neuropsychology, 7,* 377–395.

Levin, H. S., Culhane, K. A., Mendelsohn, D., Lilly, M. A., Bruce, D., Fletcher, J. M., et al. (1993). Cognition in relation to magnetic resonance imaging in head-injured children and adolescents. *Archives of Neurology, 50,* 897–905.

Loranger, A. L. (1997). Comprehension strategies instruction: Does it make a difference? *Reading Psychology, 18*(1), 31–68.

Lovett, M., Borden, S., DeLuca, T., Lacerenza, L., Benson, N., & Brackstone, D. (1994). Treating the core deficits of developmental dyslexia: Evidence of transfer of learning after phonologically- and strategy-based reading training programs. *Developmental Psychology, 30,* 805–822.

Pennington, B. F. (1991). Attention deficit hyperactivity disorder. In *Diagnosing learning disorders: A neuropsychological framework* (pp. 82–110). New York: Guilford Press.

Pennington, B. F. (1997). Dimensions of executive function in normal and abnormal development. In N. A. Krasnegor & G. R. Lyon (Eds.), *Development of the prefrontal cortex: Evolution, neurobiology and behavior* (pp. 265–281). Baltimore: Brookes.

Rosenshine, B., & Meister, C. (1997). Cognitive strategy instruction in reading. In S. Stahl & D. Hayes (Eds.), *Instructional models in reading* (pp. 85–107). Mahwah, NJ: Erlbaum.

Schuerholz, L. J., Cutting, L., Mazzocco, M. M. M., Singer, H. S., & Denckla, M. B. (1997). Neuromotor functioning in children with Tourette syndrome with and without attention deficit hyperactivity disorder. *Journal of Child Neurology, 12*(7), 438–442.

Singer, H. S., Schuerholz, L. J., & Denckla, M. B. (1995). Learning difficulties in children with Tourette syndrome. *Journal of Child Neurology, 10,* S58–S61.

Vidal-Abarca, E., & Gilabert, R. (1995). Teaching strategies to create visual representations of key ideas in content area text materials: A long-term intervention inserted in school curriculum. Special issue: Process oriented instruction: Improving student learning. *European Journal of Psychology of Education*, 10(4), 433–447.

Vygotsky, L. S. (1962). *Thought and language*. Cambridge, MA: MIT Press.

Wang, P. Y., Kaufmann, W. F., Koth, C. W., Denckla, M. B., & Barker, P. B. (2000). Thalamic involvement in Neurofibromatosis type 1: Evaluation with proton magnetic resonance spectroscopic imaging. *Annals of Neurology*, 47, 477–484.

CHAPTER 2

"Hill, Skill, and Will"

Executive Function
from a Multiple-Intelligences Perspective

SEANA MORAN
HOWARD GARDNER

A toddler forming a sentence. A kindergartner reciting the alphabet in order. A ninth-grader staying in sync with her clique. A college senior interviewing for a job. A writer formulating his next newspaper column. An entrepreneur strategizing the company's initial public stock offering. Despite the vast array of ages, tasks, and situations, these events all involve executive function, the mental process of planning and organizing flexible, strategic, appropriate actions.

Executive function regulates a person's goal-directed behavior. It contextualizes intended actions in light of past knowledge and experience, current situational cues, expectations of the future, and personally relevant values and purposes. It provides a sense of readiness, agency, flexibility, and coherence. Researchers have conceptualized executive function in terms of metacognition, inhibiting habitual responses, delay of gratification, adjusting to changing rules, and making decisions under uncertain conditions (see review in Zelazo, Carter, Reznick, & Frye, 1997).

In this chapter, we examine executive function from a multiple-intelligences and a developmental perspective. We propose that executive function emerges from intrapersonal intelligence, the computational capacity to discern and use information about oneself. Executive function regulates a person's behavior by orchestrating the other intelligences toward self-relevant purposes within and across temporal, social, and psychological contexts. Drawing on long-established categories of human psychology, we construe executive function as the integration of three parameters: *hill*—the establishment of a clear goal; *skill*—the requisite abilities and techniques for attaining that goal; and *will*—the volition to begin and persevere until the goal has been reached.

These parameters become more complexly integrated with age and experience. We propose that executive function operates differently at different stages in life as a result of the ways these parameters affect each other. In an admitted simplification, we address two broad stages: the apprentice stage, in which executive function comprises primarily internalized, culture-driven control over one's identity; and the master stage, in which executive function comprises primarily personally defined or idiosyncratically driven control over one's productivity.

To explore these ideas, we provide an overview of intrapersonal intelligence and executive function followed by vignettes of how executive function works at the different stages. We conclude with implications for how educators might influence the development of executive function.

INTRAPERSONAL INTELLIGENCE

Except in cases of severe congenital or acquired brain damage, everyone exhibits some level of each of the eight intelligences: musical, bodily-kinesthetic, naturalistic, linguistic, logical–mathematical, spatial, interpersonal, and intrapersonal. Many individuals have "searchlight" profiles composed of a relatively equal balance of several intelligences, but many others, especially those who work in creative areas like the arts and sciences, have "laser" profiles composed of one or two dominant intelligences. These different profiles provide different dispositions and capabilities for learning within various domains; as a result, one encounters individual differences among performances within a domain as well as differential developmental trajectories, such as career paths (Gardner, 2006).

According to multiple-intelligences theory, an intelligence (1) is a biopsychological potential sensitive to a particular type of information; (2) draws on particular brain regions; (3) can be assessed to show individual differences in realization, including extreme cases such as savants, prodigies, and grand masters; and (4) has a distinctive developmental pathway and evolutionary history (Gardner, 1983, 2006). We address each of these criteria for intrapersonal intelligence.

Intrapersonal intelligence is a cognitive capacity that processes self-relevant information. It analyzes and provides coherence to abilities, emotions, beliefs, aspirations, bodily sensations, and self-related representations in two ways: increasingly complex understandings of oneself (self-awareness) and increasingly complex orchestration of aspects of oneself within situations (executive function). Intrapersonal intelligence simplifies the vast amounts of information a person receives or generates by subjectifying it, turning "it is" information into "I want/need" or "for me" information.

Intrapersonal functions are typically believed to be mediated in the brain's frontal lobes, especially the right hemisphere. Damage to these areas can alter one's personality, self-esteem, moral perspective, and ability to make sense of one's emotions. It can lead to lack of insight into one's condition as well as general problems of self-planning, self-organization, and self-regulation (e.g., Damasio, 1999). These same regions are implicated in neuroimaging studies of executive function (e.g., Goldberg, 2001).

People vary greatly in how well they can immerse themselves in, distinguish among, monitor, evaluate, express, and grow from self-relevant kinds of information (e.g., Wilson & Dunn, 2004). Autism is considered the extreme condition for impaired intrapersonal intelligence; autistic individuals have difficulty framing their own (and others') emotions, thoughts, and behaviors in terms of a self. Although we are aware of no study of intrapersonal prodigies or "early bloomers," there are records—especially diaries and journals—of people who seem to be exceptional in their self-awareness and self-reflection (e.g., Virginia Woolf in Gardner, 1997; see Wilson & Dunn, 2004) and self-orchestration toward highly ambitious purposes (e.g., Colby & Damon, 1994).

Intrapersonal intelligence is one of the most recent intelligences to evolve phylogenetically and one of the latest faculties to mature in individuals. Its adaptive advantage became clear as humans needed strategies for living together harmoniously within a society (Baumeister, DeWall, Ciarocco, & Twenge, 2005; Terrace & Metcalfe, 2005). The self-relevance loop provided by intrapersonal intelligence helps simplify the complexity that results from social interaction and future orientation (e.g., Goldberg, 2001). This loop is not built in from birth; rather, intrapersonal intelligence emerges in the second year of life and develops well into middle adulthood. Infants' sensations come to convey reliable information about needs and desires; young toddlers understand that the images in the mirror are themselves; older toddlers use personal pronouns and develop a theory of mind; and school-age children, adolescents, and adults increasingly devise appropriate ways to interpret, express, and project themselves into social contexts and future scenarios (see Higgins, 2005; Kochanska, Coy, & Murray, 2001).

Intrapersonal intelligence has been less directly studied from cognitive and educational perspectives than have the other intelligences. Although some cognitive research has been done related to episodic memory (Tulving, 2005), autobiographical memory (Gilboa, 2004), and metacognition (Kuhn, 2000), research related to intrapersonal intelligence functions is found more often in personality psychology (e.g., McAdams, 1993), social psychology (e.g., Bandura, 1986), psychoanalysis (e.g., Schore, 2002), positive psychology (e.g., Robinson & Clore, 2002), developmental psychology (e.g., Gopnik & Meltzoff, 1994), and cultural psychology (e.g., Markus & Kitayama, 1991). As a result, our analysis also draws on these other self-related literatures.

EXECUTIVE FUNCTION

Executive function is a cognitive process involved in controlling behavior and readying the person for situations. More important in real-life decision making and everyday reasoning than in responding to questions on standardized tests, executive function comprises the ability to be mentally and behaviorally flexible to changing conditions and to provide coherence and smoothness in one's responses (see Zelazo et al., 1997, for review).

If the self involves paths within a social landscape, then intrapersonal intelligence is the map that conceptually organizes the self, and executive function is the orienteer who figures out routes to express, enhance, or develop the self. Executive function computes the appropriate next step: Should one keep going or change course? Once fully developed, it interpolates, connecting dispositions, preferences, interests, and self-concept to new encounters with the environment: "How does this relate to *me*?" and "What should I do now?"

To determine routes, executive function entails the integration of three parameters, which we label hills, skills, and will. A person's *hill* is the goal, aspirational self, or possible self—who the person wants to be or the destination toward which he or she directs abilities and efforts. A goal is an internally generated representation that extends the self beyond the here and now, making current perceptions and actions instrumental to some future purpose. One's *skills* are learned sequences of behavior in a societal domain or discipline that draw on one or more intelligences. Skills constitute what a person can do—the know-how to accomplish some task with relative certainty. One's *will* involves the effort, motivation, and wherewithal that connect skills to hills.

DEVELOPMENT

How does the differential coordination of goals, abilities, and motivation lead to different manifestations of executive function over the lifespan? Support for assuming a developmental perspective comes from several sources. Neuro-imaging literature posits that executive function may recruit different parts of the brain over time (e.g., brain regions children use to solve problems calling for executive function differ from those adults use; Bunge, Dudokovic, Thomason, Vaidya, & Gabrieli, 2002); hence, executive function may operate differently at discrete developmental points. In addition, several studies show that performance on executive function tasks or demonstration of executive function behaviors develops with age (see Zelazo et al., 1997, for review). Finally, many aspects or attributes of the self (e.g., self-concept, self-reflective ability, emotional maturity) as well as the ability to process and use self-information (intrapersonal intelligence) develop across the lifespan (see Damon & Hart, 1982; Loevinger, 1976). Accordingly, it makes sense that the ability to control aspects of the self in light of one's purposes and changing environment (executive function) should also develop.

In the early months of life, for the most part, a biological and emotional control system is in charge (Schore, 2002). The temporal horizon is immediate; planning extends no longer than it takes to reach and grasp or to capture an adult's attention. During the preschool years, the child develops a nascent theory of mind, slowly abandons egocentrism, and acquires an instrumental self based on attachment to, resonance with, and responses from others (e.g., Trevarthen, 1993). Toddlers can recognize themselves in pictures or mirrors, hold information in mind over a time delay, find a hidden object moved to a different location (the A-not-B task) (see Damon & Hart, 1982; Lehto, Juujarvi, Kooistra, & Pulkkinen, 2003), and coordinate their behavior with others' expectations (Kochanska et al., 2001). This age is usually considered the beginning of executive function. Hill, skill, and will are only loosely tied to each other; they are composed primarily of innate or congenital capacities that meet immediate needs. Once this foundation has been laid, we suggest there are two stages of executive function development.

During the *apprentice* stage, the self is differentiated from others yet calibrated to a larger, cultural "ideal self" model. Skill development predominates as children master the knowledge and know-how their societies and cultures require for them to become full participants. Hills usually relate to the development of specific skills and are given by authorities such as parents or teachers. Goals and associated know-how gradually increase from do-now chores to longer-term projects. Will is personal energy that can be harnessed to achieve goals deemed worthy by the culture.

During the *master* stage, the self is fully integrated and owned by the person; it is calibrated to a sense of authenticity. The three parameters are nearly seamless. Hills are paramount and often complex in terms of interconnected long-term umbrella goals and shorter-term subgoals. These goals tend to be self-chosen, as the person has sufficient experience to recombine cultural opportunities and requirements into personally meaningful, often idiosyncratic possibilities. Skill development and skill usage follow goals and may become increasingly automated so that the person feels, phenomenologically, that little effort need be exerted. Will is called upon only in times of turbulence, uncertainty, or abrupt change.

Although these stages correspond prototypically to specific age ranges, they are not tied tightly to age. We anticipate that for many people the apprentice stage starts somewhere between ages 2 and 5, when parents begin to socialize their children in earnest, and lasts until ages 20 to 35 (kindergarten through one's first job, be it after high school or graduate school). Many people may never leave the apprentice stage, as they ensconce themselves in institutional jobs with extensive external support and little need for personal initiative or agendas. We anticipate the master stage is calibrated less to age and more to experiences—especially experiences involving surprise, frustration, or perhaps even trauma—that jolt some individuals into recognizing the limits of the culture's ideal self.

THE APPRENTICE

Jessica carefully writes down her schedule using the table her mother set up for her—times, classroom locations, teacher names, subjects, and supplies needed. It is her first day of middle school, an overwhelmingly different environment from the comfort of Mrs. Anderson's fifth-grade class. Today she must contend with multiple classes and teachers, more homework, cliques, and, of course, puberty. She has always been a good student, but how will she keep from saying the wrong thing if called on in class? She has been able to make friends before, but will she know how to "act cool"? What is she supposed to do with the butterflies that invade her stomach when the popular boys walk by?

At the apprentice stage, Jessica is increasing her regulation of emotions, thoughts, and behavior in light of cultural norms regarding how she *should* act. The self comprises less one's physical features and more one's status in relation to others—first regarding such characteristics as age or sex, later regarding activities or interests (e.g., "I like dinosaurs" or "I am a good pitcher"; see Damon & Hart, 1982). The self is preoccupied with identity—one's own and others' perceptions of self that remain relatively consistent over time. Intrapersonal intelligence expands to process social comparison data as well as the bodily and emotional information available in infancy. Personally relevant is one's performance relative to standards: Do I live up to expectations? Am I better or worse than the other person?

Because humans live together in cultural groups, performance stems from learning the rules, values, and norms of the culture into which one is born, usually categorized into disciplines or domains. Through parental and school socialization, children's intrapersonal intelligence is trained in the appropriate ways to interpret emotions, express and inhibit feelings and actions, and consider others' perspectives. The growing self can understand its place within social realms more abstractly and can project itself into the future to make realistic plans (see Higgins, 2005; Kochanska et al., 2001).

At this stage, a person is clear on the difference between what goes on inside her mind versus out there in the world. A person fully recognizes how she is distinctive from other people in a variety of dimensions, including dimensions that cannot be observed directly by others. She is aware that she knows herself differently from the way that others know her because she can have thoughts or feelings others are not aware of and because she can deceive. She also understands that her goals, skills, and motivation can differ from what others expect her to have: her parents want her to learn strong academic skills and go to college, whereas she wants to learn journalism and photography and travel the world. Intense pressure to coordinate these differences can build up, calling for more complex executive functioning.

Apprentice executive function involves keeping oneself in line with expectations. It is fundamentally conscientious, becoming increasingly considerate—both positively (e.g., cooperation) and negatively (e.g., deception)—of one's effect on others and of the group on oneself. Executive function helps individuals stay abreast of themselves within the less stable, more dynamic social environment beyond the family. Individuals need to be able to change in a timely manner: understanding one's place in different milieus (Anderson, Bechara, Damasio, Tranel, & Damasio, 1999); inhibiting habitual responses that are counterproductive to appropriate goals and self-concepts (Happaney, Zelazo, & Stuss, 2004);

and updating information about oneself based on feedback from others, observation of one's own behavior, past experience, and reflection (e.g., Gomez-Beldarrain, Harries, Garcia-Monco, Ballus, & Grafman, 2004; Wilson & Dunn, 2004).

As education is a fundamental aspect of enculturation, the apprentice is the executive function stage most often studied (usually assumed as the only stage) in cognitive and educational research. Such studies focus on how the child or adult is *supposed* to behave, what the *proper* goals to reach for are, how the person *should* be skilled and direct his or her energy. Skills and skill development predominate in this stage, goals tend to be handed down by authorities, and will is often problematic—a force that must be directed toward proper cultural ends. As Plato remarked, the purpose of education is to make the person want to do what he is supposed to do.

Skills invoke the eight intelligences, to varying degrees, in culturally prescribed patterns of behavior (Gardner, 2006). These patterns of behavior are coordinated socially into domains, crafts, and disciplines, such as the arts, medicine, or carpentry. Both skills and domains are prioritized by the culture in terms of social value. In earlier eras, a premium was placed on physical prowess or aesthetic expression; hunting, farming, and the arts were held in high standing. In 21st-century Western culture, skills such as literacy, numeracy, technological savvy, and social finesse are highly prized; using one's intelligences within the domains of medicine or law is considered more prestigious than using them in taxi driving or clerical work.

This prestige continuum is important at the apprentice stage as a person tries to find a niche in society that matches his or her intelligence profile and skills. That is, the role of executive function at this stage is to focus attention and resources on developing those skills that the culture has deemed useful for "getting ahead" in life. These skills arise through taking on roles (student, sports player, volunteer) within one's community. Preferably, the person will enjoy these roles and skills, calibrating his or her self-esteem and personal meaning to exerting effort in them (Bandura, 1986; Csikszentmihalyi, Rathunde, & Whalen, 1993).

By the end of the apprentice stage, skills should be proficient, or, better yet, expert: the person can execute a behavioral pattern flawlessly and automatically, without conscious control or thought (Bargh & Chartrand, 1999). The person is in sync with others' expectations and well practiced in tasks calling on the skill. When one is in alignment with cultural environments and relationships, there is less cognitive work to be done to maintain appropriate behaviors. Nothing more than low-level monitoring for errors or change is required (Vohs, Baumeister, &

Ciarocco, 2005). As skills are automated, energy expenditure may be reduced or redirected to figuring out what one should be doing and why.

Hills (formal goals) become more prominent over the course of this stage. With the development of skills that can provide a sense of control, people can project themselves into and connect current actions to future states of being. Although individuals choose among an array of potential goals in contemporary society, for the most part these goals are constrained by authorities of the culture. Parents give their children marching orders for behavior, chores, and the like. Teachers give students assignments, deadlines, and instructions. Employers give workers benchmarks, deadlines, and specifications. Goals are provided for apprentices and internalized through role models, feedback, punishment, reward, and instruction.

Will at this stage is motivation in the classic research tradition: the impulse to act toward proper incentives presented by cultural authorities. Yet, the use of the term "will" is often confusing: "motivated" children are desired by the culture, but "willful" children are not. Motivated children, whose hearts are in the right place, are unproblematic and well behaved. Willful children are defiant, stubborn, and go against the grain. There is an inherent tension regarding will at this stage: from the "inside" it is the force that meets one's goals, but if one's goals are not in line with what the culture deems appropriate, then from the "outside" it represents a force of disobedience that must be reckoned with.

As a result of this tension, some energy at this stage must be used to balance competing forces felt within oneself before executive function can address the situation, decision, or action at hand. Thus, apprentices may be more susceptible than those at other stages to interference by immediate stimuli (Bechara, Damasio, & Damasio, 2000; Bunge, Ochsner, Desmond, Glover, & Gabrieli, 2001), suffering a higher cognitive load, and being caught in a lie by their own subtle inconsistencies (see also Vohs et al., 2005). These inside/outside tensions relating to goals and will may contribute to the wide individual differences seen among youth regarding future orientation and motivation (Csikszentmihalyi et al., 1993).

At the apprentice stage, one's culture is in charge—an ideological and cognitive control system. Executive function involves coordination of biological and cultural, internal and external sources of information toward culturally appropriate goals using culturally appropriate tools. The apprentice can delay gratification, inhibit his or her automatic responses, and adapt to rules. The temporal horizon increases as the apprentice takes on long-term and short-term, super- and subgoals. Planning ranges from how to get to the next class or business appointment to how to go on vacation next summer or become a successful Wall Street investor.

By the time she graduates from college, Jessica has joined a community of friends, chosen a career in law, developed an interest in photography, and committed herself to her boyfriend, Barry. She identifies herself in terms of accomplishments that distinguish her yet connect her to others: an English major, a Notre Dame alumna, her first-place ribbon from the state fair photography competition. Although she feels somewhat in control of her choices and activities, she still relies on cultural norms and institutions to keep her on track. She has mastered her culture's expectations. This is the stage at which many people stop: they are comfortably settled within the social structure. A few, however, perhaps including Jessica, enter a further stage of executive function that involves more reflective strategies to delineate an idiosyncratic or even unique developmental trajectory (see Feldman, 1994).

THE MASTER

> Pablo reviews the proposal one last time. Tomorrow morning he is making a sales presentation to the state's government for a $10 million contract. Despite his industry's insistence on function-specific hardware and software, Pablo devised a way for computerized gadgets (like cell phones) to reprogram themselves based on the user's immediate need—for example, the same gadget could be a cell phone, Palm Pilot, or voice recorder. His products could increase the flexibility of police, politicians, and regulators without them having to buy expensive new equipment every year. He has been patiently and persistently pursuing this account for more than a year. All he has to do is keep his eye on the ball. This account could be the tipping point for his tools to become the new industry standard.

At the master stage, Pablo has integrated his current self, future vision, and personal resources to be both authentic to his values and goals and responsive to the situation's specifics. The self moves beyond bodily sensations and movements as well as inherited cultural scripts and roles to enact one's more idiosyncratic story. The self is understood as one's dispositions, preferences, and biases built up through experience and reflection. What is personally relevant is generativity and integrity—leaving one's unique mark on the world through self-initiated, expressive productivity (Erikson, 1959; McAdams, Diamond, de St. Aubin, & Mansfield, 1997).

During infancy, the person mostly focused on taking in information from the outside; during the apprentice stage, the person coordinated internal and external information about the self. In contrast, during the master stage, the emphasis is on generating from the inside out. The person has developed a deeply personal knowledge of self, including long-term goals and idiosyncratic styles. In addition, the person has become able to integrate his or her hills, skills, and will into a personally meaningful agenda beyond the ordained program of the society in which he or she lives. Intrapersonal intelligence at this stage is most associated with concepts such as maturity, wisdom, and creativity via self-expression. Wiser, more mature people see and accept themselves as changing; they are more aware of the *process* of self (e.g., King, 2001).

Master-stage executive function involves a more complex orchestration of hill, skill, and will that can maintain progress despite the uncertainty of external support or outcome. It entails responsibility, or being the source or cause of one's actions without appeal to external authority. Setting one's own goals, reconfiguring cultural resources, and staying limber as unexpected obstacles arise become the hallmarks of executive function. Goals come into ascendance and involve more initiative and autonomy; skills increasingly involve stronger interpolation and may extend beyond those that are culturally valued; and will coordinates intercalation between goals and skills.

Masters increasingly demonstrate the ability to posit and pursue individually conceived goals. They do not limit themselves to climbing hills offered by their culture, but instead scale hills that may not have existed before (see Csikszentmihalyi, 1996). Authentic agency emerges— self-directed, intentional goal setting, decision making, and action, rather than simply behavior responding to environmental cues (e.g., Greve, 2001). Although one's culture remains an important reference, at this stage one does not just *reproduce* cultural norms and standard behaviors; one now has the capacity to *produce* culture, a variation or novelty from which new lines of thought and behavior can grow.

The master seizes initiative, a step that is difficult and risky for most people. People can keep themselves from doing the wrong thing (which the apprentice stage emphasizes) but have a harder time initiating doing the right thing without some environmental input (see Kochanska et al., 2001). Perhaps the clearest indicator of these self-initiated goals is how one allocates time that is not accounted for by family, work, household, or other obligations. These goals stem from intrinsic interest, which may or may not be in prestigious domains (e.g., a person may focus on cooking, gardening, art, or woodworking). By focusing on the challenge of the task rather than comparative performance or consumption, mastery goals seem to provide the flexibility and potential for unlimited growth (Dweck, 1999).

Skills are not just for getting ahead of comparable others, as in the apprentice stage; they are for forging toward a personal goal. Skills at this stage may become more idiosyncratic. They are no longer the genetically programmed instincts nor the learned cultural behaviors of earlier ages. Rather than focusing on executing skills well to predetermined standards, masters hone their skill repertoire in light of a personal agenda. They create their own skills, or patterns of behavior, to address their goals through interpolation.

Interpolation is the meta-skill of bringing self-knowledge to bear on other information already highly processed by the other intelligences (Badre & Wagner, 2004). It infuses personal relevance: "What is the best way *for me* to do this?" Some may say this process is not a skill in the same way as boat building or joke writing or accordion playing. In general, people do not speak in terms of "practicing" at being oneself or finding coaches to make oneself better, but more self-aware and self-reflective individuals do. They envision who they want to be, keeping reflective journals, and asking others for feedback and insight (see Wallace & Gruber, 1989). For example, Virginia Woolf's diaries and novels both examine herself and the selves of her characters with a clarity and freshness of insight few have mastered (Gardner, 1997).

This interpolation process further strengthens executive function's ability to integrate. With the strong interpolation meta-skill of the master stage, there is not a sexual self, work self, and family self; there is just one self that can harbor contradictions as told in a coherent life story with various interwoven subplots (Csikszentmihalyi, 1996; Erikson, 1959; McAdams, 1993). The more or better one interpolates, the easier integration of experiences, cognitions, emotions, contexts, and goals is. The better integrated oneself is, the easier it is to interpolate self-relevance with incoming information.

Will is the energy reserved for occasions of misalignment and turbulence—when self-initiated hills and skills do not lead to the expected result (Vohs et al., 2005). Although will is often strong in masters, as they expend considerable energy toward their personally meaningful goals, paradoxically masters may not *feel* as if they are exerting their will as much as apprentices. Better self-regulation stems from a more complex understanding of their selves' aspects. Creators, wise persons, and moral exemplars report they do not have to think about the options; the choice or action unfolds as part of their being (e.g., Colby & Damon, 1994). Masters report "losing themselves" in the task because they do not have to expend cognitive effort to figure themselves out. They better understand when they do and do not need to, can and cannot exert control (Csikszentmihalyi, 1996). Energy is not needed to determine what the right thing to do is, as in the apprentice stage, so more energy is directed toward how to do it (see Vohs et al., 2005). The focus is on achievement: mastery is its own self-perpetuating reward.

At the master stage, one's individuality is in charge—an idiosyncratic control system. Executive function involves not coordination, but integration, of various experiences and information. Reformulating the abilities to delay gratification, inhibit one's behavior, and adapt to rules in light of one's unique self, the master can now add the ability to regulate "online" without a pre-known outcome. He or she can finally face the future on its own uncertain terms and not artificially stabilize it. The temporal horizon and variety of contexts are more flexible and interactive. Planning need not be linear but can become multidimensional as the master recognizes the interdependence of different experiences, projects, and relationships. The "fit" one seeks is no longer between self and cultural expectation but between self and one's freely chosen actions. Each thought, emotion, and response is "owned" by the self in terms of authenticity and meaningfulness.

Years later, one of Pablo's favorite pastimes is to tell stories of his life to his granddaughter. The stories are full of struggles and conflicts, but, he comforts her, these obstacles were lessons that made him stronger. He identifies with these stories, even as their emphasis may change with each telling. Control is no longer a focus for Pablo: he realizes he cannot control everything, yet he is responsible for himself. He still may have bouts of doubt and insecurity, but that doubt is not the most pertinent. He continues to make the most of the experiences he has to develop himself as far as he can.

SUMMARY AND IMPLICATIONS

Executive function—the ability to regulate behavior within a fluctuating and unpredictable environment—entails an integration of what the person wants to accomplish (hill), can do (skill), and directs energy toward (will). This ability emerges from the person's capacity to access and use self-relevant information, or intrapersonal intelligence. People exhibit wide individual differences in their executive functioning. These differences are in part developmental, stemming from differential interactions over time among hill, skill, and will.

For the apprentice, executive function focuses on control of cultural symbolic resources. Skill development is preeminent as school-age children, adolescents, and young adults strive to increase their abilities, especially those capacities deemed most valuable in their society. Goals at first are set by others, but, over time and with skill mastery, the responsibility for several aspects of goal setting gradually transfers to the individual. The will is socially tamed to constrain use of energy toward societally preferred goals. Executive function's primary focus is behavioral inhibition and adaptation to rules.

For the master, executive function focuses on control of one's individuality: "Who am I?" "What is my unique contribution?" Goals are initiated rather than accepted from the culture; they become more idiosyncratic and oriented more toward the process than the end. Skills and will also become more flexible as they are used and perhaps reconceptualized depending on the goal toward which they are oriented. Executive function's primary focus is the attainment of authentic personal meaning.

What does our analysis mean in educational terms? What occurs for a person to be considered a strong "executive" at each stage? What occurs for a person to move to the next stage?

The apprentice stage provides the arena *par excellence* for the educator. To support strong executive function within this stage, the current models of schooling are generally appropriate. The format is lessons. The focus is on understanding: "What are you talking about?" The goal is to provide ways for apprentices to take in cultural knowledge, skills, and goals, then assess how well they have internalized them. Ideally, internalizing means more than just getting the right answer on a test; it also involves connecting the material to the person's self and life so it will be useful to him or her.

The apprentice stage continues for many people beyond schooling in their discipline into their adult work lives. Adults enter a workplace where, in most cases, goal setting (hill) is a management function, whereas skill use is an employee function. That is, authorities decide "what" through job assignments or job specs, and employees decide "how." Performance reviews provide feedback from outside to help employees regulate their behavior the following year. A question arises that requires research: Why do people stay in the apprentice stage? It may be because of individual differences or because the cultural norm for many communities and occupations is for this stage to be the end point. In either of these cases, the educator's job is done once apprentices can understand what is expected of them.

The educators' scope could be enlarged, however, to play a role in aiding transformation from the apprentice to the master stage. The challenge involves setting up conditions under which apprentices can (1) take risks that go beyond the socially scaffolded cultural norms for performance, expression, or understanding; (2) reflect on their current self-regulation, especially its limits; and (3) become more sensitive to nuances within themselves or the environment that might signal an opportunity to take risks or reflect.

For example, if a parent or teacher or employer does not provide real choices, if everything is mandatory and compulsory, there is no impetus to develop mental flexibility or cope with uncertainty. If one's environment is kept stable, if fluctuations are hidden from the child, there is no impetus to develop updating faculties. If freedom to fail in minor situations is not allowed, children do not have opportunities to develop response inhibition or a new repertoire of responses. That is, if people feel *too* comfortable, there is little stimulus for development. Practical advice to help educators provide bridges to the master stage has included modeling strong master-level executive function themselves; using conditional (e.g., "it could be") rather than absolute ("it is") statements when introducing concepts so that apprentices are aware of alternatives (Langer, 1997); making sure apprentices are aware of the sources of their knowledge (e.g., "How do you know that?"; Langer, 1997) and their assumptions (e.g., as Socrates does in *Meno*); and understanding the sometimes productive roles of confusion, frustration, and anxiety as motivators for apprentices to voice their own puzzlement, learn to question, and perhaps create richer systems of understanding and self-regulation (Stacey, 1996).

We focus on setting up conditions rather than teaching. If apprentices are increasingly to take responsibility for their own goal setting, skill development, and energy direction, then educators probably should avoid direct instruction or interventions. Pertaining to this issue, Powell and Voeller (2004) propose a "prosthetic frontal lobe" to help children with low executive function by having parents and teachers anticipate consequences for and give guidelines to them. Early in the apprentice stage or for certain purposes, this prosthetic may be advisable, but in the long term, excessive prosthetics can hamper the development of executive function. If care is not taken to think through the implications for developing responsibility, the apprentice may learn to perform well to task specifications or to the expectations of others (Fischer & Bidell, 1998), yet not understand what is right for his or her particular persona and niche.

Finally, what role might educators play within the master stage? Compared to the apprentice's "intake, then test" model, the master stage adheres more to one of "express, then gather feedback." Others serve as resources, not mentors. The impetus for an "educational moment" must come from the master, not the educator. Compared to the apprentice's focus on understanding what people are talking about, the master focuses on what people are *not* talking about but that might be worth asking. The format is not lessons, but endeavors. Since usually the master stage is achieved after formal schooling is completed, we focus on the workplace as a setting.

Whereas the apprentice has an attitude of "I'm the employee. You're the boss. I work for you," the master has an independent contractor perspective: "I'm the boss of me. I am here to help you solve some issue or complete some task." Some people in certain roles (e.g., entrepreneurs, actors, software developers, and professors) tend to have this attitude regardless of whether they work within an institutionalized setting. The client provides boundaries for a job, not a recipe of specifications—opportunities, not duties. The master figures out not only how, but also what, to do. For example, at least ideally, professors set up their own courses (what to teach) and research programs (what questions to explore) as well as determine pedagogy or methodology (how); actors flesh out the contours of their character (what the person is about) as well as their behavior (how to act). Feedback is provided through proposal, not performance, review, often done in tandem *with*, not *for*, the master. The educator becomes less a director and more a collaborator; he or she is on call for educational moments that the master brings to light.

Part of the struggle for educators at the master stage is relinquishing cultural control and granting freedom to the mature individuals. Although some scholars suggest increased freedom leads to a "tyranny of choice" (Schwartz, 2000), at the master stage freedom parallels Dewey's (1938) notion of "acting with purpose" rather than "acting on impulse." The master is responsible for foreseeing the consequences of his or her impulses and regulating appropriately. The role of the educator is to support the master's formation of purposes.

We suspect that executive function has become a hot scholarly topic at the start of the 21st century because its aims are becoming more important. Education reform has stimulated a call for students to take more responsibility for their learning (e.g., Miller & Brickman, 2004). Workplace changes away from stability toward more dynamic models have stressed the need for leaders-as-facilitators and for people to manage their own careers (e.g., Halbesleben, Novicevic, Harvey, & Buckley, 2003). Social mobility, diversity initiatives, globalization, and technology require people to coordinate more varied types of information and adapt to a wider array of situations than ever before, often with considerably less time for deliberation. Within a more turbulent environment, we face a dual challenge: (1) to maintain continuity and consistency in behavior so that others consider us reliable and trustworthy; and (2) to develop fluidity and innovation so that we will not become obsolete in our work, relationships, and communities.

CONCLUSION

Returning at last to the riddle posed in our title, How does one think of executive function in terms of multiple-intelligences theory? Each of the intelligences has its own trajectory, which is heavily, even decisively, influenced by the inherent abilities of the individual on the one hand, and the priorities, opportunities, and limitations of the ambient culture on the other. For all human beings, the core of intrapersonal intelligence is a sense of self, one that begins to emerge between ages 1 and 2 and continues to deepen throughout life. The more differentiated the individual and the more options in the society, the more extensive and individualized the sense of self is likely to be. At the master level, the sense of self includes detailed knowledge of one's characteristics and idiosyncrasies, along with intimate knowledge of how best to act in terms of one's profile.

The expression of self involves the second aspect of intrapersonal intelligence—the executive capacity to integrate one's goals, skills, and motivation. Incipient signs of executive function emerge in one's early years, and every normal individual develops this integration and orchestration capacity throughout life. The crucial differences across individuals and cultures inhere in how closely the culture's agenda matches the individual's agenda. To the extent that one's life is largely controlled by external circumstances, cultural models, and deeply entrenched rewards and punishments, the model for executive control comes from without. A person's socialization becomes his or her executive function. If, on the other hand, an individual lives in a society with more latitude or elects for whatever reason to venture forth on his or her own, then the integration and orchestration become far more personal. In the latter case, development of executive function involves the gradual fading away of external models and the perennial fashioning of a personal model that allows a person to achieve what he or she wants to achieve in the way that he or she wants to achieve it.

REFERENCES

Anderson, S. W., Bechara, A., Damasio, H., Tranel, D., & Damasio, A. R. (1999). Impairment of social and moral behavior related to early damage in human prefrontal cortex. *Nature Neuroscience, 2*(11), 1032–1037.

Badre, D., & Wagner, A. D. (2004). Selection, integration and conflict monitoring: Assessing the nature and generality of prefrontal cognitive control mechanisms. *Neuron, 41*, 473–487.

Bandura, A. (1986). *Social foundations of thought and action: A social cognitive theory.* Englewood Cliffs, NJ: Prentice-Hall.

Bargh, J. A., & Chartrand, T. L. (1999). The unbearable automaticity of being. *American Psychologist, 54*, 462–479.

Baumeister, R. F., DeWall, C. N., Ciarocco, N. J., & Twenge, J. M. (2005). Social exclusion impairs self-regulation. *Journal of Personality and Social Psychology, 88*(4), 589–604.

Bechara, A., Damasio, H., & Damasio, A. R. (2000). Emotion, decision making and the orbitofrontal cortex. *Cerebral Cortex, 10*, 295–307.

Bunge, S. A., Dudokovic, N. M., Thomason, M. E., Vaidya, C. J., & Gabrieli, J. D. E. (2002). Immature frontal lobe contributions to cognitive control in children: Evidence from fMRI. *Neuron, 33*, 301–311.

Bunge, S. A., Ochsner, K. N., Desmond, J. E., Glover, G. H., & Gabrieli, J. D. E. (2001). Prefrontal regions involved in keeping information in and out of mind. *Brain, 124*, 2074–2086.

Colby, A., & Damon, W. (1994). *Some do care: Contemporary lives of moral commitment.* New York: Free Press–Macmillan.

Csikszentmihalyi, M. (1996). *Creativity.* New York: HarperCollins.

Csikszentmihalyi, M., Rathunde, K., & Whalen, S. (1993). *Talented teenagers: The roots of success and failure.* New York: Cambridge University Press.

Damasio, A. (1999). *The feeling of what happens: Body and emotion in the making of consciousness.* San Diego, CA: Harcourt.

Damon, W., & Hart, D. (1982). The development of self-understanding from infancy through adolescence. *Child Development, 53*, 841–864.

Dewey, J. (1938). *Experience and education.* New York: Collier Books.

Dweck, C. S. (1999). *Self-theories: Their role in motivation, personality, and development.* Philadelphia: Psychology Press.

Erikson, E. (1959). *Identity and the life cycle.* New York: International Universities Press.

Feldman, D. H. (1994). *Beyond the universals of cognitive development* (2nd ed.). Norwood, NJ: Ablex.

Fischer, K. W., & Bidell, T. R. (1998). Dynamic development of psychological structures in action and thought. In W. Damon (Series Ed.) & R. M. Lerner (Vol. Ed.), *Handbook of child psychology, vol. 1: Theoretical models of human development* (5th ed., pp. 467–561). New York: Wiley.

Gardner, H. (1983). *Frames of mind.* New York: Basic Books.

Gardner, H. (1997). *Extraordinary minds.* New York: Basic Books.

Gardner, H. (2006). *Multiple intelligences: New horizons.* New York: Basic Books.

Gilboa, A. (2004). Autobiographical and episodic memory—One and the same? Evidence from prefrontal activation in neuroimaging studies. *Neuropsychologia, 42*, 1336–1349.

Goldberg, E. (2001). *The executive brain: Frontal lobes and the civilized mind.* New York: Oxford University Press.

Gomez-Beldarrain, M., Harries, C., Garcia-Monco, J. C., Ballus, E., & Grafman, J. (2004). Patients with right frontal lesions are unable to assess and use advice to make predictive judgments. *Journal of Cognitive Neuroscience, 16*(1), 74–89.

Gopnik, A., & Meltzoff, A. N. (1994). Mind, bodies and persons: Young children's understanding of the self and others as reflected in imitation and theory of mind research. In S. T. Parker & R. W. Mitchell (Eds.), *Self-awareness in animals and humans: Developmental perspectives* (pp. 166–186). New York: Cambridge University Press.

Greve, W. (2001). Traps and gaps in action explanation: Theoretical problems of a psychology of human action. *Psychological Review, 108*(2), 435–451.

Halbesleben, J. R. B., Novicevic, M. M., Harvey, M. G., & Buckley, M. R. (2003). Awareness of temporal complexity in leadership of creativity and innovation: A competency-based model. *The Leadership Quarterly, 14*, 433–454.

Happaney, K., Zelazo, P. D., & Stuss, D. T. (2004). Development of orbitofrontal function: Current themes and future directions. *Brain and Cognition, 55*, 1–10.

Higgins, E. T. (2005). Humans as applied motivation scientists: Self-consciousness from "shared reality" to "becoming." In H. S. Terrace & J. Metcalfe (Eds.), *The missing link in cognition: Origins of self-reflective consciousness* (pp. 157–173). New York: Oxford University Press.

King, L. A. (2001). The hard road to the good life: The happy, mature person. *Journal of Humanistic Psychology, 41*(1), 51–72.

Kochanska, G., Coy, K. C., & Murray, K. T. (2001). The development of self-regulation in the first four years of life. *Child Development, 72*(4), 1091–1111.

Kuhn, D. (2000). Metacognitive development. *Current Directions in Psychological Science, 9*(5), 178–181.

Langer, E. (1997). *The power of mindful learning*. Reading, MA: Addison-Wesley.

Lehto, J. E., Juujarvi, P., Kooistra, L., & Pulkkinen, L. (2003). Dimensions of executive functioning: Evidence from children. *British Journal of Developmental Psychology, 21*, 59–80.

Loevinger, J. (1976). *Ego development*. San Francisco: Jossey-Bass.

Markus, H. R., & Kitayama, S. (1991). Culture and the self: Implications for cognition, emotion, and motivation. *Psychological Review, 98*(2), 234–253.

McAdams, D. P. (1993). *The stories we live by*. New York: Guilford Press.

McAdams, D. P., Diamond, A., de St. Aubin, E., & Mansfield, E. (1997). Stories of commitment: The psychosocial construction of generative lives. *Journal of Personality and Social Psychology, 72*(3), 678–694.

Miller, R. B., & Brickman, S. J. (2004). A model of future-oriented motivation and self-regulation. *Educational Psychology Review, 16*(2), 9–33.

Powell, K. B., & Voeller, K. K. S. (2004). Prefrontal executive function syndromes in children. *Journal of Child Neurology, 10*(10), 785–797.

Robinson, M. D., & Clore, G. L. (2002). Belief and feeling: Evidence for an accessibility model of emotional self-report. *Psychological Bulletin, 128*(6), 934–960.

Schore, A. N. (2002). Advances in neuropsychoanalysis, attachment theory, and trauma research: Implications for self psychology. *Psychoanalytic Inquiry,* *22*(3), 433–484.

Schwartz, B. (2000). Self-determination: The tyranny of freedom. *American Psychologist, 55*(1), 79–88.

Stacey, R. D. (1996). *Complexity and creativity in organizations.* San Francisco: Berrett-Koehler.

Terrace, H. S., & Metcalfe, J. (Eds.). (2005). *The missing link in cognition: Origins of self-reflective consciousness.* New York: Oxford University Press.

Trevarthen, C. (1993). The self born in intersubjectivity: The psychology of an infant communicating. In U. Neisser (Ed.), *The perceived self* (pp. 121–173). New York: Cambridge University Press.

Tulving, E. (2005). Episodic memory and autonoesis: Uniquely human? In H. S. Terrace & J. Metcalfe (Eds.), *The missing link in cognition: Origins of self-reflective consciousness* (pp. 3–56). New York: Oxford University Press.

Vohs, K. D., Baumeister, R. F., & Ciarocco, N. J. (2005). Self-regulation and self-presentation: Regulatory resource depletion impairs impression management and effortful self-presentation depletes regulatory resources. *Journal of Personality and Social Psychology, 88*(4), 632–657.

Wallace, D. B., & Gruber, H. E. (1989). *Creative people at work.* New York: Oxford University Press.

Wilson, T. D., & Dunn, E. W. (2004). Self-knowledge: Its limits, value and potential for improvement. *Annual Review of Psychology, 55,* 493–518.

Zelazo, P. D., Carter, A., Reznick, J. S., & Frye, D. (1997). Early development of executive function: A problem-solving framework. *Review of General Psychology, 1*(2), 198–226.

CHAPTER 3

Executive Capacities from a Developmental Perspective

JANE HOLMES BERNSTEIN
DEBORAH P. WABER

As this book attests, the role of executive function in children's cognition and behavior has become a focus of intense and growing interest. A PsychINFO QuickSearch using the search terms "executive function" and "children" yielded 5 citations for 1985, 14 for 1995, and a cumulative 501 by 2005, with 485 of these identified by the search term "development of executive function." Such enthusiasm can enhance scientific productivity; it can also be seductive and constrain critical thinking.

As our contribution to this volume, we discuss some important caveats to the consideration of frontal systems, "executive functions," and the relationship between them, especially in the context of the developing child. These comments are organized around three themes: modularity and the plausibility of executive functions as an isolatable set of skills; developmental considerations and distinctions between adult and child; and the role of factors intrinsic or extrinsic to the child. We consider some implications for clinical practice. Finally, we suggest some useful ways to think about processes that are referred to under the rubric of "executive function" in the developing child and highlight implications for future research.

As a preamble to our discussion, we note that, of several challenges to attempts to elucidate the nature of "executive functions," a significant one is their assumed association with the frontal lobes. Two issues are relevant here. One is the range and appropriacy of the "frontal metaphor" as dissected by Pennington (1997). The metaphor is based on "finding a similarity between the behavioral symptoms or cognitive test performances, or both, of some group of individuals, either at a particular developmental stage or with a given behavioral disorder, and the behavioral symptoms or cognitive test performances, or both, of humans or other animals with acquired frontal lesions" (Pennington, 1997, p. 265). It has potential for integrating different research traditions, but has important limitations (discussed later in this chapter).

The other relevant issue is the often privileged position of the frontal lobes—and, by extension, executive functions—in thinking about the brain–behavior relationships of frontal systems. This sense of privilege appears to derive from an appeal to evolutionary development. The frontal lobes in humans are frequently understood to be the "most recently evolved and especially human part of the brain . . . the latest achievement in the evolution of the nervous system; it is only in human beings (and great apes, to some extent) that they reach so great a development" (Sacks, 2001, pp. vii, ix) . But, the frontal lobes are neither new in evolutionary terms nor special to humans: they have been part of the neural apparatus of the mammalian line for 176 million years (Jerison, 1997). The goal-oriented behavior that these neural systems support is not only common to all mammals, but also critical to their survival and to the evolutionary success of the whole mammalian enterprise. No animal could adapt flexibly to changing environments without the capacity for coordination, integration, and control (executive control processes) of the complex mechanisms supporting its behavioral repertoire. Such control processes are—indeed, must be—inextricably embedded in the total package of biological systems that all animals need to obtain food, reproductive partners, and other critical resources. Looks notwithstanding, frontal brain systems are not bigger in humans than in other primates, given the size and complexity of the body for which they contribute control processes (Jerison, 1997). Both the frontal metaphor and any sense of evolutionarily based "privilege" must be approached with caution.

MODULARITY OF EXECUTIVE FUNCTIONS

In neuropsychology, the term "modularity" refers to the proposition that functions are organized in relatively discrete modules. These modules are believed to be distinct from one another and, thus, able to be validly examined in isolation, without necessary consideration of other coexistent functions or a broader systemic context, which is theoretically spared (but see Farah, 1994). This modular orientation derives in large part from the fact that the neuropsychology is rooted historically in the systematic observation of adults with focal brain lesions, where a primary clinical goal was to localize function, since imaging techniques were not yet available.

This reductionist approach continues to influence contemporary cognitive neuroscience and is particularly influential in clinical neuropsychology. Thus, there is an implicit assumption that functions are organized in discrete packages. In this context, it is assumed that a "central executive" (Baddeley, 1998), typically referred to as executive function, can be distinguished from other functions, such as visuospatial skills, language, and motor planning. Further, it is assumed that executive function can itself be reliably parsed into discrete functional modules. Thus, neuropsychological test batteries are constructed with parallel sets of measures for each function, including executive, which are frequently further parcelated into specific executive capacities, often linked to specific tests (e.g., Wisconsin Card Sort = set shifting).

It can be argued that the term "executive function(s)" gives precedence to this modular conceptualization. The term "functions" not only embodies modular assumptions, but also tends to put executive systems on an equal footing with language functions, visuospatial functions, and so forth. This is in striking contrast to the evolutionarily based account and to other theoretical perspectives that view executive capacities as more domain general (Denckla, 1996).

Indeed, the executive function construct is not nearly as tidy as the modular account would suggest, a problem that may be especially troublesome where children are concerned. Attempts to derive subsets of executive functions have yet to yield consistency or consensus. The boundaries of what constitutes a measure of executive function are often indistinct, since virtually any goal-oriented behavior or task entails an executive component. Moreover, laboratory- and ecologically derived measures of executive functions are consistent only in their inconsistency (Anderson, Anderson, Northam, Jacobs, & Mikiewicz, 2002; Vriezen & Pigott, 2002; Waber, Gerber, Turcios, Wagner, & Forbes, 2006). How then can we conceptualize this obviously important yet elusive construct?

Recent explorations made possible by functional neuroimaging may provide some clarification. Duncan and Owen (2000) have argued that "a specific network of prefrontal regions is recruited to solve many diverse cognitive problems" (2000, p. 475). They analyzed functional studies of five different cognitive demands that are thought to represent diverse executive functions: response conflict, novelty, working memory: number of elements, working memory: delay, and perceptual difficulty. Surprisingly, despite the apparent diversity of these tasks, they consistently recruited the same three specific regions in mid-dorsolateral and mid-ventrolateral prefrontal cortex and dorsal anterior cingulate cortex. Duncan and Owen suggest that these tasks, diverse though they may be, recruit a similar network that is sufficiently abstract and general to adapt to a variety of executive demands. They comment that "the very generality of activity in these regions helps explain why most conceptions of prefrontal functions are themselves so general and ill defined" (2000, p. 481).

Further expanding on this observation, Duncan (2001) proposed an "adaptive coding model," which suggests that prefrontal cortex adjusts its function in an on-line fashion to match the requirements of a particular task. Single-cell studies in monkeys suggest that prefrontal neurons are "tuned" by specific task demands and that this tuning is flexible and on-line, shaped by the current demands of the task. Expanding on this set of controlled observations, he goes on to suggest that in the prefrontal cortex, response properties of single neurons are highly adaptable. Cells become tuned to code information relevant to specific tasks as they arise and must be highly flexible to meet shifting demands of specific tasks. Such a flexible and ad hoc system would be more likely to represent a highly dynamic process than a discrete function or set of discrete functions. Duncan characterizes prefrontal cortex "not so much as the seat of particular cognitive operations, but as a *resource* that gives such operations greater focus, power, or flexibility" (2001, p. 827, emphasis added). Such a model would account for the great difficulty in characterizing executive functions with specificity as well as the highly context- and situation-dependent nature of whatever cognitive functions are referenced by the term.

Although this model remains speculative and demands further experimental investigation, it nonetheless provides a powerful metaphor for understanding the nature of executive functions, control processes, and the like. The processes are fluid and best instantiated in on-line contexts, and they are likely to be highly dependent on contextual factors, both internal and external to the organism. Such a model may eventually provide a better account for the perplexing inconsistency in measurement across settings and events than do approaches that are explicitly or implicitly more static and modular. Measurement of behavior within the framework of such a model, however, may call for the development of novel assessment approaches.

DEVELOPMENTAL VERSUS ADULT MODELS

As the above discussion indicates, arriving at a clear understanding of what executive functions are or even how to refer to these processes is a challenge. Doing so in a developmental context can be even more difficult. In the developmental setting, constructs such as executive function must be understood in the context of the powerful forces of development, which are not inherently linear but are more typically characterized by repeated reorganization and restructuring. It is against this developmental backdrop that individual differences of greatest clinical interest must be appreciated and interpreted.

Although we tend to think of individual differences in relation to executive functions, the lion's share of the variability among children is accounted for by maturational processes. Executive capacities are present from very early on, evident from the time the infant begins to engage in volitional activities. The changes in capacities for self-regulation and planful behavior are dramatic, beginning in infancy and continuing beyond adolescence. Indeed, much of typical cognitive, social, and emotional development can be referenced to the overwhelming evolution of these capacities. Any differences among individuals are subservient to these overriding developmental processes, whereas the reverse tends to be the case in adults, at least until the more advanced years.

Adult neuropsychology has documented clear and consistent links between executive capacities and the integrity of the frontal lobes; lesions to the frontal lobes are typically associated with disorganization and dysregulation of behavior. Conceptualization of executive functions in children, however, has several sources. Historically, the concept of executive control processes arose from cognitive psychology. Atkinson and Shiffrin (1968) proposed a model of memory that distinguished control processes from structural features. Structural features are viewed as hard-wired; control processes are more optional and strategic. This model was adapted to the developmental context by theorists such as Brown (Campione & Brown, 1977), who used the term "control processes," and Belmont and Butterfield (1971), who referred to "executive control" as they applied cognitive models to learning, particularly among individuals with mental retardation. In the developmental literature, therefore, the cognitive and neuropsychological strands came together as the development of executive controls became linked to frontal cortex, especially prefrontal cortex.

Although the clinical issues presented by children rarely involve discrete lesions to frontal cortex, they very frequently involve executive processes, and so the focus in children has necessarily been on behavioral manifestations rather than focal damage. Because of the correlation in adults between frontal lesions and dysexecutive behavior, executive functioning in children has often been viewed as indicative of the development and integrity of frontal lobes and their function.

The risks of such downwards-extension strategies in neuropsychological investigations of the child were highlighted more than 20 years ago by Fletcher and Taylor (1984). They pointed out that measures that correlate reliably with specific regions of brain damage in adults will not necessarily have the same significance for children and that tests developed and normed for adults may be sensitive to different functions in children. Fletcher and Taylor's cautions are even more applicable to the challenge of the executive functions/frontal systems brain–behavior relationship. As noted above, Pennington (1997) finds potential in the "frontal metaphor" to "integrate phenomena ordinarily studied by separate research traditions" (p. 266), noting that the broad scope of application of the metaphor can be partially justified by the diversity of behaviors and cognitive tests that are found to be impaired after frontal lesions. He warns, however, of important limitations, noting that the fruitfulness of the metaphor will depend on the success with which these limitations can be addressed by future research. These limitations include overextension of the metaphor to most special needs populations and the associated lack of specificity differentiating among these groups, lack of specifiable early lesions in populations exhibiting the "frontal" deficits, failure to consider whether executive deficits are primary or secondary, heterogeneity of manifestations, and the fact that diffuse neuropathological processes, which are more typical in children, are so frequently associated with executive deficits.

These various issues stem in large part from the fact that in children, cognition has not yet assumed the more modular architecture of the adult but tends to be more global, dynamic, and undifferentiated. Indeed, one of the hallmarks of cognitive development is progressive differentiation of functions (and increasing limitations in terms of plasticity and recovery of function). Hence, in children, even focal brain injury will not necessarily result in relatively isolated impairment of a specific cognitive function. The perturbations caused by the injury will be incorporated into the ongoing developmental course and can be expected to yield more wide-ranging effects under the influence of the powerful processes of development.

Again, the emerging functional imaging literature may help refine our conceptual models. Although studies comparing functional networks associated with executive-type tasks in adults and children are few, those that exist are suggestive. Working memory performance, for example, is typically associated with a fronto-parietal network. Kwon, Reiss, and Menon (2002) reported age-related (from 7 to 22) increases in activation in response to a spatial working memory task bilaterally in both prefrontal and posterior parietal cortex. This result suggests in a relatively straightforward sense that with age there is increasing maturation and functional specialization of both of these regions.

More intriguing is a study by Olesen, Nagy, Westerberg, and Klingberg (2003), who also studied spatial working memory, correlating structural and functional changes from 8 to 18 years. Using diffusion tensor imaging (DTI) to visualize white matter tracts, they correlated maturation of white matter microstructure with brain functional activation during a working memory task. The general hypothesis is that maturation of white matter, which provides connectivity in the brain, is associated with increased processing capacity of gray matter. Regions of correlation were indeed prominent in frontal lobes but were also detected in multiple sites throughout the brain, including parietal cortex and anterior corpus callosum. They comment, "If we assume that it is development of axonal thickness and myelination that is responsible for the age-related increase in FA (fractional anisotrophy, that is, white matter organization), this would mean that an increase in FA may possibly be associated with enhanced effectiveness of the communication between regions" (Olesen et al., 2003, p. 54). This work, which must be considered exploratory at this point, provides support for the position that cognitive developmental processes do not reflect the maturation of specific regions or functional modules so much as the assembly, integration, and refinement of functional networks, as Johnson proposes in his interactive specialization model of development (Johnson & Munakata, 2005). Hence, a task such as working memory, while certainly dependent on the integrity of key areas such as dorsolateral prefrontal cortex, presumably also reflects the integrity of a disseminated network that develops in relation to both intrinsic and extrinsic influences.

Developmental abilities and disabilities, therefore, are likely to reflect processes associated with the construction, integration, and establishment of functional networks, rather than the functions of specific brain regions. From this perspective, the developmental terrain is far more complex and forbidding than that of the adult. The dramatic changes in executive capacities that occur over developmental time may well reflect these processes of construction of functional networks. How such networks might behave in individuals with developmental disorders (in most of which executive capacities are affected) is of primary interest. Moreover, it follows from this more systemic view that behavioral manifestations of executive functions can reflect a multiplicity of underlying factors that can influence the effectiveness and integrity of the network on which task execution depends rather than the integrity of a specific region or regions, as a more modular approach would suggest.

EXTRINSIC AND INTRINSIC INFLUENCES
ON EXECUTIVE CAPACITIES

Executive capacities may be thought of as the interface between the child and the social and physical world within which he or she interacts. Perspective on this relationship can be found in evolutionary terms. Evolutionary explanations of behavior seek ultimate causes, not proximate ones; the question is framed not as "What *is* this system," but as "What is this system *for?*" One answer to this question with respect to executive systems is that the associated neural circuitry supports the flexible organization and reorganization of attention (control of sensory input), intention (control of behavioral output), and thought (memory and processing) (Pribram, 1997) that permit the integration of past with present to guide future action and behavior. In order for this to occur, frontal circuitry (which is not limited to frontal regions but comprises connectivity of frontal regions to other relevant cortical and subcortical loci) and the control systems it supports function and are shaped in a bidirectional fashion by contextual processes both extrinsic and intrinsic to the individual. In this framework, understanding of cognitive development in general will not be advanced by tallying the acquisition of separate abilities but will need to characterize changing patterns of use of multifaceted abilities (Carlson, 2005; Schneider, Schumann-Hengsteler, & Sodian, 2005).

We have emphasized elsewhere the critical role of context in neurobehavioral development and function (Bernstein, 2000; Bernstein & Waber, 2003). The ontogeny of neural circuitry is crucial to these continual brain–context transactions. As this circuitry matures, the transactions between it and the external context deliver the young child from the tyranny of internal biology (in the form of reflexive action patterns) and permits ever more precise selection of differing response options with respect to the child's environment. Maturation of the frontal circuitry necessarily involves ever-increasing interface with the context as executive control systems continually select behavioral options that promote the adaptive match. The developing brain has an increasing ability to differentiate contextual variables, which most likely feeds back to promote increased differentiation at the neural level and then feeds forward to promote further differentiation of context and so forth. Because contextual interaction is so critical to the successful ontogeny of brain function, the brain can—indeed, must—be exquisitely sensitive to contextual variables. The symbolic power of language, moreover, dramatically extends the range of possible contexts far beyond those available to nonhuman animals.

The bidirectional influence of context on the development of executive skills is not only a function of the child learning from his or her own activities as an increasingly autonomous agent in goal-oriented problem solving, but also results from the equally active shaping of the child's behavior (via limits, cues, prompts, scaffolding, scripts) in transactions with other agents in the environment whose goal is to socialize the child to group norms and expectations. Thus, effortful control and delay-of–gratification abilities are predicted by the quality of parent–child interaction when children were toddlers (Kochanska, Murray, & Harlan, 2000; Sethi, Mischel, Aber, Shoda, & Rodriguez, 2000). Language input from adults is an important influence on development of executive skills (Barkley, 1997). In the academic setting, success is influenced in large part by the degree to which students become self-regulators of their own learning (Blair, 2002; Zimmerman & Schunk, 1989), with intentional control over one's learning being related both to achievement in school and to self-concept (Dweck, 1986; Skinner, Zimmer-Gembeck, & Connell, 1998).

This bidirectional interaction is reflected in the structural development of the brain as well. Myelination of white matter tracts is thought to be protracted across development, extending past adolescence in prefrontal cortex (Paus et al., 2000; Sowell, Thompson, Holmes, Jernigan, & Toga, 1999). Such development, however, is not automatic and preprogrammed but seems to be sensitive to extrinsic factors (Fields, 2005). Once the basic plan of the brain is laid down, neural network connectivity may be enhanced by the complexity of experience. Imaging studies of nonhuman primates with sensory deprivation (Manger, Woods, & Jones, 1996) and of human adults with highly developed musical talent (Elbert, Pantev, Wienbruch, Rockstroh, & Taub, 1995; Gaser & Schlaug, 2003; Hashimoto et al., 2004), with and without exposure to reading (Castro-Caldas, Petersson, Reis, Stone-Elander, & Ingvar, 1998) or skilled in Braille following loss of sight (Buchel, Price, Frackowiak, & Friston, 1998), clearly document the ability of the brain to forge new connections in response to experience. One can speculate that the neural systems that support executive capacities, being so intimately connected to external demands, are similarly influenced by extrinsic environmental factors. Mezzacappa (2004), for example, has demonstrated associations between salient environmental factors early in life and executive capacities of young children as demonstrated on computer-based information-processing tasks.

The sensitivity to contextual variables that is the hallmark of intact (frontal network-supported) executive functioning has relevant clinical implications. Behavioral organization can be highly sensitive to procedure and local conditions. In the clinical context, this sensitivity influences assessment methodology, diagnosis, and intervention. Methodologically, how executive capacities are conceptualized influences how they are measured: by specific tasks or by behavioral ratings? And if by means of tasks, what sort? Tasks that are novel will elicit very different executive capacities from those that are familiar. Diagnostically, the meaning of given behaviors will need to be scrutinized as a function of the conditions under which they were elicited, ranging from the overall setting to the social transactions occurring at the time to the demand characteristics of specific psychological tasks and maneuvers. The diagnostic meaning of observed behaviors will also change with development. As children mature, they are expected to engage with changing contexts in an appropriate and adaptive fashion. To the extent that the child is too sensitive to extrinsic influences, or not sensitive enough, executive functions may be viewed as disordered. Even here, there is considerable variation in the manifestation of sensitivity, depending upon various extrinsic considerations. A child who may be well regulated and attentive in the well-structured classroom setting may become silly and dysregulated at a sleepover. Children in general may be less well regulated in a culture that is permissive with respect to discipline and highly regulated in a culture that is more strictly regimented. Not surprisingly, interventions will need to be developed with reference to the actual conditions under which a given child is expected to function. A strategy of remediation of a given executive function will be of little use to child or family if its effects are limited to the setting and/or conditions in which the functional skill was learned. A more holistic intervention approach will be necessary to address contextual and situational variables as a critical component of the overall management plan. To maximize the match (Bernstein & Waber, 2003) between child and context, such a plan may require not only remedial instruction, change in teaching strategy, the provision of modifications or accommodations for typical expectations, and/or change in instructional setting, but even a change in the school itself.

Given the central role of extrinsic environmental factors in the development of executive capacities, it is tempting to consider the potential impact of the informational environments in which children in the developed world, especially the United States, are now raised. Their experiences in this regard are vastly different from those encountered by their parents or even children growing up 15 years ago. Children in our information age are flooded with stimulation from multiple media sources and exposed to an intensity of technology-assisted multitasking that was not required of earlier generations. It seems reasonable to speculate that such experience could be reflected in the quality of neural connectivity, especially for those brain systems that are most involved in interface with the environmental context. The flood of information may stimulate the development of more efficient and finely tuned executive systems, or it may result in less well-regulated executive systems as children lack highly structured environments that are crucial in shaping behaviors. Moreover, there are presumably individual differences in the "goodness of fit" between the informational environment and optimal development of executive systems, with some children thriving and others foundering.

Factors intrinsic to the child are also contextually relevant. A child whose language competence is diminished may not have the cognitive tools to build developmentally appropriate executive capacities. By the same token, developmental language disorders often occur in the context of more systemic effects on information processing, such that language and executive capacities come to be diminished because developmental processes build on variations in initial state that may themselves be relatively subtle (Karmiloff-Smith, 1998). Thus, both language and executive processes could be affected, albeit to differing degrees, by a variation in a relatively subtle, lower-level aspect of processing on which higher-order functioning builds. Diminished regulatory capacities at a relatively low level could thus increase a impact of the language dysfunction on the elaboration of higher-order executive and regulatory capacities.

In some instances, cognitive compromises may exert a situational impact on executive capacities because of the systemic nature of these functions. For example, the child who struggles to process language in the classroom may become fidgety and inattentive not because of a primary executive problem but because he or she is overwhelmed or confused. Similarly, a very bright child may become fidgety or inattentive because of boredom and disengage in the classroom. A child who is internally distracted by stressful social events at home or in school may exhibit diminished executive capacities to attend, organize, and function in an efficient goal-directed fashion, again not because of a primary executive problem but because the frontal circuitry cannot be effectively engaged.

Executive processes are exquisitely sensitive to extrinsic, environmental factors and most likely to intrinsic factors as well. These can vary from moment to moment as situations change. Measuring executive functions, therefore, can be a treacherous undertaking, since they are so pre-eminently situationally dependent and fluid and vary depending upon the context.

HOW SHOULD WE THINK ABOUT EXECUTIVE FUNCTIONS IN THE DEVELOPMENTAL CONTEXT?

Based on the above discussion, several points are clear as we consider how to consider executive capacities in developmental neuropsychology and especially in the assessment and understanding of the individual child.

1. In the developmental context, the modular approach should be viewed critically. Although the developmental process points toward increasing differentiation and hence modularity of the cognitive architecture as children make the transition to adolescence and adulthood, how the young brain progresses from its less differentiated state to modularity is not well understood nor is there agreement on the nature of the questions to be asked. This being the case, the definition of "executive functions"—essentially a modular concept—is itself problematic. What does it mean when executive functions are so frequently affected by so many conditions and circumstances? And when the same behavior can have different significance for different children and different age groups in different cultures?

2. In development, executive processes are best understood in the context of functional networks constructed over the course of development. Whereas in the adult, disorders of executive processes are regularly associated with discrete lesions to regions of frontal cortex, executive functions in the child can be adversely affected by any influences that affect not only components of the network but also, its construction. Importantly, this may include experiential influences or context, which are intimately involved in the construction of these more differentiated networks. Understanding executive functions requires scrutiny of contextual variables as well as neural correlates of behavior.

3. As a metaphor, it may be useful to think of executive capacities as a resource and not a set of functions that can themselves be meaningfully and reliably parsed. If Duncan's (2001) adaptive coding model ultimately has merit, these processes themselves must be constructed and become more efficient. It should be a goal of research to understand how the construction occurs and why it sometimes fails to occur as expected.

4. Executive capacities are best seen in on-line contexts, a resource summoned in relation to specific task demands. They are likely, therefore, to be variable and somewhat inconsistent between tasks and to be highly context- and situation-dependent. Measurement of such capacities within the current framework of psychological assessment tools, which presume to measure static characteristics or competencies, presents a challenge.

5. Caution should be exercised in drawing inferences from so-called tests of executive functions, which typically are based on modular assumptions. More profitable approaches should include task analysis and clinical limit testing to describe executive capacities in a variety of tasks and settings. The true challenge of assessment in this regard is to understand how the frontal circuitry actually might work in supporting the executive skills that underlie the capacity to manage novelty and to

be flexible in response to unknown, unpredictable, on-line behavioral responses that may not be captured by static psychological tests.

6. Developmental processes are oriented toward increasing differentiation and integration, and individual differences or variations become integrated into this process. Executive capacities can be expected to improve as these developmental forces come into play. Assessment approaches that are limited to the single "snapshot in time" will be inadequate to the task of providing the comprehensive description of a child that is needed to maximize both current well-being and future outcomes, a description that can only be understood in the context of the broader developmental trajectory as it projects across time.

7. Because of the context dependence of executive functions, it is not surprising that children can perform adequately on laboratory-type tasks given in a one-on-one clinical setting yet encounter difficulty in a busy classroom setting or on the playing field. Performance under all conditions must be integrated into the clinical diagnosis and management plan.

8. Problems with organization and self-regulation in children may have many sources. For executive capacities more than any other component of the neuropsychological evaluation, a whole-child approach is mandatory: specific tests of executive function will be informative but not conclusive.

CONCLUSION

In this chapter, we have considered the development of executive functions with regard to three primary issues: assumptions of modularity; contrasting considerations with adults and developing children; and the role of extrinsic and intrinsic factors in the development and expression of executive capacities. We suggest that assumptions of modularity in the developing child lead to models of neurobehavioral function that are not a good fit with the observed phenomena. Executive capacities in children, and possibly in adults as well, may be better understood as a relatively domain general resource that can be implemented in an ad hoc fashion, "tuned" by a specific task and/or environmental demand. Inconsistencies are thus expectable and meaningful. Moreover, the network metaphor is likely to be more useful in evaluating children than the adult lesion metaphor, shifting the emphasis to processes of construction and integration as well as refinement of capacities. Developmental forces will exert themselves and help shape these executive capacities as will sensitivity to context. Because executive functions lie at the interface between the child and the environment and are necessarily exquisitely sensitive to context, these capacities can be expected both to orchestrate complex and creative behaviors in new settings and to be vulnerable to disruption when contextual factors prove overwhelming. They are, however, equally likely to be highly amenable to intervention.

REFERENCES

Anderson, V. A., Anderson, P., Northam, E., Jacobs, R., & Mikiewicz, O. (2002). Relationships between cognitive and behavioral measures of executive function in children with brain disease. *Child Neuropsychology, 8*(4), 231–240.

Atkinson, R. C., & Shiffrin, R. M. (1968). Human memory: A proposed system and its control processes. In K. W. Spence & J. T. Spence (Eds.), *The psychology of learning and motivation: II* (pp. 89–195). New York: Academic Press.

Baddeley, A. (1998). The central executive: A concept and some misconceptions. *Journal of the International Neuropsychological Society, 4*(5), 523–526.

Barkley, R. A. (1997). *ADHD and the nature of self-control.* New York: Guilford Press.

Belmont, J. M., & Butterfield, E. C. (1971). Learning strategies as determinants of memory deficiencies. *Cognitive Psychology, 2,* 411–420.

Bernstein, J. H. (2000). Developmental neuropsychological assessment. In K. O. Yeates, D. M. Ris, & H. G. Taylor (Eds.), *Pediatric neuropsychology: Research, theory, and practice.* New York: Guilford Press.

Bernstein, J. H., & Waber, D. P. (2003). Pediatric neuropsychological assessment. In T. E. Feinberg & M. J. Farah (Eds.), *Behavioral neurology and neuropsychology* (2nd ed., pp. 773–781). New York: McGraw-Hill.

Blair, C. (2002). School readiness: Integrating cognition and emotion in a neurobiological conceptualization of children's functioning at school entry. *American Psychologist, 57*(2), 111–127.

Buchel, C., Price, C., Frackowiak, R., & Friston, K. (1998). Different activation patterns in the visual cortex of late and congenitally blind subjects. *Brain, 121*(3), 409–419.

Campione, J. C., & Brown, A. L. (1977). Memory and metamemory development in educable retarded children. In R. V. Kail & J. W. Hagen (Eds.), *Perspectives on the development of memory and cognition* (pp. 367–406). Hillsdale, NJ: Erlbaum.

Carlson, S. M. (2005). Developmentally sensitive measures of executive function in preschool children. *Developmental Neuropsychology, 28*(2), 595–616.

Castro-Caldas, A., Petersson, K. M., Reis, A., Stone-Elander, S., & Ingvar, M. (1998). The illiterate brain. Learning to read and write during childhood influences the functional organization of the adult brain. *Brain, 121*(6), 1053–1063.

Denckla, M. B. (1996). A theory and model of executive function: A neuropsychological perspective. In G. R. Lyon & N. A. Krasnegor (Eds.), *Attention, memory, and executive function* (pp. 263–278). Baltimore: Brookes.

Duncan, J. (2001). An adaptive coding model of neural function in prefrontal cortex. *Nature Reviews Neuroscience, 2,* 820–829.

Duncan, J., & Owen, A. M. (2000). Common regions of the human frontal lobe recruited by diverse cognitive demands. *Trends in Neurosciences, 23*(10), 475–483.

Dweck, C. S. (1986). Motivational processes affecting learning. *American Psychologist, 41*(10), 1040–1048.

Elbert, T., Pantev, C., Wienbruch, C., Rockstroh, B., & Taub, E. (1995). Increased cortical representation of the fingers of the left hand in string players. *Science, 270,* 305–307.

Farah, M. J. (1994). Neuropsychological inference with an interactive brain: A critique of the "locality" assumption. *Behavioral and Brain Sciences, 17,* 43–104.

Fields, R. (2005). Myelination: An overlooked mechanism of synaptic plasticity. *The Neuroscientist, 11*(6), 528–531.

Fletcher, J. M., & Taylor, H. G. (1984). Neuropsychological approaches to children: Towards a developmental neuropsychology. *Journal of Clinical Neuropsychology, 6*(1), 39–56.

Gaser, C., & Schlaug, G. (2003). Brain structures differ between musicians and non-musicians. *Journal of Neuroscience, 23,* 9240–9245.

Hashimoto, I., Suzuki, A., Kimura, T., Iguchi, Y., Tanosaki, M., Takino, R., et al. (2004). Is there training-dependent reorganization of digit representations in area 3b of string players? *Clinical Neurophysiology, 115*(2), 435–447.

Jerison, H. J. (1997). Evolution of prefrontal cortex. In N. A. Krasnegor, G. R. Lyon, & P. S. Goldman-Rakic (Eds.), *Development of the prefrontal cortex* (pp. 9–26). Baltimore: Brookes.

Johnson, M. H., & Munakata, Y. (2005). Processes of change in brain and cognitive development. *Trends in Cognitive Sciences, 9*(3), 152–158.

Karmiloff-Smith, A. (1998). Is atypical development necessarily a window on the normal mind/brain?: The case of Williams syndrome. *Developmental Science, 1*(2), 273–277.

Kochanska, G., Murray, K. T., & Harlan, E. T. (2000). Effortful control in early childhood: Continuity and change, antecedents, and implications for social development. *Developmental Psychology, 36*(2), 220–232.

Kwon, H., Reiss, A. L., & Menon, V. (2002). Neural basis of protracted developmental changes in visuo–spatial working memory. *Proceedings of the National Academy of Sciences of the United States of America, 99*(20), 13336–13341.

Manger, P., Woods, T., & Jones, E. (1996). Plasticity of the somatosensory cortical map in macaque monkeys after chronic partial amputation of a digit. *Proceedings of Biological Sciences, 263*(1372), 933–939.

Mezzacappa, E. (2004). Alerting, orienting, and executive attention: Developmental properties and sociodemographic correlates in an epidemiological sample of young, urban children. *Child Development, 75*(5), 1373–1386.

Olesen, P. J., Nagy, Z., Westerberg, H., & Klingberg, T. (2003). Combined analysis of DTI and fMRI data reveals a joint maturation of white and grey matter in a fronto-parietal network. *Cognitive Brain Research, 18*(1), 48–57.

Paus, T., Zijdenbos, A., Worsley, K., Collins, D. L., Blumenthal, J., Giedd, J. N., et al. (2000). Structural maturation of neural pathways in children and adolescents: In vivo study. *Science, 283,* 1908–1911.

Pennington, B. (1997). Dimensions of executive functions in normal and abnormal development. In N. A. Krasnegor, G. R. Lyon, & P. S. Goldman-Rakic (Eds.), *Development of the prefrontal cortex* (pp. 265–281). Baltimore: Brookes.

Pribram, K. (1997). The work in working memory: Implications for development. In N. A. Krasnegor, G. R. Lyon, & P. S. Goldman-Rakic (Eds.), *Development of the prefrontal cortex* (pp. 359–378). Baltimore: Brookes.

Sacks, O. (2001). Foreword. In E. Goldberg (Ed.), *The executive brain.* New York: Oxford University Press.

Schneider, W., Schumann-Hengsteler, R., & Sodian, B. (2005). *Young children's cognitive development: Interrelationships among executive functioning, working memory, verbal ability, and theory of mind.* Hillsdale, NJ: Erlbaum.

Sethi, A., Mischel, W., Aber, J. L., Shoda, Y., & Rodriguez, M. L. (2000). The role of strategic attention deployment in development of self-regulation: Predicting preschoolers' delay of gratification from mother–toddler interactions. *Developmental Psychology, 36*(6), 767–777.

Skinner, E. A., Zimmer-Gembeck, M. J., & Connell, J. P. (1998). *Individual differences and the development of perceived control* (Vol. 63). Oxford, UK: Blackwell Publishing.

Sowell, E. R., Thompson, P., Holmes, C. J., Jernigan, T. L., & Toga, A. W. (1999). In vivo evidence for post-adolescent brain maturation in frontal and striatal regions. *Nature Neuroscience, 2*(10), 859–861.

Vriezen, E. R., & Pigott, S. E. (2002). The relationship between parental report on the BRIEF and performance-based measures of executive function in children with moderate to severe traumatic brain injury. *Child Neuropsychology, 8*(4), 296–303.

Waber, D., Gerber, E. B., Turcios, V., Wagner, E. R., & Forbes, P. W. (2006). Executive functions and performance on high-stakes testing in children from urban schools. *Developmental Neuropsychology, 29*(3), 459–477.

Zimmerman, B. J., & Schunk, D. H. (Eds.). (1989). *Self-regulated learning and academic achievement: Theory, research, and practice.* New York: Springer-Verlag.

CHAPTER 4

Connecting Cognitive Science and Neuroscience to Education

Potentials and Pitfalls
in Inferring Executive Processes

KURT W. FISCHER
SAMANTHA G. DALEY

Scientific understanding of mind and brain is advancing quickly and energetically, and society's need to improve the quality of education makes headlines every day. Naturally, these two trends create a broad interest in using research about the brain and mind to guide educational practice. Knowing how our minds/brains function, how we use the brain and body to process and store new information, how our minds/brains change and develop, and how damage to our brains contributes to disabilities and other problems—all these research efforts have great potential for moving forward the science and practice of learning.

This move to make educational practice more scientific has properties that are similar to the history of medical practice. Medicine once relied on the collected wisdom of culture but had no systematic procedure for testing which medical practices were actually effective. In the last 200 years, especially since the innovations of Louis Pasteur in France, medicine has established a powerful base in research in the biological sciences. Medical practice is now guided by what the biological sciences know about the body, and the biological sciences conduct research that is informed by what is important to medicine. This process is interactive and reciprocal. Scientists do not dictate medical practice, but they contribute to investigating and understanding innovative treatments and techniques that often derive from the clinical skills and experiences of practitioners. In parallel fashion, education must clarify and strengthen its relationship with the research disciplines that study development, learning, and the brain. This relationship should be a reciprocal one in which educational practice and scientific research inform and learn from each other, as medicine and biology act symbiotically.

Although this relationship is still emerging, the growth in knowledge of development, learning, and the brain already provides potentially productive connections between educational practice and scientific research. One particularly promising arena is analysis of possible general abilities that are proposed as an important focus for educational practice, such as the teaching of executive function, the topic of this book. Based on both research and practice—scientific knowledge about how children learn and develop and the history of efforts in education to teach a broad, general ability—we will argue that there is no tightly organized executive function but only loosely coupled, diverse executive skills. A closer relationship between educational practice and research can provide a more accurate and practically useful view of executive function and other candidates for general abilities, such as metamemory, metacognition, and theory of mind (Fischer & Immordino-Yang, 2002; Fischer, Immordino-Yang, & Waber, 2006).

Commonly in human development and in learning in schools, researchers and teachers observe the regular occurrence of similar behaviors and changes that suggest a unified entity, such as executive function. Careful research and practical observation typically find that these behaviors are more diverse than unified. This widely occurring pattern pervades all aspects of human learning and development, including motor functioning, cognitive development, and brain development, as well as executive function. We argue that, like the other cases, executive function has important general characteristics that make it seem to be a unified entity, but at the level of detail important for educational practice it is diverse and variable, not unified. The practical implications of such an interpretation are many.

A RECIPROCAL PARTNERSHIP: DEVELOPMENT, NEUROSCIENCE, AND EDUCATION

Over the last two centuries, the biological sciences have come to form a natural partner for the improvement of medical practice. What fields might play a similar role in relation to education? The complex nature of educational practice means that several types of research can produce educationally usable knowledge (Fischer & Katzir, in press). In this chapter, we focus particularly on knowledge about human development, the learning process, and brain functioning.

The study of how human beings develop and learn falls under the umbrella of the discipline of human development and its sibling, developmental psychology. This is the field of research that investigates how learning takes place and how people change as they grow from infancy through adulthood. Its research methods have traditionally involved controlled experiments in laboratories as well as studies of naturally occurring changes in behavior with age and setting. Research questions have often focused on narrow inquiries related to (1) normative patterns for particular ages or social groups and (2) species-general human characteristics of thought, memory, attention, emotion, and learning. The field is now experiencing major efforts to move it toward a broader framework that examines development as a function of the many components that affect human behavior, including biology, context, culture, and individual variation. Indeed, the first volume of the influential *Handbook of Child Psychology* highlights this important shift in emphasis (Damon & Lerner, 2006).

Neuroscience involves the study of the brain, especially its organization, functioning, and underlying physiology, including the neurons, synapses, and neural networks that it comprises. Neuroscience emphasizes brain functioning but not necessarily outwardly noticeable behavior. Most questions in neuroscience focus on specific, experimentally tractable hypotheses about the brain's response to simple stimuli (Turk et al., 2002). Study of the brain often requires combinations of fields in permutations such as cognitive neuroscience, behavior genetics, and behavioral neurochemistry. Our focus in this chapter is on research that makes connections between the brain's activity and people's actions and thoughts.

Education is different from development and neuroscience, as it is not only an academic area of study, but also a practical field. We consider education broadly to include traditional classroom learning, adult learning, and informal learning activities.

Education, human development, and neuroscience have yet to establish a truly reciprocal partnership despite continually increasing interactions tending in that direction. A handful of cases show the enormous potential of reciprocal interactions for benefiting educational practice. For example, research in dyslexia has led to major advances not only in understanding the bases of specific reading disabilities, but also in the design of interventions to help students with dyslexia learn to read and write effectively. Maryanne Wolf and her colleagues (Wolf & Bowers, 1999; Wolf & Katzir-Cohen, 2001; Wolf, Miller, & Donnelly, 2000) have developed a curriculum to support students with dyslexia that integrates knowledge from neuroscience, development, cognitive science, and education in innovative and meaningful ways. David Rose and his colleagues use principles from these disciplines to inform the development of software and other educational tools that support reading, writing, and instruction that is flexible enough for a variety of learners, following the principles of what they call "universal design" (Rose, Meyer, Strangman, & Rappolt, 2002; Rose, Chapter 13, this volume). These are but two examples that show what is possible when expert scientists and educators from different disciplines work together to study and inform educational activities.

Such efforts move forward the reciprocal relationships of education with cognitive developmental science and neuroscience, producing major advances and innovations in educational practice. Yet caution remains imperative in basing education-related decisions on basic research, especially when there are one-sided relationships rather than reciprocal partnerships. For example, concepts about executive function in cognitive science have led to educational practices that are overly simple and do not engage the variability that teachers encounter every day with students in their classrooms.

SIMILARITIES ACROSS DOMAINS: SIMILAR PATTERNS DO NOT SIGNIFY A UNITARY ABILITY

In a common type of unwarranted leap, researchers uncover similar patterns of behavior or brain functioning and assume that the similarities reflect a single underlying process or structure. The discovery of these similarities, such as parallel patterns of learning or development, provides the basis for many important scientific discoveries, so researchers should seek them, but the interpretation of the parallels requires caution: Even when the similarities point to some common process or function, they typically do not imply a unified or singular capacity, so implications for educational practice are not simple (Fischer & Bidell, 2006). One of the most general characteristics of human functioning (both body and behavior) is that many components operate mostly independently while at the same time having some important links and similarities.

In medicine, when a person experiences a sudden high fever, doctors dare not assume that this symptom indicates a singular cause. A fever can come from bacterial infection, viral infection, overheating of the body, insufficient cooling of the body, malfunction of the immune system, and many other diverse causes. In every case, the body's temperature regulation system is involved, but there is no single cause across cases. A veterinarian can build her practice on the understanding that both poodles and schnauzers are dogs, but she dare not assume that the various dogs are identical, or she will make critical mistakes in treatment. We will now discuss several examples of similarities in patterns of biological and cognitive development and then how to interpret the similarities and what the insights from these examples imply for analyzing executive function.

Motor System(s)

The motor system—the functions of the body that allow and control movement—can in many ways be viewed as a single entity. Like the digestive system or the respiratory system, students tend to study the motor system as a unit. Understanding the functioning of muscles, tendons, ligaments, and the rest will provide a solid foundation for understanding how people can tap their toes, nod their heads, or throw a baseball. Given the common functions and the strong connections of some components, it makes sense to view the motor functions as a system.

At the same time, the shared functions of the motor system do not make it unitary or uniform, and assuming such a unity leads to critical misunderstanding. For example, an impairment or injury in one aspect of motor activity often has little or no influence on another aspect. The motor system is highly differentiated into gross and fine motor activities, voluntary and involuntary muscles, distinct organs (arms, legs, heart, stomach, motor cortex, cerebellum, etc.) and even further specialized within each of these categories.

Any basic anatomy and physiology textbook makes clear the complexity of the processes that enable human movement. In any one part of the motor system, such as muscles, crucial distinctions must be made. One textbook highlights the need to consider both differences and similarities among types of muscles (Marieb, 2006). There are three types of muscle tissue, which differ in cell structure, body location, and type of stimulation to cause contraction, but all types have the same kinds of filaments that participate in contraction. In another piece of the motor system, different joints are capable of different types of rotation, each with different implications for injury and treatment (Mader, 2005). Regarding how components work together, there are distinct categories that specify characteristic patterns of coordination, such as voluntary and involuntary movements and gross and fine motor skills.

Viewing the motor system as a unified entity, then, is useful for analyzing how bodily movement happens, but the system is composed of many different parts and processes. It cannot be treated as a unitary structure. The parts function independently in most ways, although they are partly connected and coordinated. The same is true of behavioral systems.

Cognitive Development

The traditional view of development assumes that components that show similar growth functions involve the same unitary underlying process or capacity—a single stage of logic for Piaget's (1983) theory or a single buffer of short-term memory for classical information-processing views (Case, 1974; Klahr & Wallace, 1976). This traditional view treats development as a ladder on which people move upward step by step to successively higher general cognitive stages in a linear fashion. An individual functions at a single general stage across domains and no longer uses earlier ones, according to this view. The stages on this metaphorical ladder assume a common state of development across all domains of learning and behavior, from the ability to solve arithmetic problems to the maturity to respond to social challenges. A 5-year-old will show the same (pre-operational) stage of cognitive development in arithmetic and social understanding, and an adult will show the same (formal operational) stage in both domains.

People do not show this kind of consistency. Research strongly documents that the ladder metaphor is wrong when applied across domains (Fischer & Bidell, 2006), and any experienced teacher or observer of children knows that students show different capacities in different domains. Only within a domain do children develop along a relatively unified, consistent pathway.

A dynamic view of development moves from the traditional ladder view to a different metaphor that includes both consistency and variability, consistent pathways within a domain and different pathways among different domains. Development proceeds along the strands of a web as shown in Figure 4.1. Each strand in the web represents a different specific domain of development. Depending on the breadth of the content one chooses, the strands might represent broad domains such as motor skills, arithmetic knowledge, and literacy, or they might represent specific subdomains within a narrower domain such as simple arithmetic problems, with addition on one strand, subtraction on another, and multiplication on a third. The strands in the figure specify domains in the development of executive processes. Development proceeds from the top of the diagram to the bottom, but a person can develop along different strands at different paces. While the ladder metaphor and the theory behind it emphasize the normative commonalities in development across domains, the web and the dynamic view capture variations in development across domains, as well as connections and separations (represented by intersections and branches).

Besides this variability *across* domains of functioning, the web metaphor also allows for variability *within* domains for individual learners. A person working on a specific task does not stay fixed at one point on a

Domains

Regulating   Monitoring   Reflective
learning   comprehension   judgment

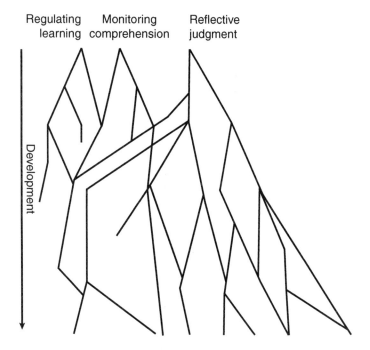

FIGURE 4.1. A developmental web for domains of executive function.

strand but varies his or her activity depending on context and state (Fischer & Bidell, 2006; Fischer, Bullock, Rotenberg, & Raya, 1993). A 1-year-old learns to walk on a level carpet inside the home but is unable to make a few steps across the grass in the backyard. Everyone has experienced situations such as being able in practice to remember lines for a play or shoot a free throw and then failing with the same behavior in the performance that matters. What does it mean to "know" material or to have "mastered" a skill? On any particular task, a person acts at a wide variety of levels, ranging from the functional, or typical, level to the optimal level (what can be done with contextual support). The role of a supportive environment in causing variation along a strand in the web has been widely documented for tasks as diverse as telling a story about social interactions or predicting whether objects will sink or float.

The variability in behavior captured by the web helps illuminate the uniformity seen in some developmental changes. Children demonstrate rapid changes in performance in specific age regions for optimal conditions in familiar domains—changes that have some of the properties of stages. Such spurts have been documented in studies of, for example, reflective judgment in adolescents and adults (Kitchener, Lynch, Fischer, & Wood, 1993) and use of pronouns in the early speech of Dutch children (Ruhland & van Geert, 1998), as shown in Figure 4.2. These spurts and other kinds of discontinuities tend to cluster at particular age regions for optimal performance, such as approximately 2 years for spurts in vocabulary, use of sentences, and pretend play. In Figure 4.1, look carefully at when the strands change direction, branch, or join, and you will see that these discontinuities cluster in specific regions.

People develop in spurts under optimal conditions, but typically not under ordinary conditions, which lack contextual support and/or extensive familiarity and practice (Fischer et al., 1993). Figure 4.3 illustrates a typical pattern for development of optimal and functional (ordinary) levels in a domain such as reflective judgment or representation of social interactions. Skills develop in spurts for optimal level (high support, top line) but more slowly and smoothly for functional level (low support, bottom line). The same person shows both optimal and functional levels, which come and go with variations in contextual support and state. In this way, each person acts at multiple levels from moment to moment, even for a single domain (strand in the web), moving up and down within in a range of skill levels as a function of support and state.

When observers note only the spurts and other discontinuities, which cluster at a specific age region in the developmental web, they see what appears to be a single ability emerging at that age. Examined more

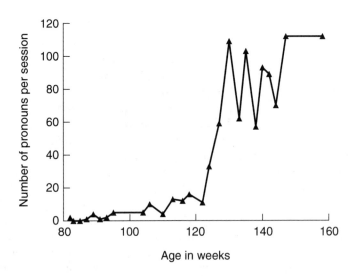

FIGURE 4.2. Developmental spurt in pronoun use by Tomas, a Dutch boy.

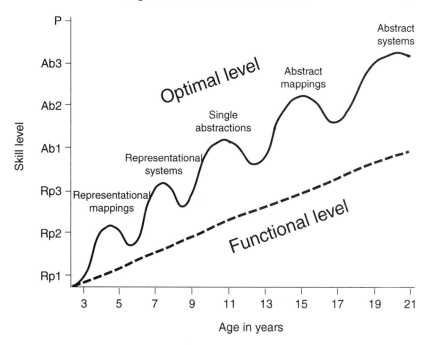

FIGURE 4.3. Optimal and functional levels in cognitive development. Skills develop along a common complexity scale marked by a series of skill levels. With high support, they grow in spurts for optimal level. Without support, they grow more continuously for functional level.

broadly (in the whole web), this pattern becomes one regularity within the broader picture of variability. There is clearly no single, unitary ability emerging across all skills and domains at one age. Instead, a person builds skills along each strand, following its domain-specific developmental progression, and at certain points along the strand, spurts ahead. This spurt is a local process in the domain, not a shift in a single, unitary new ability.

Development is a complex phenomenon that encompasses both (1) elements of uniformity, such as regions of common change across strands or domains, and (2) elements of individuality and variation. As with motor functioning, assuming unity neglects the variation that is present in cognitive development and, thus, oversimplifies and distorts the nature of development, making it seem like a ladder. An accurate view of development must account for both uniformity and variability.

The uniform aspects of cognitive development provide a valuable heuristic based on large-scale patterns of developmental change. Indeed, they have led to the identification of a general developmental scale underlying both cognitive development and learning (Dawson-Tunik, Commons, Wilson, & Fischer, 2005; Fischer & Bidell, 2006; Fischer & Immordino-Yang, 2002). At the same time, focus on only the uniformity leads to distortions, especially in education. The unitary view produces an emphasis on norms and a neglect of the variation that is inevitably present in educational settings. Children within a classroom will not all reach the same reading level at the same time, despite ladder-like views of reading that mark a text as at one specific grade level. This perspective makes individual variation appear abnormal and problematic rather than a phenomenon to be explored and explained. If a student is able to complete a page of algebra problems one day but seems to have forgotten everything the next day, the behavior appears abnormal and inexplicable (although sensitive teachers know to expect such variation). With the dynamic view of development, such variation is understandable and potentially predictable from context and emotional state (e.g., Did he skip breakfast so he cannot concentrate today? Is a test next period causing anxiety? Did he have a supportive algebra lesson right before he did the problems yesterday?).

A dynamic view of development recognizes the similarities in development across different domains and simultaneously interprets them in terms of the patterns of variation. This dynamic view is more useful and accurate than a traditional view that assumes a unitary process because it deals directly with the complexities of human learning and action. Educators and developmental scientists working together can (1) illuminate the understanding of development by connecting it to variations in students' behaviors in schools and families and (2) simultaneously create research that feeds back to practitioners to help them use cognitive and developmental analysis to facilitate learning and teaching in schools.

Brain Development

The science of brain development is much less mature than that of cognitive development. Yet early evidence suggests that the model for cognitive development applies straightforwardly to important aspects of brain development as well. Brain growth and cognitive growth seem to show the same kind of web pattern and the same type of recurring growth cycle, with multiple developing strands and spurts and other discontinuities in growth along each strand. For instance, the part of the prefrontal cortex that supports working memory (holding information on-line for a time) develops separately from the part of the occipital cortex that analyzes visual information, although both develop with similar discontinuities (Fischer & Rose, 1996). (Scholars frequently nominate the prefrontal cortex as the key brain region for executive function.)

The strongest empirical evidence of these brain growth patterns comes from research on the development of electrical activity in the cortex, measured through the electroencephalogram (EEG). The most studied property of the EEG is its energy (called "power"), which develops through fits and starts at specific ages that correspond to the ages of emergence of optimal levels in cognitive capacity from infancy through early adulthood (Fischer & Bidell, 2006; Somsen, van 't Klooster, van der Molen, van Leeuwen, & Licht, 1997; Thatcher, 1994). Figure 4.4 shows the results of one normative study (Matousek & Petersén, 1973) for the relative energy in the alpha band of EEG in the back of the cortex, with spurts and plateaus clearly evident at approximately 4, 8, 12, 15, and 20 years of age, apparently marking the cognitive levels that are most relevant for the school years. Note the similarity to the growth curve for optimal level in Figure 4.3.

The similarity of growth curves for EEG energy and cognitive performance suggest a connection between development of brain and behavior, but few studies have looked at brain and behavior concurrently to test the correspondence directly. For the current argument, assume that the correspondence is real—that growth spurts in the EEG

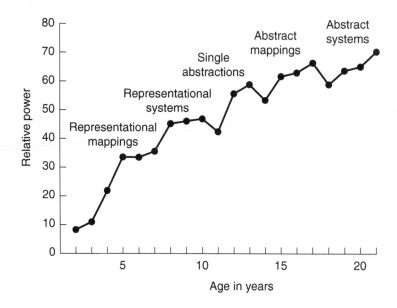

FIGURE 4.4. Development of relative power in alpha EEG in occipito-parietal area in Swedish children and adolescents. The energy (relative power) in the EEG grows in spurts that parallel the pattern for optimal level in Figure 4.3. This graph shows relative power in the occipital–parietal area of the cortex for the alpha band of the EEG in Swedish subjects (Matousek & Petersén, 1973).

indeed reflect brain reorganizations that relate to the new capacities that emerge at specific ages. Even if this scientific hypothesis proves true, there are major issues about the implications for educational practice. Caution is required in drawing conclusions about the nature of learning and development.

In the 1970s and 1980s, several American biologists and educators used evidence about age-related spurts in head circumference and EEG energy, which they called "phrenoblysis" (Epstein, 1974, 1978) to draw conclusions about how schoolchildren learn (Fischer & Lazerson, 1984). They treated these conclusions as facts and used them to make extensive recommendations to school boards, teachers, and parents. For example, the scholars went directly from their findings about spurts in head growth and EEG to conclusions that when the head is in a growth plateau (a period of little change, not a spurt), no learning can occur. They told educators that instruction in new concepts should focus on periods of growth because that was when new learning could occur. Yet there was absolutely no research testing how learning related to periods of brain and head growth, and there was substantial evidence that children learn new material at all ages during the school years, with no flat periods where learning does not occur.

One reason for the popularity of these recommendations in education was that few educators knew much about the biology of the brain, so many of them simply accepted the claims of phrenoblysis as scientific fact. With stronger reciprocal connections between neuroscience, cognitive developmental science, and education, the scientists' hypothesis about the relation of spurts and plateaus to learning would have been subject to empirical test before being used to make recommendations for educational policy and practice.

The model of phrenoblysis assumed that the brain and cognition worked together as a unitary system instead of being composed of many parts, most of which are only loosely coupled. Contrary to that assumption, development does not happen in a single process across all regions of the brain, although there are important similarities in some aspects of brain development across many brain regions. An overly simple look at the EEG evidence can lead to the conclusion that the entire brain is developing during a growth spurt. In reality, development takes place along separate strands (in a developmental web), and one of the goals of neuroscientific research is to characterize relations among the growing strands. Early evidence indicates that the growth process occurs in cycles, moving systematically around locations in the brain, not as a single spurt at the same time across all brain regions (Thatcher, 1994). The left and right hemispheres seem to develop in different sequences, which appear to repeat for each cycle of cortical reorganization (Fischer &

Rose, 1996). Again, what at first appears like a unified process is in fact a diverse set of individual processes acting in concert with each other. Scientists and educators can understand how the "system" works only by examining the parts and how they vary, which will eventually lead to an explanation of the neuroscientific principles of brain development and learning.

Executive Function Is Not Unitary

Executive function is typically conceived as a broad cognitive capacity and is subject to the same kinds of pitfalls in interpretation as other concepts about cognition and brain. The idea of a single, unified executive function falls into the same trap as concepts of unitary motor abilities, cognitive development, and brain development. The continuing lack of consensus regarding a definition of executive function arises in large part from the problems that result from treating it as a single, unitary cognitive ability. Teuber (1972) was one of the first to address the question directly, in his article entitled "Unity and Diversity of Frontal Lobe Functions," and a number of researchers have taken up the issue more recently (Duncan, Johnson, Swales, & Freer, 1997; Miyake, Friedman, Emerson, Witzki, & Howerter, 2000). As Baddeley (1996) puts it, the question remains whether it will "prove more appropriate to regard the executive as a unified system with multiple functions, or simply as an agglomeration of independent though interacting control processes" (p. 5).

Analyses of executive function have taken positions of both unity and divergence and various stances in between. The Norman and Shallice (1986) model of the control of action posits a relatively unified system during completion of non-routine activities. It posits two modes of control, one responsible for routine activities and one for non-routine ones. Routine tasks are triggered whenever appropriate stimuli are present, and the system proceeds automatically without further monitoring. Tasks that are more complex or novel require higher-order control by an executive system that regulates the execution of the activities. While the early version of this model was strongly unitary, it has moved toward differentiation in revised versions (Miyake et al., 2000).

Toward the other end of the spectrum from unified to independent is Pennington and Ozonoff's (1996) model, which treats executive function as a useful functional construct but moves away from the broad frontal cortex metaphor, in which all types of executive tasks are seen as reflecting a single brain function. The authors interpret the metaphor as a logical outgrowth of findings about deficits in patients with frontal lobe damage. Many patients have difficulty with planning or problem solving, but their intelligence is often preserved. Pennington and Ozonoff propose a cluster of weakly coupled functions converging upon "planning or programming future actions, holding those plans or programs on-line until executed, and inhibiting irrelevant actions" (p. 55).

A clear indication of the shift even further toward separate processes is to refer to executive functions in the plural (Burmeister et al., 2005; Fischer, Barkley, Smallish, & Fletcher, 2005; Manchester, Priestley, & Jackson, 2004). Recall from the discussions of the motor system, cognitive development, and brain development that this kind of model of separate components that work together is pervasive in cognitive science and biology. A unified executive function may be useful as a construct (Zelazo, Mueller, Frye, & Marcovitch, 2003), but it is misleading as a representation of the true nature of the system. Several pieces of evidence support the stance that executive functioning consists of diverse components that function independently in many ways.

First, people perform differentially on measures of separate aspects of executive function. Just as a theory of unitary stages of cognitive development predicts similar capabilities across domains, a unitary view of executive function predicts similar performance in different components, such as planning and inhibition. Several studies show distinct differences in these components.

For example, Carlson, Moses, and Claxton (2004) found that 3- and 4-year-olds performed differently on tests of planning and inhibitory control, showing largely independent processes. In a landmark study, Miyake and colleagues (2000) focused on differential performance on elements of executive function in college students. Most research uses simple correlations between tasks, which could reflect differences in aspects of the task that do not involve executive functioning, such as language use. Miyake and colleagues used a more powerful statistical analysis, a latent variable approach, to investigate three separate elements of executive function: shifting, updating, and inhibition. With confirmatory factor analysis, they found that the three constructs were clearly distinguishable and that they demonstrated some underlying commonality. They concluded that the results indicated "both unity and diversity of executive functions" (Miyake et al., 2000, p. 87). Just like the strands in the developmental web, they are mostly independent but loosely coupled.

The hypothesized components of executive function neither appear at the same level of mastery within individuals nor do they necessarily develop together. Anderson (2002) suggests that individual elements of executive function show different developmental trajectories, including attentional control, cognitive flexibility, goal setting, and information processing. Each domain involves a distinct developmental strand in the web for executive function, as shown in Figure 4.1, and evidence suggests that separate processes develop at different rates, reaching skilled levels at different ages. The precise nature of these trajectories needs to be investigated empirically, but clearly the evidence points to diversity in executive functions throughout development.

EDUCATIONAL IMPLICATIONS

Does the debate and confusion about the definition of executive function make any difference for educational practice? Yes. As in the examples of motor functioning, cognitive development, and brain development, assumption of a unity that is not present leads quickly to dangers in practical implications. One of the most potent pitfalls involves decisions about how to support students with deficits in executive function, whose profiles vary dramatically.

Many developmental disabilities, such as attention-deficit/hyperactivity disorder (ADHD) and autism, involve deficits in executive function (Pennington & Ozonoff, 1996). Although these deficits make the disorders appear similar, the executive dysfunction manifests differently in distinct disorders, and diverse interventions are required. For example, the process of inhibition shows less impairment in many individuals with autism than in those with ADHD, even though the impairment in other executive functions, such as planning, is more severe in autism (Hill, 2004; Pennington & Ozonoff, 1996). Following the web model in Figure 4.1, different aspects of executive function develop along separate strands (which sometimes intersect or branch).

Profiles of executive function deficits can even be unique and undetectable by traditional measures. Multiple studies have reported cases of individuals with frontal lobe damage who performed well on executive tasks in a laboratory setting but had clear difficulty with executive tasks in real life (Burgess, Alderman, Evans, Emslie, & Wilson, 1998). Profiles of executive function performance are highly variable and do not warrant a unitary concept.

Recognizing that executive function has multiple aspects and is not unitary thus has practical implications in the classroom. Research and practice that separate distinct aspects of a phenomenon, moving beyond the vague frontal metaphor for executive function, will help educators devise more useful, differentiated diagnoses and interventions. Blanket statements of deficits in executive function are certainly less useful than focused ones highlighting particular component skills like attention, inhibition, and planning. The remarkable success of research and practice that specify the particular functions underlying dyslexia and other reading difficulties, described early in this chapter, provides an excellent model for this endeavor (Fischer et al., 2006).

An interactive relationship between education and the learning, brain, and developmental sciences will foster this type of nuanced understanding and improve the work of both educators and researchers. Just as doctors facing a particular challenge or novel discovery in patients can inform the work of biological scientists, educators can help foster useful and productive research in complementary disciplines. The benefits are reciprocal because innovative research findings can be appropriately translated into educational practice.

REFERENCES

Anderson, J. R. (2002). Spanning seven orders of magnitude: A challenge for cognitive modeling. *Cognitive Science, 26,* 85–112.

Baddeley, A. (1996). Exploring the central executive. *Quarterly Journal of Experimental Psychology: Section A, 49,* 5–28.

Burgess, P. W., Alderman, N., Evans, J., Emslie, H., & Wilson, B. A. (1998). The ecological validity of tests of executive function. *Journal of the International Neuropsychological Society, 4,* 547–558.

Burmeister, R., Hannay, H. J., Copeland, K., Fletcher, J. M., Boudousquie, A., & Dennis, M. (2005). Attention problems and executive functions in children with spina bifida and hydrocephalus. *Child Neuropsychology, 11,* 265–283.

Carlson, S. M., Moses, L. J., & Claxton, L. J. (2004). Individual differences in executive functioning and theory of mind: An investigation of inhibitory control and planning ability. *Journal of Experimental Child Psychology, 87,* 299–319.

Case, R. (1974). Structures and strictures: Some functional limitations on the course of cognitive growth. *Cognitive Psychology, 6,* 544–574.

Damon, W., & Lerner, R. M. (Eds.). (2006). *Handbook of child psychology: Theoretical models of human development* (6th ed., Vol. 1). New York: Wiley.

Dawson-Tunik, T. L., Commons, M., Wilson, M., & Fischer, K. W. (2005). The shape of development. *European Journal of Developmental Psychology, 2,* 163–195.

Duncan, J., Johnson, R., Swales, M., & Freer, C. (1997). Frontal lobe deficits after head injury: Unity and diversity of function. *Cognitive Neuropsychology, 14,* 713–741.

Epstein, H. T. (1974). Phrenoblysis: Special brain and mind growth periods. *Developmental Psychobiology, 7,* 207–224.

Epstein, H. T. (1978). Growth spurts during brain development: Implications for educational policy and practice. In J. S. Chall & A. F. Mirsky (Eds.), *Education and the brain* (Yearbook of the National Society for the Study of Education). Chicago: University of Chicago Press.

Fischer, K. W., & Bidell, T. R. (2006). Dynamic development of action, thought, and emotion. In W. Damon & R. M. Lerner (Ed.), *Handbook of child psychology: Theoretical models of human development* (6th ed., vol. 1, pp. 313–399). New York: Wiley.

Fischer, K. W., Bullock, D. H., Rotenberg, E. J., & Raya, P. (1993). The dynamics of competence: How context contributes directly to skill. In R. H. Wozniak & K. W. Fischer (Eds.), *Development in context: Acting and thinking in specific environments* (pp. 93–117). Hillsdale, NJ: Erlbaum.

Fischer, K. W., & Immordino-Yang, M. H. (2002). Cognitive development and education: From dynamic general structure to specific learning and teaching. In E. Lagemann (Ed.), *Traditions of scholarship in education*. Chicago: Spencer Foundation.

Fischer, K. W., Immordino-Yang, M. H., & Waber, D. P. (2006). Toward a grounded synthesis of mind, brain, and education for reading disorders: An introduction to the field and this book. In K. W. Fischer, J. H. Bernstein, & M. H. Immordino-Yang (Eds.), *Mind, brain, and education in reading disorders*. Cambridge, UK: Cambridge University Press.

Fischer, K. W., & Katzir, T. (Eds.). (in press). *Building usable knowledge in mind, brain, and education*. Cambridge, UK: Cambridge University Press.

Fischer, K. W., & Lazerson, A. (1984). Research: Brain spurts and Piagetian periods. *Educational Leadership, 41*(5), 70.

Fischer, K. W., & Rose, S. P. (1996). Dynamic growth cycles of brain and cognitive development. In R. Thatcher, G. R. Lyon, J. Rumsey, & N. Krasnegor (Eds.), *Developmental neuroimaging: Mapping the development of brain and behavior* (pp. 263–279). New York: Academic Press.

Fischer, M., Barkley, R. A., Smallish, L., & Fletcher, K. (2005). Executive functioning in hyperactive children as young adults: Attention, inhibition, response perseveration, and the impact of comorbidity. *Developmental Neuropsychology, 27*, 107–133.

Hill, E. L. (2004). Executive dysfunction in autism. *Trends in Cognitive Sciences, 8*, 26–32.

Kitchener, K. S., Lynch, C. L., Fischer, K. W., & Wood, P. K. (1993). Developmental range of reflective judgment: The effect of contextual support and practice on developmental stage. *Developmental Psychology, 29*, 893–906.

Klahr, D., & Wallace, J. G. (1976). *Cognitive development: An information-processing view*. Hillsdale, NJ: Erlbaum.

Mader, S. S. (2005). *Understanding human anatomy and physiology* (5th ed.). New York: McGraw-Hill.

Manchester, D., Priestley, N., & Jackson, H. (2004). The assessment of executive functions: Coming out of the office. *Brain Injury, 18*, 1067–1081.

Marieb, E. N. (2006). *Essentials of human anatomy and physiology* (8th ed.). New York: Pearson Benjamin Cummings.

Matousek, M., & Petersén, I. (1973). Frequency analysis of the EEG in normal children and adolescents. In P. Kellaway & I. Petersén (Eds.), *Automation of clinical electroencephalography* (pp. 75–102). New York: Raven Press.

Miyake, A., Friedman, N. P., Emerson, M. J., Witzki, A. H., & Howerter, A. (2000). The unity and diversity of executive functions and their contributions to complex "frontal lobe" tasks: A latent variable analysis. *Cognitive Psychology, 41*, 49–100.

Norman, D. A., & Shallice, T. (1986). Attention to action: Willed and automatic control of behavior. In R. J. Davidson, G. E. Schwartz, & D. Shapiro (Eds.), *Consciousness and self-regulation: Advances in research and theory* (Vol. 4, pp. 1–18). New York: Plenum.

Pennington, B. F., & Ozonoff, S. (1996). Executive functions and developmental psychopathology. *Journal of Child Psychology and Psychiatry, 37*, 51–87.

Piaget, J. (1983). Piaget's theory. In P. H. Mussen & W. Kessen (Ed.), *Handbook of child psychology: History, theory, and methods* (4th ed., vol. 1, pp. 103–126). New York: Wiley.

Rose, D. H., Meyer, A., Strangman, N., & Rappolt, G. (2002). *Teaching every student in the digital age: Universal design for learning.* Alexandria, VA: ASCD.

Ruhland, R., & van Geert, P. (1998). Jumping into syntax: Transitions in the development of closed class words. *British Journal of Developmental Psychology, 16*(Pt. 1), 65–95.

Somsen, R. J. M., van 't Klooster, B. J., van der Molen, M. W., van Leeuwen, H. M. P., & Licht, R. (1997). Growth spurts in brain maturation during middle childhood as indexed by EEG power spectra. *Biological Psychology, 44*, 187–209.

Teuber, H.-L. (1972). Unity and diversity of frontal lobe functions. *Acta Neurobiologiae Experimentalis, 32*, 615–656.

Thatcher, R. W. (1994). Cyclic cortical reorganization: Origins of human cognitive development. In G. Dawson & K. W. Fischer (Eds.), *Human behavior and the developing brain* (pp. 232–266). New York: Guilford Press.

Turk, D. J., Heatherton, T. F., Kelley, W. M., Funnell, M. G., Gazzaniga, M. S., & Macrae, C. N. (2002). Mike or me? Self-recognition in a split-brain patient. *Nature Neuroscience, 5*, 841–842.

Wolf, M., & Bowers, P. (1999). The "double-deficit hypothesis" for the developmental dyslexias. *Journal of Educational Psychology, 91*, 1–24.

Wolf, M., & Katzir-Cohen, T. (2001). Reading fluency and its intervention. *Scientific Studies of Reading, 5*, 211–239.

Wolf, M., Miller, L., & Donnelly, K. (2000). Retrieval, Automaticity, Vocabulary Elaboration-Orthography (RAVE-O): A comprehensive fluency-based reading intervention program. *Journal of Learning Disabilities, 33*, 375–386.

Zelazo, P. D., Mueller, U., Frye, D., & Marcovitch, S. (2003). The development of executive function in early childhood. *Monographs of the Society for Research in Child Development, 68*(3).

PART II

Executive Function Difficulties in Different Diagnostic Groups
Challenges of Identification and Treatment

In high school, my grades kept a D average. It seemed like nothing I did, however hard I tried, would improve my grades. My teachers all said I just wasn't trying and wasn't putting in the effort. I couldn't believe it. Was I stupid? . . .

—SEAN, COLLEGE SOPHOMORE

The terms "executive function disorder" and "executive dysfunction" are being used increasingly to describe a broad range of weaknesses in students like Sean. As was discussed in previous chapters, these labels are used differently by theoreticians, diagnosticians, and educators, and the lack of consensus at the theoretical level is also evident in the clinical domain. In fact, there is still considerable disagreement about whether these labels should be used as stand-alone diagnostic terms or whether they can simply be used to describe deficits in a broad range of executive function processes.

The chapters in this section extend the discussion by Denckla in chapter 1 and provide an overview of current assessment and treatment methods for addressing executive function weaknesses in a number of clinically diagnosed populations. One common theme that emerges from

73

these chapters is that a number of clinical populations exhibit weaknesses in one or more of the following executive function processes:

- Selecting relevant task goals
- Planning and organizing information and ideas
- Prioritizing and focusing on relevant themes rather than irrelevant details
- Initiating and sustaining activities
- Holding information in working memory
- Shifting strategies flexibly
- Inhibiting competing actions
- Self-monitoring, checking, and regulating behavior

Another theme that is addressed in these chapters is the lack of specificity that characterizes the measures used to assess executive function processes. The authors note that in psychology and education, discussions of executive function and metacognition generally address cognitive components that are domain-general, whereas the neurosciences focus on the role of the frontal lobes. In this section of the book, it is suggested that the mixing of the psychological construct of "executive function" and the neuroanatomical term "frontal lobe" may explain some of the conceptual confusion surrounding these constructs. This lack of clarity in the definition of executive function makes it difficult to design accurate diagnostic methods for evaluating students who exhibit weaknesses in these processes.

In Chapter 5, Meltzer and Krishnan provide an overview of the current understandings and misunderstandings about executive function, metacognition, and strategic learning in individuals with learning disabilities. They address the challenges of appropriate diagnosis of executive and self-regulatory processes and discuss the interconnections among executive function processes, effort, motivation, and self-concept in students with learning disabilities. Implications for effective treatment and teaching are also discussed in this chapter. These difficulties with accurate assessment are explored further in Chapter 6, where Stein and Krishnan discuss the challenges associated with the assessment of students with nonverbal learning disabilities. They stress the influence of executive function processes on the educational and social skills of these students and the importance of consistent structure, scaffolding, and verbal mediation. In Chapter 7, Ozonoff and Schetter discuss the burgeoning literature that examines executive function difficulties in children with Asperger syndrome and high-functioning autism (a group they refer to collectively as having autism spectrum disorders). These groups often display behaviors that are considered indicators of executive function deficits and are possibly mediated by frontal dysfunction. Again, questions relating to definitions, assessment, and treatment are addressed.

All three chapters in this section emphasize the limitations of the current measurement systems for providing accurate descriptions of deficits in executive function processes. Clearly, there is a need to develop more accurate tests that can identify these weaknesses in those diagnostic groups that exhibit executive function difficulties. Most important, these chapters point out the ongoing link between assessment and treatment and the need for intervention research that identifies specific methods for teaching students so that they can perform at the level of their potential.

CHAPTER 5

Executive Function Difficulties and Learning Disabilities

Understandings and Misunderstandings

LYNN MELTZER
KALYANI KRISHNAN

My mind is like a cloud of gas and inside the cloud are a million different little molecules speeding around, colliding with each other. There's no structure to it.

—BRANDON, COLLEGE GRADUATE

Over the past decade, the term "executive function disorder" has been used increasingly by diagnosticians and educators to describe students like Brandon who struggle with those components of the academic curriculum that require the integration and organization of multiple subprocesses. Many students who exhibit these difficulties do not meet the criteria for a learning disability because they readily succeed with the narrowly defined subskills that are measured on most widely accepted test inventories. Nevertheless, they often struggle to perform at an academic level that reflects their cognitive potential when open-ended projects and papers are assigned that require them to access executive function processes.

This chapter provides an overview of current understandings and misunderstandings about executive function, metacognition, and strategic learning in individuals with learning disabilities and attention-deficit disorders. There is also an emphasis on the challenges of assessing executive and self-regulatory processes in students with learning disabilities. The discussion focuses on the interactions among executive function processes, self-awareness, effort, and persistence in these students. Finally, the major principles of intervention and treatment are addressed.

EXECUTIVE FUNCTION PROCESSES: CURRENT UNDERSTANDINGS

How are executive function processes associated with learning disabilities? In the context of understanding learning disabilities, what is meant by the term "executive function"? Descriptions of executive function processes originally focused on the orchestration of basic cognitive processes during goal-oriented problem solving and had no direct application to the classroom (Flavell, Friedrichs, & Hoyt, 1970). Brown (1978, 1997) and Brown and Campione (1983) extended this theoretical paradigm to the classroom setting in their seminal work on metacognition and began to differentiate executive processes from self-regulation. They also investigated methods of teaching these processes and addressing the individual's knowledge, understanding, and regulation of his or her own cognitive processes. Since then, a broad range of definitions and models of executive function have been proposed (Gioia, Isquith, Kenworthy, & Barton, 2002). Nevertheless, the concepts of executive function and metacognition are not clearly differentiated, and there is still a lack of clarity about their shared and unique characteristics, especially in students with learning disabilities and attention-deficit disorders.

To understand the relationship between executive function difficulties and learning disabilities, it is important to discuss the definitions of executive function provided by the most influential researchers and theorists in this area (see Part I of this volume for additional information). Denckla (1996 and Chapter 1, this volume), one of the first researchers to use this concept clinically, defined executive processes as "a set of domain-general control processes that involve inhibition and delay of responding (p. 265) for the goal of organization and integration of cognitive and output processes over time" (Denckla, 1996, p. 265). Executive function processes have also been construed as the "supervisory and self-regulatory functions that organize and direct cognitive activity, emotional response, and overt behavior" (Gioia et al., 2002, p. 122). Although these definitions differ in their specific details, there is overlap and general agreement that executive function is an all-encompassing construct or "an umbrella term" (Anderson, 2002, p. 71) for the complex cognitive processes that underlie flexible, goal-directed behavior responses to novel or difficult situations. Furthermore, as is emphasized by Anderson (2002), numerous processes are associated with executive function, with the major elements comprising anticipation, goal selection, planning, initiation of activity, self-regulation, mental flexibility, deployment of attention, and use of feedback. More specifically, on the basis of his review of a wide range of definitions, Eslinger (1996) concluded that executive function processes include the following:

- Metacognitive knowledge about tasks and strategies
- Flexible use of strategies
- Attention and memory systems that guide these processes (e.g., working memory)
- Explicit and implicit learning
- Self-regulatory processes such as planning and self-monitoring

The premise of this chapter is that executive function processes are global and broader than metacognitive strategies and that "executive function" is an umbrella term that incorporates a collection of interrelated processes responsible for purposeful, goal-directed behavior (Anderson, 2002; Gioia, Isquith, Guy, & Kenworthy, 2000).

EXECUTIVE FUNCTION DYSFUNCTION: A LEARNING DISABILITY PARADIGM WITH A NEW TWIST?

I feel like a bottle of ginger ale—I need the fizzle to settle before I can do what I need to do.
—CHRIS, AGE 11 YEARS

What is the impact of executive function processes on the performance of students like Chris, whose learning disabilities affect their output on a wide range of academic tasks? These students have been characterized as "actively inefficient learners" (Swanson, 1989; Torgesen, 1982) because of their difficulties accessing, organizing, and coordinating multiple mental activities simultaneously in academic areas including reading comprehension and written expression. These students are viewed as inefficient because they often struggle to use self-regulatory strategies such as checking, monitoring, and revising during learning tasks. Students with learning disabilities may also show limited awareness of the usefulness of particular strategies for efficient problem solving and effective learning as well as weaknesses in cognitive flexibility (Meltzer, 1993; Meltzer & Montague, 2001). More specifically, students with learning and attention problems often have difficulty sorting, organizing, and prioritizing information and overfocus on details while struggling to identify major themes. As a result, information may become "clogged," and they may become "stuck" so that they cannot easily initiate new tasks or shift flexibly among alternative approaches. These weaknesses, characterized as executive function difficulties, often emerge as the academic curriculum becomes more complex and conceptually demanding, requiring students to organize and synthesize large amounts of information.

Academic tasks that involve written output, summarizing, taking notes, or reading complex text for meaning may be particularly challenging for students with learning disabilities, who often exhibit symptoms that can be likened to a clogged funnel (Meltzer, 2004; see Figure 5.1).

In other words, their strong conceptual reasoning abilities may not match their output and productivity because of their difficulties organizing and prioritizing numerous details, juggling these details in working memory, and shifting flexibly between abstract concepts and literal details as well as from the major themes to the details. Exceptionally bright students with learning and attention problems often experience

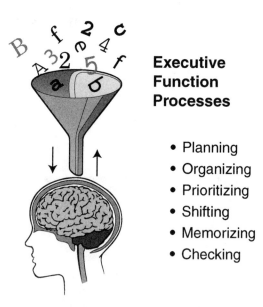

FIGURE 5.1. Executive function: The funnel model (Meltzer, 2004).

significant difficulties in the middle and high school grades because the complexity and volume of information can be overwhelming. More specifically, executive function weaknesses interfere with a range of processes, including planning, organizing, prioritizing, accessing information in working memory, shifting strategies, and self-monitoring (see Figure 5.2), and typically affect output rather than input.

THE IMPACT OF EXECUTIVE FUNCTION PROCESSES ON SPECIFIC ACADEMIC DOMAINS

For students with learning disabilities, performance on complex academic tasks is often inefficient due to weaknesses in the core executive processes shown in Figure 5.2. Although these students frequently succeed with the sophisticated problem solving and conceptual reasoning that underlie these tasks, they may have difficulty initiating work, organizing, prioritizing, selecting appropriate goals, shifting strategies, and self-monitoring. The effects of executive function weaknesses on academic performance in these different domains are discussed below in the context of reading comprehension, written expression, studying, completion of long-term projects, and test taking.

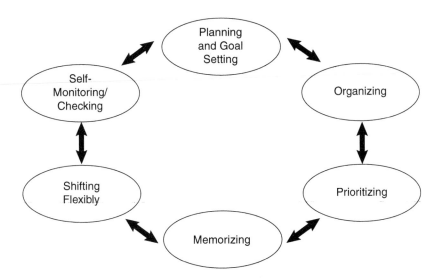

FIGURE 5.2. Core executive function processes that affect academic performance.

Reading comprehension requires students to decode text while allocating and managing their cognitive and attentional resources so that they can also focus on the meaning of the text. Students with learning disabilities often lack reading fluency because they have difficulty decoding words accurately, monitoring their performance to ensure that they are tracking the text correctly, and synthesizing the content in order to "build meaning." In order to construct meaning successfully, students need to draw on prior knowledge. They need to shift flexibly from retrieving and interpreting background knowledge to attending to and interpreting print and new content. Coordinating these dual processes also requires them to integrate known information with new content. Flexibility of thinking is also called into play when students interpret words or language that may be ambiguous, draw inferences and conclusions, and process redundant information, actions required to process most written texts. Students need to prioritize and reprioritize information in an effort to make the text useful for their particular purpose, an executive process that is often extremely challenging for students with learning disabilities. For instance, in an effort to make history accessible and enjoyable, authors of textbooks may write in a dramatic and imaginative way rather than presenting content in a dry, sequential manner. In order to understand the cause–effect nature of the information, however, students will need to reorganize events from such texts in order to place them in the correct chronology. Each time students are asked to respond to questions such as "What was the most important event in this book?" or "What were the key factors that contributed to World War I?" they are being asked to prioritize and synthesize information. In summary, students with learning disabilities often struggle with the executive function processes that affect a broad array of reading skills.

Written language involves numerous executive function processes. For many students with learning disabilities, the writing process is seldom automatic. They often struggle to initiate written tasks because of their difficulties with executive function processes such as planning and defining the first step (Graham & Harris, 1993). In order to plan their thoughts in preparation for writing, they need to evaluate and to rephrase or paraphrase the assigned topic, a task that presupposes the ability to think flexibly. Organization and prioritization are also integral to written expression, which requires the crafting of a complete thought that is independent of context and accessible to the "absent audience." Many students with learning disabilities struggle with the organization of a broad range of processes and subskills, including the spatial organization of writing on a page, using accurate syntax at the level of the sentence, organizing arguments in order to persuade the reader, and using the traditional structure of introduction, body, and conclusion in an essay (Graham & Harris, 1993; Graham, Harris, & McArthur, 2004; Graham, Harris, & Olinghouse, Chapter 10, this volume).

Independent studying, homework, and long-term projects are also challenging for many students with learning disabilities as they advance to the higher grades. These tasks are highly dependent on executive function processes and require students to plan ahead, predict outcomes, and set long-term goals. Self-regulation and self-monitoring play critical roles in these independent and higher-order learning pursuits, as does cognitive flexibility. Independent projects, a major component of our 21st-century curriculum, are particularly challenging for students with weak executive function processes, as they involve several aspects of organization, including time management, sequencing information, acquiring the materials and information needed to complete tasks, bringing tasks to completion, and remembering to submit them in time to earn credit.

Test taking is another academic task that places demands on a student's ability to plan and execute specific responses on demand. Successful test takers are alert, actively engaged, and thoughtful throughout the learning process. Students with learning disabilities frequently struggle to perform appropriately on tests and cannot easily "show what they know" (Meltzer & Montague, 1995; Scruggs & Mastropieri, 1995). They may not listen to cues from teachers such as "This is important," or "Listen carefully, now!" They may not easily understand the format of textbooks and may not recognize sidebars, diagrams, or tables of contents as tools for organizing and prioritizing information. They may not use cues from the classroom and from print to predict possible questions on upcoming tests and to plan potential responses. When faced with an assignment to study for a test within a specified time period, many students with learning disabilities do not easily manage their time, struggle to identify the most important information for studying, and do not prioritize their tasks. If they have prior information relevant to the format of the test they will be taking, such as study guides prepared by the teacher, they do not always use this information to direct the process of studying. When they are actually taking a test, these students may not easily allocate time, plan their responses, self-monitor, or complete the test efficiently. All of these tasks require considerable reliance on executive function processes. Determining which students are at risk for executive function difficulties is an important step for ensuring their continued academic success; however, accurate assessment of these executive function processes is challenging, as is discussed below.

ASSESSMENT OF EXECUTIVE FUNCTION PROCESSES: MOVING BEYOND STRUCTURED TASKS

I was trying hard and everyone else got A's and I got a C. What was wrong with me?

—SEAN, COLLEGE SOPHOMORE

The goals of assessment for students like Sean are twofold: *identification* (or description) and *prescription*. The identification goal is focused on discovering and explaining *what* the student knows and can do, *how* the student learns and processes information, and *why* learning may be delayed (Meltzer, 1993). This goal requires an analysis of the student's profile of cognitive, educational, and affective processes. The prescriptive goal of assessment is to provide specific recommendations for teaching strategies that closely match a student's profile of strengths and weaknesses. In light of these twin objectives, the assessment of executive function processes in children and adults poses unique challenges. Executive function processes may be delayed or disrupted for a variety of reasons. Because these processes are intimately linked to the functioning of frontal and prefrontal cortices (Barkley, 1996; Denckla, 2005; Pennington, 1991, 1997). Therefore, these processes may be compromised by a number of different factors, including attention, fatigue, anxiety, stress, or depression, all of which rely on intact prefrontal processing. On the other hand, students may show primary weaknesses in one or more executive function processes that may underlie their learning difficulties. Thus, it is important to determine the origins and the primacy of the weak executive function processes. In those cases where the executive function processing weaknesses are secondary to attention-deficit/hyperactivity disorder (ADHD), depression, or anxiety, interventions include medication and/or psychotherapy. These interventions are, however, likely to have a limited impact on a primary weakness in organization or cognitive flexibility, which may be more amenable to strategic teaching and cognitive-behavioral training. Thus, in order to evaluate *why* learning may be delayed as well as how executive function weaknesses may be contributing to the student's learning difficulties, the assessment process needs to include a detailed background history and specific steps to rule out a variety of alternate explanations. Consequently, interpreting the results of any executive function assessment battery is a complex task. Some of the challenges to the accurate assessment of executive function processes are discussed below.

Diagnostic Fuzziness

A major challenge to the accurate identification of executive function difficulties in students with learning disabilities and ADHD relates to the lack of consensus regarding the definition of these disorders. Confusion in the field regarding the concept of executive function has been long-standing, as pointed out by Morris (1996), who characterized researchers and clinicians in the field as a "community . . . without clear *community standards*." The literature shows fuzzy boundaries regarding the overlap between executive function difficulties, attention-deficit disorders, and learning disabilities (Barkley, 1996; Denckla, 2005; Eslinger, 1996; Pennington, 1991, 1997). Many affective states, such as motivation, effort, and persistence also impact executive function processes, which further complicates assessment. As a result of this lack of clarity, tests have been used variably as measures of attention, memory, or executive function processes, depending on the perspective of a particular test administrator. For example, many researchers have used tasks such as the Wechsler Digit Span subtest as a measure of attention, whereas others have used it as a measure of working memory or auditory short-term memory. By the same token, tests such as the Stroop and the Trail Making Test have been used as measures of attention in some settings and as measures of executive function processes in others. These overlaps occur for multiple reasons, one of which is diagnostic fuzziness. On the other hand, task analyses of these tests show that, in fact, they do require this multiplicity of processes. For example, although measures such as the Wechsler Coding subtest or the NEPSY Visual Attention tasks assess selective and sustained attention, they also measure learning and memory. In addition, they require the student to maintain "set," to execute a series of planned responses, and to self-monitor, all processes that are associated with executive function. Such analysis reflects what has long been known in the field of learning disabilities: that a majority of tests described as measuring a single process actually sample a multiplicity of processes across the attentional, cognitive, and emotional domains.

Impact of Developmental Changes and Curriculum Demands

The concept of a developmental progression in these executive processes is still an open question (see Bernstein & Waber, Chapter 3, this volume). The academic demands at different ages and grade levels require increasing levels of independence, organization, synthesis, and self-monitoring, thus suggesting a curriculum effect to the identification and diagnosis of executive function process difficulties. Referrals for the assessment of executive function processes typically include middle school and high school students who are struggling with the demands for independence, speed, and integration that the curriculum requires. Many of these students may have been successful in early elementary school, where the focus has been on developing isolated skills (e.g., decoding, spelling, math facts, and computation). They begin to experience academic difficulties in the upper grades when they are required to integrate many skills in order to complete complex, open-ended tasks independently (e.g., reading comprehension, summarizing, math problem solving, essay writing). Often, what seems to be at issue is the *requirement to coordinate and integrate multiple skills independently*, particularly for students with mild academic difficulties. Subtle weaknesses in one or more of the executive function processes interact to affect students' performance on open-ended tasks even when weaknesses are not evident on discrete tasks that measure each of these processes individually.

Recent changes in public education have inadvertently compounded the problems of identification and diagnosis by placing a strong emphasis on high-stakes testing and, consequently, shifting the curriculum toward what appear to be highly challenging, developmentally demanding goals. First-graders are assigned increasingly challenging homework, and the literacy expectations have risen to include the ability to write simple book reports. At the middle and high school levels, complex multistep projects are assigned that require weeks of independent research in multiple domains and involve numerous executive function processes, including setting goals, planning, prioritizing, accessing working memory, and shifting mindsets. Many students may therefore be required to complete academic tasks that are developmentally and cognitively too challenging. The curriculum emphasis may, therefore, be fuelling a surplus of referrals of students of all ages for assessment of executive function processes, the implication being that more and more students display deficits in this area.

Multidimensionality of Executive Function Processes

The multidimensional nature of the construct of executive function also creates unique obstacles for assessment and compromises the reliability of identification. Marlowe (2000) noted, "the measurement of executive functions is still quite limited and translation of test scores to real world competencies is problematic"(p. 446). A frequent observation in the clinical setting is that even the most complex clinical task, in the end, is far less complex than typical situations in the real world that place demands on the executive function processes of individuals. It is not unusual for a child to navigate clinical tasks with no appreciable difficulty but struggle with the open-ended choices presented by a rainy Saturday afternoon. The child who cannot respond to the challenge presented in "Please clean your room" may be able to succeed with discrete measures of visual attention, planning, and flexibility on standardized batteries. Furthermore, as noted by Dawson and Guare (2004), results from these highly specific and structured tasks also do not align themselves easily with the experiences of students who struggle when working independently or focusing on long-term projects.

As discussed above, the need to integrate and coordinate multiple subskills, some of which may be disproportionately or unexpectedly weak, appears to be one of the major difficulties facing students with learning disabilities who present with executive function weaknesses. Test batteries that are commonly used to assess executive function processes yield scores along a number of dimensions; however, they do not provide a framework for interpreting the implications of specific clusters of low or "lowish" scores. What might a student who achieves borderline scores on multiple subtests of one of these batteries experience when he or she is assigned an open-ended, long-term research project? What are the educational implications of having subtle weaknesses in cognitive flexibility, planning, and visual scanning when none of these scores is actually in the below-average range? The interpretation of profiles such as these requires a deep understanding of the interrelationship among these executive function processes and the curriculum demands. On the other hand, the delivery of special education services requires the identification of clear and incontrovertible areas of weakness. Discussions of placement often revolve around the interpretation of borderline scores and the lack of definitional clarity. A student who does not begin a complex diagnostic task immediately may experience difficulties with the interpretation of multistep directions as well as with planning and prioritizing. If these factors are not linked clearly and unambiguously with weak task initiation through a comprehensive and well-constructed theoretical model, they may be erroneously dismissed as indicative of a lack of motivation and effort.

Interactions of Skills, Strategies, Motivation, and Effort

As Moran and Gardner (Chapter 2, this volume) note, "we construe executive function as the integration of three parameters: *hill*—the establishment of a clear goal; *skill*—the requisite abilities and techniques for attaining that goal; and *will*—the volition to begin and persevere until the goal has been reached." The coordination and integration of all three sets of complex, multistep processes is often challenging for many students with learning disabilities, who are frequently unable to "show what they know" on tests. Students with weak executive function processes often experience marked levels of frustration and anxiety in their attempts to respond to these challenges (Barkley, 1997; Stein & Krishnan, Chapter 6, this volume). This can result in reduced feelings of self-efficacy and resilience, which in turn lead to lowered motivation, effort, and persistence. Similarly, a large body of literature suggests a cyclical relationship among high levels of motivation, effort, and strong academic performance (Brunstein, Schultheiss, & Grassman, Helliwell, 2003; Kasser & Ryan, 1996; Meltzer, Katzer, Miller, Reddy, & Roditi, 2004; Meltzer, Reddy, Pollica, & Roditi, 2004; Pajares & Schunk, 2001; Sheldon & Elliot, 1999). Individuals who are resilient select meaningful and realistic goals, exert the effort needed to attain these goals, and self-regulate their cognitive and emotional processes effectively (Raskind, Goldberg, Higgins, & Herman, 1999). The learning environment, including the choice of instructional methods and materials, plays a significant role in mediating this cyclical relationship among self-perceptions, emotions, self-regulation, goal setting, and motivation (Barnard, 1995). In particular, effective cognitive strategies help students bridge the gap between their weak executive function skills and the academic demands they face. For these students, academic performance is often dependent on their use of effective strategies that help them bypass their weak skills and shift flexibly among different approaches and mindsets so as to attain their goals, or "climb the hill," using Moran and Gardner's terminology (Chapter 2, this volume).

The need for a variety of tests that assess the complex interactions among "hill, skill, and will" is evident if we consider the cyclical relationship that characterizes strategy use, effort, self-concept, and academic performance (Meltzer, Katzir-Cohen, Miller, & Roditi, 2001; Miller, Meltzer, Katzir-Cohen, & Houser, 2001). In fact, strategy use mediates the relationship between students' self-reported levels of effort and their academic self-concepts, indicating a reciprocal strategy–effort interaction. As is suggested by the paradigm in Figure 5.3 (Meltzer et al., 2004b), a self-sustaining cycle is put into motion when students use strategies and succeed academically. Their experience of academic success results in higher levels of motivation, even greater effort, better use of strategies, and continued academic success. The academic self-perceptions of students with learning disabilities appear to be influenced by the effort they make to use effective strategies in their schoolwork. When they are successful academically as a result of their hard work and

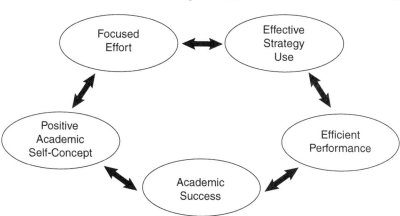

FIGURE 5.3. The relationship between strategy use, effort, self-concept, and academic performance. From Meltzer, Reddy, Pollica, and Roditi (2004). Copyright 2004 by International Academy for Research in Learning Disabilities. Reprinted by permission.

strategy use, students with learning disabilities usually value the strategies they use and feel empowered to work hard as they recognize that their persistence will lead to improved academic performance. For some, the learning process may have been especially negative and demoralizing, leading to negative academic self-concepts and a sense of learned helplessness. For these students, goal setting and prioritizing provide a concrete way of increasing their effort and strategy use so that a positive cycle of strategy use, effort, and academic self-concept can begin to be established.

With regard to identification and diagnosis of executive function difficulties, strong resilience and self-efficacy, coupled with effective compensatory strategies, may mask weaknesses in executive function processes. Understanding a student's motivation and effort informs the choice of the intervention as well as the prognosis. Therefore, effective assessment needs to address all components of this effort cycle and identify the specific cognitive or emotional processes that may be interfering with students' efficient academic performance. In other words, assessment procedures must identify whether or not students are able to set reasonable and meaningful goals, to deploy effective strategies, and to recognize the importance of investing the effort to use strategies as a means of attaining academic success. These interacting processes are particularly important when students need to succeed on complex tasks that involve the core executive function processes such as planning, prioritizing, shifting approaches, and self-monitoring.

EXECUTIVE FUNCTION MEASURES: THEIR SCOPE AND LIMITATIONS

Neuropsychological testing is usually administered in a distraction-free clinical setting by an adult who structures the tasks by explaining the rules, setting goals, and prompting the student, thus eliminating the need for multitasking or prioritizing (Manchester, Priestly, & Jackson, 2004). Standardized tests do not assess critical executive function processes, such as task initiation and sustained attention, as the examiner cues the students and presents tasks that are brief (Dawson & Guare, 2004). Furthermore, standardized tests rarely present students with independently executed, open-ended tasks. Instead, these situations require the presence of an adult performing and monitoring in an executive role. The highly structured nature of standardized tasks also eliminates the need to plan and organize independently. As Dawson and Guare (2004) point out, "Standardized tests are designed to be easily scored with a catalog of right and wrong answers that are straightforward and invariant, again minimizing demands on executive function." Thus, the more precisely we try to measure executive function processes through discrete clinical tasks, the less we evaluate actual executive function processes and the less we can generalize these results to real-life situations.

Norm-Referenced Tests

As is clear from the above, executive function processes constitute a complex, multidimensional construct. Therefore, the ongoing challenge is to replace discrete, isolated tasks with multidimensional tasks that assess the student's ability to integrate multiple processes in open-ended situations, to narrow broad tasks into manageable chunks, and to work independently on self-imposed goals. What about the test batteries that are currently used to assess executive function processes? A brief overview of the most widely used assessment batteries is provided below:

    The *Developmental Neuropsychological Assessment* (NEPSY; Korkman, Kirk, & Kemp, 1998; PsychCorp) and the *Delis–Kaplan Executive Function System* (D-KEFS; Delis, Kaplan, & Kramer, 2001; PsychCorp) are the most widely used assessment batteries. They comprise several tasks that assess various executive function processes, including selective attention, working memory, planning, organization, and cognitive flexibility. For example, the Trail Making Test on the D-KEFS involves five conditions, including visual scanning and motor speed. This allows the examiner to assess cognitive flexibility when the student switches between numerical and alphabetic sequences. Another open-ended task that focuses on a number of these executive function processes is the *Tower test*, which is included on both the NEPSY and the D-KEFS. This test assesses goal setting, planning, prioritizing, and self-monitoring.

Many of the difficulties discussed above apply to these standardized batteries. The tasks are brief, structured, and mediated by an examiner. Given the multidimensional nature of executive function processes, it is difficult to interpret the results of these discrete tasks and to link them directly to instructional strategies that help students improve on tasks that require the application of executive function processes (Elliot, 2003).

The *Wisconsin Card Sorting Test* (WCST; Heaton, 1981; Psychological Assessment Resources) is a widely used neuropsychological test of prefrontal cortex processes and is often considered a prototypical measure of executive function. Although it has been used to assess perseveration and abstract thinking, it is also used as a neuropsychological instrument because of its reported sensitivity to frontal lobe dysfunction. As the name suggests, this is a sorting task in which the student is directed to match a test card to one of four target categories based on shape, color, or number of stimuli. Once 10 consecutive correct matches have been achieved, the examiner changes the sorting criterion without warning. Thus, the WCST allows the clinician to assess a variety of executive function processes, including strategic planning, organized searching, the ability to use and integrate environmental feedback to shift cognitive sets, directing behavior toward achieving a goal, and modulating impulsive responding. The complexity of administering and scoring this task often affects the reliability of the assessment findings.

The *Rey Complex Figure Test* (Myers & Myers, 1995; Psychological Assessment Resources), a widely used measure of visual–spatial organization and visual memory, provides a useful analysis of an individual's executive function processes. Here, the student is presented with a complex, detailed, geometric figure to copy and reproduce from memory. Because the task is open-ended and complex and because individuals can select numerous pathways for solving the task, the RCFT provides a window into students' ability to structure information, to plan, and to problem-solve. Accurate reproduction of the RCFT figure is generally considered to require intact executive function processes as assessed through goal orientation, planning, the ability to hold a goal in working memory, and the ability to monitor performance (Anderson, Anderson, & Garth, 2001). As emphasized by Anderson and colleagues (2001), the Rey also assesses many other processes, including perceptual organization, visual–motor coordination, and fine-motor skills. Overall, the Rey is regarded as one of the few measures that can provide a meaningful assessment of the complexity of the executive function processes and the individual's ability to coordinate multiple subprocesses to achieve a particular goal.

The Rey and the WCST do not eliminate all the confounding factors involved in the assessment of executive function processes. In particular, the results of these tasks do not link logically and easily with appropriate teaching and treatment recommendations for students with learning disabilities. This is partly because of the conceptual distance between these tasks and actual academic tasks such as reading, spelling, writing, and math problem solving. The other challenge in interpreting and generalizing these data to academic achievement difficulties or accomplishments relates to the lack of a comprehensive theory of executive function processes and their impact on educational performance. An alternative approach to the assessment of executive function processes is the use of criterion-referenced, process measures.

Criterion-Referenced, Process Measures

Effective assessment of executive function processes requires process measures that assess the *how* and *why* of performance in combination with product measures that assess the end product, or *what*, of performance. To understand the impact of higher-order executive function processes on the efficiency of a student's academic performance, assessments need to evaluate these processes along with the basic skills that must be accessed automatically for efficient academic performance. Process-oriented assessment procedures allow identification of the processes and strategies used by students to solve particular problems. These invaluable procedures provide insights into a student's learning strengths and weaknesses, which can contribute to a broader understanding of his or her learning disability. Process-oriented assessments also help identify students who have learned to compensate for weaknesses in automaticity and basic skill deficits through effective problem-solving strategies. Such holistic evaluation systems, if anchored in a well-informed developmental context, can account for the changing abilities, skills, needs, and motivational states of each child (Meltzer, 1993). Process-oriented assessments can also explain how these characteristics interact with the instructional requirements of the curriculum. Thus, instructional strategies can be matched with each student's specific learning profile.

One example of a process-oriented assessment measure is the *Survey of Problem-Solving and Educational Skills* (SPES), a criterion-referenced assessment system for evaluating problem-solving strategies and educational skills (Meltzer, 1986). The SPES comprises two sections, the Survey of Problem-Solving Skills (SPRS) and the Survey of Educational Skills (SEDS). The SPRS consists of six tasks, three predominantly nonlinguistic tasks that incorporate geometric patterns as stimuli and three linguistic tasks. These six tasks assess two major areas: (1) problem-solving accuracy and (2) the student's ability to reflect on his or her own strategies and to explain these processes. The SEDS is a systematic procedure for isolating processing weaknesses and strengths in the four basic academic skill areas: reading, writing, spelling, and mathematics. Tasks are designed to identify the processes and strategies that a student uses to approach various educational tasks. The resulting profile of strengths and weaknesses is based on criterion-referenced information rather than grade equivalents or standard scores.

At the core of this assessment system is a theoretical framework for systematically evaluating the processes that students use across all the tasks presented. Although the SPES was not developed as a specific measure of executive function processes, it does provide a window into the student's ability to organize, prioritize, shift mindsets, integrate details, and self-monitor. In the clinical setting, administration of tasks like the SPES, coupled with an in-depth understanding of the underlying theoretical model, allows the examiner to track converging evidence of specific processing strengths and weaknesses. This facilitates the gathering of essential diagnostic impressions and descriptive data that are critically important for complementing the standardized scores that the evaluation may produce. An additional benefit of using a measure such as the SPES is the thread of process ratings that runs through both problem-solving and educational tasks. The SPRS and the SEDS result in Summary Processing Profiles that represent the approach and learning strategies that the child applies to a range of problem-solving and learning tasks. This profile can help provide a foundation for constructing an appropriate prescriptive educational plan.

Behavior Rating Scales

In view of the limited ecological validity of brief standardized tests for assessing executive function processes, alternative methods of evaluation have been increasingly emphasized (Gioia et al., 2002). In fact, a combination of clinical tests with ecologically valid behavior rating scales is considered the best method of assessing executive function processes. The clinical criteria are similar to those used for assessing attention-deficit disorders, where agreement among two to three observers across different settings (home, school, and a clinical setting) is still considered more reliable than complex computer assessment systems. A number of potentially useful behavior rating scales are discussed briefly below.

Behavior Rating Inventory of Executive Function (BRIEF)

The BRIEF (Gioia, Isquith, Guy, & Kenworthy, 2000) is a widely used questionnaire system consisting of multiple rating forms, a parent questionnaire, a teacher questionnaire, and a self-rating form for students above the age of 12. The BRIEF includes 86 items, such as: "Forgets to hand in homework, even when completed"; "Gets caught up in details and misses the big picture"; "Becomes overwhelmed by large assignments"; "Underestimates the time needed to finish tasks." This assesses processes associated with the core executive function processes: Behavioral Regulation (scales: Inhibit, Shift, Emotional Control) and Metacognition (scales: Initiate, Working Memory, Plan/Organize, Organization of Materials, Monitor). Overall, the BRIEF provides a reliable measure of parent, teacher, and self-reports of executive function processes, with high internal consistency (alphas = .80–.98) and test–retest reliability (r's = .82 for parents and .88 for teachers) as well as moderate correlations between teacher and parent ratings (r = .32–.34). The BRIEF cannot be the sole measure of executive function processes, however, and must be interpreted in the context of a comprehensive neuropsychological evaluation, which includes a direct sampling of students' processing and behavior, as well as a detailed developmental and educational history.

Metacognitive Awareness System (MetaCOG)

The MetaCOG (Meltzer, Reddy, Pollica, & Roditi, 2004) comprises five rating scales that assess students' and teachers' perceptions of strategy use, metacognitive awareness, motivation, and effort, all critical for academic performance on tasks that rely on executive function processes (see Table 5.1) (Meltzer, Katzir-Cohen, et al., 2001; Miller et al., 2001). These are described below.

METACOG STUDENT SURVEYS

Motivation and Effort Survey (ME). The ME consists of 38 items that assess students' self-ratings of their effort on different academic tasks that require the use of executive function processes (alpha = .91) (Meltzer, Reddy, Pollica, Roditi, Sayer, et al., 2004). Students rate how hard they work on a 5-point scale in various academic areas such as reading, writing, math, homework, studying for tests, and long-term

TABLE 5.1. Metacognitive Awareness System (MetaCOG)

Student questionnaires
- ME—Motivation and Effort Survey
- STRATUS—Strategy Use Survey
- MAQ—Metacognitive Awareness Questionnaire

Teacher questionnaires
- TPSE—Teacher Perceptions of Student Effort
- TIQ—Teacher Information Questionnaire

Parent questionnaires
- PPSE—Parent Perceptions of Student Effort

Note. Five-point rating for all surveys.

projects. Effort in nonacademic areas such as sports, music, art, and hobbies is also rated.

Strategy Use Survey (STRATUS). The STRATUS consists of 40 items that assess students' self-reported strategy use in reading, writing, spelling, math, studying, and test taking (alpha = .945). Items focus on students' perceptions of their use of strategies for planning, organizing, memorizing, shifting, and self-checking strategies when they approach their schoolwork (e.g., "When I have to remember new things in school, I make up acronyms to help me. Before I write, I plan out my ideas in some way that works for me [outline, list, map]. When I do math, I ask if my answers make sense").

Metacognitive Awareness Questionnaire (MAQ). The MAQ consists of 18 items that assess students' understanding of what strategies are and how they can apply them to their schoolwork (e.g., "When you begin something new, do you try to connect it to something you already know? When you begin something new, do you try to think about how long it will take you and make sure you have enough time? When you are working at school or at home, do you think about different ways you could do your work?").

METACOG TEACHER SURVEYS

Teacher Perceptions of Student Effort (TPSE). The TPSE consists of 38 items that assess teachers' ratings of students' behaviors when working hard and the effort they apply in different academic domains (alpha

= .98, Meltzer, Reddy, Pollica, et al., 2004b). Teachers rate students' effort and performance in reading, writing, math, homework, tests, and long-term projects that rely on executive function processes (e.g., "He spends as much time as needed to get his work done," "She does not give up even when the work is difficult"). Teachers also rate students' overall strategy use and academic performance in response to the question, "If you had to assign a grade for this student's overall academic performance, what would it be?"

Teacher Information Questionnaire (TIQ). This survey assesses teachers' understanding of the terms *metacognitive, strategy,* and *effort,* as well as their understanding of effective ways to promote students' strategy use and executive function processes in the classroom (e.g., "Students use strategies effectively without being taught these strategies directly. Teaching the curriculum is more important than teaching strategies. It is possible to motivate every student to work hard").

METACOG PARENT SURVEYS

Parent Perceptions of Student Effort (PPSE). The PPSE consists of 38 items that assess parents' ratings of students' behaviors when working hard and the effort they apply in different academic domains that require the use of executive function processes. Items are identical to those used on the student self-report survey (ME) and the teacher survey (TPSE).

As discussed above, student, teacher, and parent reports can be directly compared to determine overall consistency in their ratings of many of the core components of executive function processes across different settings. In summary, the multidimensionality of executive function processes and the interactions among individual students' profiles, their developmental status, and the curriculum pose challenges for assessment. A broad approach to the assessment of executive function processes is critical and should include a detailed developmental and educational history, questionnaires completed by parents and teachers, behavior rating scales, standardized tests, and theoretically grounded process measures. A comprehensive theoretical model provides a critically important framework for integrating and synthesizing data from these different sources to develop a coherent processing profile and an appropriate diagnosis, particularly in the case of students with subtle difficulties.

INTERVENTION APPROACHES

One of my greatest weaknesses in school was my organization. I could never find anything and did not know where my papers were. Today, thanks to the strategies I learned, I am able to organize my writing and to organize my life.

—LINDSEY, SEVENTH GRADER

As discussed, executive function processes are the underpinning for most academic work from the fourth grade on, when the curriculum increasingly emphasizes performance on tasks that require coordination, integration, and synthesis of the many processes and subskills needed for effective performance. Reading comprehension, homework, note taking, long-term projects, studying, and test taking all require students like Lindsey to integrate and organize multiple subprocesses simultaneously and to shift approaches constantly. Academic success in all these content areas is dependent on students' ability to plan their time, organize and prioritize information, distinguish main ideas from details, monitor their progress, and reflect on their work. Intervention approaches typically focus on two different levels: the level of the environment and the level of the person (Dawson & Guare, 2004).

Intervention *at the level of the environment* focuses on changes that adults such as parents and teachers can implement by structuring situations and assignments. Adults can provide structure with schedules, lists, prompts, and visual cues. These systems and scaffolds are eventually reduced as students begin to learn how to set goals, plan, prioritize, organize, shift approaches, and self-monitor. Therefore, the objective is to provide modeling and scaffolding in the hope that students will eventually internalize these strategies. Specifically, tasks and school assignments need to be explicit, short, closed-ended, and structured. Scoring rubrics can be used to define the tasks in structured ways. For example, adults can modify the tasks that students are required to complete, change the cues that prompt students to finish tasks, or adjust the way in which adults interact with students with executive function problems.

Other task adjustments include scaffolds, structure, stepwise procedures, and extended time.

Intervention *at the level of the person* emphasizes explicit, systematic strategy instruction focused on these executive function processes. This strategy instruction is essential for the academic progress of students with learning disabilities and beneficial for all students (Meltzer, Katzir-Cohen, et al., 2004; Swanson & Hoskyn, 1998). To benefit optimally from strategy instruction that addresses executive function processes, students need to understand their profiles of strengths and weaknesses and to recognize which strategies match their specific learning needs. The assessment process is the first important step in this direction and helps students recognize the cyclical relationship of their strategy use, effort, self-concept, and academic success (see Figure 5.3). When students understand their profiles of strengths and weaknesses, they are more likely to invest the effort needed to use the specific strategies that address their executive function weaknesses and help them succeed academically. For students with learning and attention difficulties, strategy instruction needs to be explicit, structured, and recursive and should be a requirement for in-class and homework assignments. Frequent use of strategies allows for consolidation and generalization and ensures that students learn to use strategies flexibly in different domains and with different tasks. Small-group instruction within the larger classroom often provides opportunities for practice and mastery of strategies, whereas large-group classroom-based instruction ensures that generalization occurs.

Within the one-on-one remedial setting or the larger classroom setting, a number of principles guide the teaching of strategies that address executive function processes. The principles listed below are important for teaching all students, but are critical for those students with learning disabilities who display weaknesses in executive function processes.

- Strategies for planning, organizing, prioritizing, memorizing, shifting flexibly, and checking should be taught explicitly and systematically.
- Students should be taught *how, when,* and *why* specific strategies can be successfully used for different academic tasks.
- Strategy instruction should be embedded in the curriculum.
- Students should be taught strategies for organizing their time, materials, ideas, deadlines, and completed work.
- Students should be encouraged and taught how to modify specific strategies to match their own learning profiles.
- Strategy instruction should be spiraled so that students practice different ways of applying strategies to different academic tasks.
- Students' motivation to use strategies needs to be addressed to ensure generalization of strategy use across tasks and settings.
- Students should refine their self-monitoring and self-checking strategies by developing personalized error checklists that match their learning profiles. This helps structure the editing process, which becomes goal-oriented, so that students focus on trying to identify their most common mistakes rather than editing randomly.

- Students should experience mastery and success so that they understand the benefits of using specific strategies. This ensures that students value the strategies, use them consistently, and generalize them to other tasks and settings.
- Strategy use should be counted as a part of students' grades. Specifically, students' strategy use should be rewarded, and grades should be assigned for the process as well as the final product. When teachers make strategy use count, students' motivation and effort increases.
- Students should be helped to understand that hard work and an inordinate number of hours spent studying will not, *on their own*, result in academic success. Rather, students need to learn that hard work and use of effective strategies will help them bypass the impact of their learning difficulties so that they can show what they know in the classroom and on tests. Strategies help students learn *how* to learn and to recognize the important phases in the learning process as steps toward their final goal.

One system for systematically teaching strategies for improving students' planning, organization, memorization, shifting, and self-checking is incorporated in BrainCogs (Institutes for Learning and Development and FableVision, 2004). This interactive software program teaches students to develop strategies for learning, studying, and test taking and to use strategies that match their learning profiles. Students also learn *when* to use *which* strategies and in *what* contexts. Once students recognize the purpose and benefits of using strategies for tasks that are heavily dependent on executive function processes, they can be encouraged to personalize specific strategies, many of which can then be applied to different academic tasks across the grades. The STAR strategy (see Figures 5.4a and 5.4b) is one example of a useful strategy for summarizing reading material and organizing ideas for writing (Meltzer, Roditi, Steinberg, Biddle, Taber, Caron, & Kniffin, 2006). This strategy helps students plan, organize, prioritize, and shift approaches, whether they are writing book reports in the first few grades (see Figure 5.4a) or complex science reports in the middle school grades (see Figure 5.4b).

When students with learning disabilities use effective strategies such as this to compensate for their weak executive function processes, their academic performance often improves, which, in turn, enhances motivation and effort. This, in turn, results in more efficient and successful academic performance (Meltzer, 1996; Meltzer, Katzir-Cohen, et al., 2001; Meltzer, Reddy, Pollica, Roditi, Sayer, & Theokas, 2004). Strategy use that enhances executive function processes in conjunction with focused effort and positive self-concept helps all students attain the academic

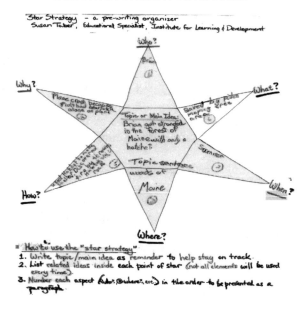

FIGURE 5.4a. The STAR strategy: An organizer for a fourth-grader's book report about *Hatchet* by Gary Paulsen.

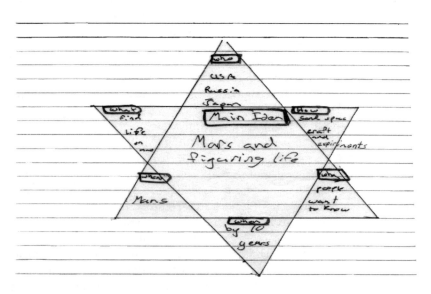

FIGURE 5.4b. The STAR strategy: An organizer for a seventh-grader's science project about space travel to Mars.

success of which they are capable and deserving (see Chapter 8, this volume, for a detailed discussion of strategy instruction).

CONCLUSIONS

Recent changes in public education have resulted in greater emphasis on high-stakes testing and have shifted the curriculum toward highly challenging, developmentally demanding goals that require students to access executive function processes rapidly and efficiently. Academic success is increasingly dependent on students' ability to plan their time, organize and prioritize information, distinguish main ideas from details, monitor their progress, and reflect on their work. Weaknesses in these core executive function processes are not easily identified, and modifications are clearly needed in our diagnostic and teaching methods. Advances in brain-based measures including fMRI and PET scans will undoubtedly help refine our methods of diagnosis and our understanding of the effects of these executive function processes on the performance of students with learning disabilities. Hopefully, these neurological measures will be coordinated with more effective educational interventions so that we can begin to narrow the gap between the medical and educational models and improve our methods of identifying and teaching students with executive function weaknesses. An improved understanding will help both educators and parents foster persistence, resilience, and academic success in students and thus improve the long-term outcomes for students with learning disabilities. These issues are best explained by a college student with a learning disability and executive function weaknesses whose performance changed dramatically after neuropsychological and educational testing helped him understand his learning profile and learn strategies for overcoming his difficulties:

I now know that my success is due to my self-understanding and the
confidence I have developed as well as the strategies I have learned.
—SEAN, COLLEGE SOPHOMORE

REFERENCES

Anderson, P. (2002). Assessment and development of executive function (EF) during childhood. *Child Neuropsychology, 8*(2), 71–82.

Anderson, P., Anderson, V., & Garth, J. (2001). Assessment and development of organizational ability: The Rey complex figure organizational strategy score (RCF-OSS). *The Clinical Neuropsychologist, 15*(1), 81–94.

Barkley, R. A. (1996). Linkages between attention and executive functions. In G. R. Lyon & N. A. Krasnegor (Eds.), *Attention, memory, and executive function* (pp. 45–56). Baltimore: Brookes.

Barkley, R. A. (1997). *ADHD and the nature of self-control.* New York: Guilford Press.

Barnard, B. (1995). Fostering resilience in children. *ERIC clearinghouse on elementary and early childhood education.* [ED386327]. Urbana, IL.

BrainCogs. (2003). *Institute for Learning and Development/ResearchILD and Fable Vision,* www.fablevision.com.

Brown, A. L. (1978). Knowing when, where, and how to remember: A problem of metacognition. In R. Glaser (Ed.), *Advances in instructional psychology.* Hillsdale, NJ: Erlbaum.

Brown, A. L. (1997). Transforming schools into communities of thinking and learning about serious matters. *American Psychologist, 52*(4), 399–413.

Brown, A. L., & Campione, J. C. (1983). Psychological theory and the study of learning disabilities. *American Psychologist, 41,* 1059–1068.

Brunstein, J. C., Schultheiss, O. C., & Grassman, R. (1998). Personal goals and emotional well-being: The moderating role of motive dispositions. *Journal of Personality and Social Psychology, 75,* 494–508.

Dawson, P., & Guare, R. (2004). *Executive skills in children and adolescents.* New York: Guilford Press.

Delis D., Kaplan, E., & Kramer, J. H. (2001). *The Delis–Kaplan Executive Function System.* San Antonio, TX: Psychological Corporation.

Denckla, M. B. (1996). A theory and model of executive function: A neuropsychological perspective. In G. R. Lyon & N. A. Krasnegor (Eds.), *Attention, memory, and executive function* (pp. 263–278). Baltimore: Brookes.

Denckla, M. B. (2005). Executive function. In D. Gozal & D. Molfese (Eds.), *Attention deficit hyperactivity disorder: From genes to patients* (pp. 165–183). Totowa, NJ: Humana Press.

Deshler, D. D., Schumaker, J. B., Lenz, B. K., Bulgren, J. A., Hock, M. F., Knight, J., et al. (2001). Ensuring content-area learning by secondary students with learning disabilities. *Learning Disabilities Research and Practice, 16*(2), 96–108.

Elliot, R. (2003). Executive functions and their disorders. *British Medical Bulletin, 65,* 49–59.

Eslinger, P. J. (1996). Conceptualizing, describing, and measuring components of executive function: A summary. In G. R. Lyon & N. A. Krasnegor (Eds.), *Attention, memory, and executive function* (pp. 367–395). Baltimore: Brookes.

Flavell, J. H., Friedrichs, A. G., & Hoyt, J. D. (1970). Developmental changes in memorization processes. *Cognitive Psychology, 1,* 324–340.

Gioia, G. A., Isquith, P. K., Guy, S. C., & Kenworthy, L. (2001). *Behavior Rating Inventory of Executive Function.* Odessa, FL: Psychological Assessment Resources.

Gioia, G. A., Isquith, P., Kenworthy, L., & Barton, R. (2002). Profiles of everyday executive function in acquired and developmental disorders. *Child Neuropsychology, 8*(2), 121–137.

Graham, S., & Harris, K. R. (1993). Teaching writing strategies to students with learning disabilities: Issues and recommendations. In L. J. Meltzer (Ed.), *Strategy assessment and instruction for students with learning disabilities: From theory to practice* (pp. 271–292). Austin, TX: PRO-ED.

Graham, S., Harris, K., & McArthur, C. (2004). Writing instruction. In B. Y. L. Wong (Ed.), *Learning about learning disabilities* (3rd ed., pp. 281–313). San Diego, CA: Academic Press.

Heaton, R. K. (1981). *Wisconsin Card Sorting Test (WCST)*. Odessa, FL: Psychological Assessment Resources.

Helliwell, J. F. (2003). How's life? Combing individual and national variations to explain subjective well being. *Economic Modeling, 20*, 331–360.

Kasser, T., & Ryan, R. M. (1996). Further examining the American dream: Differential correlates of intrinsic and extrinsic goals. *Personality and Social Psychology Bulletin, 22*, 280–287.

Korkman, M., Kirk, U., & Kemp, S. (1998). *Developmental neuropsychological assessment*. San Antonio, TX: Psychological Corporation.

Manchester, D., Priestly, N., & Jackson, H. (2004). The assessment of executive function: coming out of the office. *Brain Injury, 18*(11), 1067–1081.

Marlowe, W. (2000). An intervention for children with disorders of executive function. *Developmental Neuropsychology, 18*(3), 445–454.

Meltzer, L. (1986). *Surveys of problem-solving and educational skills*. Cambridge, MA, and Toronto: Educators Publishing Service, Inc.

Meltzer, L. (1991). Problem-solving strategies and academic performance in learning-disabled students: Do subtypes exist? In L. Feagans, B. Short, & L. Meltzer (Eds.), *Learning disability subtypes*. Hillsdale, NJ: Erlbaum.

Meltzer, L. (1993). Strategy use in children with learning disabilities: The challenge of assessment. In L. J. Meltzer (Ed.), *Strategy assessment and instruction for students with learning disabilities: From theory to practice* (pp. 93–136). Austin, TX: Pro-Ed.

Meltzer, L. (1996). Strategic learning in students with learning disabilities: The role of self-awareness and self-perception. In T. E. Scruggs & M. Mastropieri (Eds.), *Advances in learning and behavioral disabilities* (Vol. 10, pp. 181–199). Greenwich, CT: JAI Press.

Meltzer, L. (2004). *Executive function in the classroom: Metacognitive strategies for fostering academic success and resilience*. Paper presented at the Learning Differences Conference, Cambridge, MA.

Meltzer, L., Katzir-Cohen, T., Miller, L., & Roditi, B. (2001). The impact of effort and strategy use on academic performance: Student and teacher perceptions. *Learning Disabilities Quarterly, 24*(2), 85–98.

Meltzer, L., Katzir, T., Miller, L., Reddy, R., & Roditi, B. (2004a). Academic self-perceptions, effort, and strategy use in students with learning disabilities: Changes over time. *Learning Disabilities Research and Practice, 19*(2), 99–108.

Meltzer, L., & Montague, J. (2001). Strategic learning in students with learning disabilities: What have we learned? In B. Keogh & D. Hallahan (Ed.), *Research and global perspectives in learning disabilities: Essays in honor of William J. Cruickshank* (Chapter 7). Hillsdale, NJ: Erlbaum.

Meltzer, L., Reddy, R., Pollica, L., & Roditi, B. (2004). Academic success in students with learning disabilities: The roles of self-understanding, strategy use, and effort. *Thalamus*, *22*(1), 16–32.

Meltzer, L., Reddy, R., Pollica, L., Roditi, B., Sayer, J., & Theokas, C. (2004). Positive and negative self-perceptions: Is there a cyclical relationship between teachers' and students' perceptions of effort, strategy use, and academic performance? *Learning Disabilities Research and Practice*, *19*(1), 33–44.

Meltzer, L., Roditi, B., Button, K., Steinberg, J., Pollica, L., Stein, J., et al. (2005). *The Drive to Thrive program*, Lexington, MA: Research Institute for Learning & Development.

Meltzer, L., Roditi, B., Pollica, L., Steinberg, J., Stacey, W., & Krishnan (2004). *Metacognitive Awareness System (MetaCOG): Research Institute for Learning and Development (ResearchILD)*, Lexington, MA.

Meltzer, L., Roditi, B., Steinberg, J., Biddle, K. R., Taber, S., Caron, K. B., & Kniffin, L. (2005). *Strategies for success: Classroom teaching techniques for students with learning differences, 2nd Edition*. Texas: Pro-Ed.

Miller, L., Meltzer, L. J., Katzir-Cohen, T., & Houser, R. F., Jr. (2001). Academic heterogeneity in students with learning disabilities. *Thalamus*(Fall), 20–33.

Morris, R. D. (1996). Relationships and distinctions among the concepts of attention, memory, and executive function: A developmental perspective. In G. R. Lyon & N. A. Krasnegor (Eds.), *Attention, memory, and executive function*. Baltimore: Brookes.

Myers, J. E., & Myers, K. R. (1995). *Rey Complex Figure Test and recognition trial: Professional manual*. Odessa, FL: Psychological Assessment Resource, Inc.

Pajares, F., & Schunk, D. H. (2001). Self-beliefs and school success: Self-efficacy, self-concept, and school achievement. In R. Riding & S. Rayner (Eds.), *Perception* (pp. 239–266). London: Ablex Publishing.

Pennington, B. F. (1991). Attention deficit hyperactivity disorder. In *Diagnosing learning disorders: A neuropsychological framework* (pp. 82–110). New York: Guilford Press.

Pennington, B. F. (1997). Dimensions of executive function in normal and abnormal development. In N. A. Krasnegor & G. R. Lyon (Eds.), *Development of the prefrontal cortex: Evolution, neurobiology and behavior* (pp. 265–281). Baltimore: Brookes.

Raskind, M. H., Goldberg, R. J., Higgins, E. L., & Herman, K. L. (1999). Patterns of change and predictors of success in individuals with learning disabilities: Results from a twenty-year longitudinal study. *Learning Disability Quarterly*, *19*, 70–85.

Scruggs, T. E., & Mastropieri, M. (Eds.). (1998). *Teaching test-taking skills: Helping students show what they know*. Cambridge, MA: Brookline Books.

Sheldon, K. M., & Elliot, A. J. (1999). Goal striving, need satisfaction, and longitudinal well-being: The self-concordance model. *Journal of Personality and Social Psychology*, *76*, 482–497.

Swanson, H. L. (1989). Strategy instruction: Overview of principles and procedures for effective use. *Learning Disabilities Quarterly*, *12*, 3–15.

Swanson, H. L., & Hoskyn, M. (1998). Experimental intervention research on students with learning disabilities: A meta-analysis of treatment outcomes. *Review of Educational Research, 68,* 277–321.

Swanson, H. L., & Hoskyn, M. (2001). Instructing adolescents with learning disabilities: A component and composite analysis. *Learning Disabilities Research and Practice, 16*(2), 109–119.

Torgesen, J. K. (1982). The learning-disabled child as an inactive learner: Educational implications. *Topics in Learning and Learning Disabilities, 2,* 45–51.

CHAPTER 6

Nonverbal Learning Disabilities and Executive Function

The Challenges of Effective Assessment and Teaching

JUDITH A. STEIN
KALYANI KRISHNAN

This chapter focuses on identifying the executive function difficulties that characterize many students with nonverbal learning disabilities. We begin with a discussion of the characteristics of individuals with nonverbal learning disabilities followed by an overview of effective assessment and teaching practices for this population. In the remainder of the chapter, we highlight the important components of a comprehensive assessment of executive function. We also discuss teaching principles and strategies that have been shown to be effective in addressing the academic and social problems of students with nonverbal learning disabilities.

WHAT ARE THE CHARACTERISTICS OF STUDENTS WITH NONVERBAL LEARNING DISABILITIES?

The definition of a nonverbal learning disability has been rather elusive and somewhat controversial in the fields of education and psychology. The term "nonverbal learning disability" first appeared in the literature in the late 1960s when Johnson and Myklebust (1967) described a syndrome in which children had strong verbal skills and significant difficulties with visuospatial tasks, social perception (i.e., understanding the relevance of time, space, facial expressions, interpersonal actions, and other nonverbal aspects of daily living), and the mastery of mathematical concepts and procedures. Johnson and Myklebust conceptualized nonverbal learning disabilities based on a hierarchical model of cognitive processes. They noted that the primary deficits associated with nonverbal learning disabilities involved perception and imagery, which in turn affected higher levels of functioning, including symbolization and conceptualization. Common features of children with nonverbal learning disabilities included difficulties with part-to-whole perception, right–left orientation, spatial organization, motor coordination, visualization, and identification of body parts. At the time of Johnson and Myklebust's writings, little was known about the executive function deficits that characterize children with nonverbal learning disabilities.

During the 1970s and 1980s, Byron Rourke spearheaded an intensive research program in which he investigated this syndrome and published several books documenting his clinical observations and research findings (Rourke, 1989, 1995). Rourke defined nonverbal learning disabilities as a neurological syndrome that included primary deficits in tactile and visual perception, motor coordination, and the assimilation of novel material. Secondary and tertiary deficits were identified in visual attention, visual memory, concept formation, problem solving, and pragmatic language. The combination of these neuropsychological deficiencies was viewed as underlying the academic and social/behavioral difficulties that emerge as children are faced with the complexities of the academic and social demands of the late elementary years and beyond. Rourke's findings indicated that academic difficulties were experienced in the areas of writing, reading comprehension, mathematical problem solving, and science (Tanguay, 2002; Thompson, 1997). Because of their struggles with attending to and understanding nonverbal communication, their poor adaptation to novel situations, and their language idiosyncracies, children with nonverbal learning disabilities were found to have enormous difficulty interacting appropriately with peers.

In Rourke's original model of nonverbal learning disabilities, individuals were identified as having a nonverbal learning disability if they met specific neuropsychological criteria (Drummond, Ahmad, & Rourke, 2005; Pelletier, 2001; Rourke, 1995). While Rourke's criteria for defining nonverbal learning disabilities included general measures of abilities in the areas of motor coordination, tactile perception, visuospatial relationships, language, problem solving, and academic achievement, he did not include measures of executive function, although deficits in this realm may have been implied by his discussion of deficits in higher-order thinking, hypothesis testing, adaptation to novelty, and social cognition (Rourke, 1989, 1995).

In terms of assessment, then, Rourke and his colleagues emphasized the importance of evaluating primary deficits (i.e., tactile and visual perception and complex psychomotor skills) rather than the assessment of more complex neuropsychological areas, such as planning, integration, organization, social competence, and behavioral regulation. While Rourke's contributions to our understanding of this disorder have been on the cutting edge of the field of learning disabilities, the limitations of this approach have created gaps in our knowledge about the more complex features of nonverbal learning disabilities and have curtailed its application in clinical and educational settings. For example, some of the measures that Rourke utilized to determine the diagnostic criteria are no longer commonly used. Assessment measures have been updated; for example the Wechsler Intelligence Scale for Children—Fourth Edition (WISC-IV) no longer yields a Verbal and Performance IQ score and now comprises different subtests (e.g., Matrix Reasoning and Picture Concepts have taken the place of Object Assembly). In addition, some of Rourke's most discriminating tests are not well known or available in many clinical and educational settings (e.g., the Target Test and Tactual Performance Test [Reitan & Wolfson, 1993]). Finally, no measures of executive function, social competence, or performance on complex educational tasks (e.g., reading comprehension, written expression, study and test-taking skills) were included by Rourke and his colleagues.

WHAT ARE THE COMMON EXECUTIVE FUNCTION DEFICITS AMONG STUDENTS WITH NONVERBAL LEARNING DISABILITIES?

Few reports in the literature directly address the executive function processes in children and adults with nonverbal learning disabilities; however, anecdotal and clinical reports have described multiple executive function difficulties in this population (Tanguay, 2002; Thompson, 1997). Recently, Jing, Wang, Yang, and Chen (2004) investigated several components of executive function among children with nonverbal learning disabilities. They identified significant weaknesses in attention control, working memory, and cognitive shifting among these children when compared to a control group. Similarly, Cornoldi, Rigoni, Tressoldi, and Vio (1999) found that children with nonverbal learning disabilities showed deficits in the areas of visuospatial working memory and visual imagery. When compared to a control group, these children had more difficulty solving spatial problems that required visualization and reliance on working memory.

According to Howard Gardner's conceptualization of executive function (Chapter 2, this volume), two important executive processes include the ability to prepare oneself for a particular situation and the ability to regulate one's behavior. For many students with nonverbal learning disabilities, the tasks of preparing oneself for a change in activity or a novel situation and then regulating one's behavior accordingly are especially challenging. This group of students often has a limited ability to anticipate impending change and to interpret and respond to their environment in a flexible way. A prime example of this phenomenon is illustrated by the following case example:

> Sam is a 10-year-old boy who has a very difficult time transitioning into a new class at the beginning of the school year. He has trouble remembering the new classroom routine, is highly anxious about losing his papers and assignments, and frequently asks for help with even the simplest tasks ("Where do I put my lunchbox?"). Just as he is learning the ropes and getting used to his teacher and the classroom rules, a substitute teacher is assigned to the class. Suddenly, he panics (his anxiety level skyrockets), and he becomes totally confused about the day's schedule, lunchtime routines, and homework assignments. He becomes angry when the substitute teacher explains concepts differently and does not follow the typical daily schedule of activities. Sam ends up having a terrible day—getting in trouble for not listening, not completing his work, arguing with his peers ("Put your book away! We always do math before reading, stupid!"), and being disrespectful to the teacher ("That's not the right way to do it!").

Adjusting to a new environment is fraught with multiple challenges for students like Sam. Beginning with their perceptual deficits, children with nonverbal learning disabilities are especially vulnerable to misreading novel situations because their visual and tactile perception may be distorted. Until they can become familiar with the environment through verbal mediation and verbal encoding (i.e., by labeling objects and relationships using words), they may feel disoriented. They often struggle to interpret new situations because of their executive function weaknesses, which affect their ability to sort, prioritize, sequence, or organize the information in their environment efficiently. In addition, their tendency to interpret language in a literal and inflexible manner may leave them vulnerable to misunderstanding verbal instructions or written assignments, leading to further disequilibrium and stress. This emotional overload combines with the already diminished problem-solving capacities of these children, further diminishing their ability to respond flexibly. In response to this cycle, they tend to dig in their heels, rigidly relying on familiar patterns of behavior and social interactions as a way to reestablish balance. This rigidity and lack of cognitive flexibility further reflect their executive function difficulties.

Executive function difficulties have been identified as major contributors to the academic and social problems that plague students with nonverbal learning disabilities. Specifically, these individuals often demonstrate difficulties with planning, organizing, working memory, disinhibition (especially with verbal and behavioral responses), shifting (or cognitive flexibility), and self-monitoring. In addition, many students with nonverbal learning disabilities have difficulties with reading comprehension, specifically with identifying the main themes or concepts and making inferences with respect to the meaning of the text or the attributes of characters. Difficulties in this arena can partially be attributed to deficits in working memory, which, in turn, lead to problems in organizing the information into a hierarchy (details to main ideas). Moreover, weaknesses in cognitive flexibility adversely impact these students' abilities to understand the various perspectives and/or motivations of multiple characters within a literary text.

In the social arena, difficulties with social perception (i.e., the understanding of nonverbal communication and social interactions) impair the social acceptance and success that these youngsters experience. In addition, these students struggle to regulate their emotional and behavioral responses to peer interactions. Even when children with nonverbal learning disabilities understand the social context (e.g., someone is teasing), they have substantial difficulty inhibiting their initial impulse and rarely consider alternative responses before acting. These executive function deficits wreak havoc on their social lives. One case example that illustrates these difficulties is as follows:

A 10-year-old girl was running on the track with her physical education class. Having already been teased because she was the slowest runner, she decided to end her run with flair by jumping over the cones marking the end of the course. Unfortunately, her jump resulted in her landing directly on top of a cone and falling to the ground. Of course, this action provoked a great deal of laughter from her peers, and she was mortified and humiliated. While many deficits associated with her learning profile may have contributed to her downfall (including her poor motor control and weak understanding of spatial relationships), her difficulties with executive function processes (e.g., self-evaluation, self-monitoring, and poor assessment of possible consequences) were even more important. In addition, she could not understand her peers' reactions and was unable to shift her perspective to appreciate the humor of the situation.

HOW DO WE ASSESS EXECUTIVE FUNCTION DIFFICULTIES FOR CHILDREN WITH NONVERBAL LEARNING DISABILITIES?

Accurately assessing an individual's functioning in the executive function realm is challenging regardless of the population. Standard measures of executive function processes such as the Behavior Rating Inventory of Executive Function (BRIEF; Gioia, Isquith, Guy, & Kenworthy, 1996), Wisconsin Card Sort (Heaton, 1981), and Tower Test (Delis, Kaplan, & Kramer, 2001) can provide some information regarding the processes of planning, shifting mental sets, self-monitoring performance, and working memory. (See Meltzer & Krishnan, Chapter 5, this volume, for a more detailed discussion of executive function process measures.) Despite the variety of available standardized measures, including self-report questionnaires as well as structured tasks such as the Wisconsin Card Sort (Heaton, 1981), Tower Test, Stroop Color Word Test, and Trail Making Test (Delis et al., 2001), none provides an authentic assessment of an individual's ability to plan, organize, shift, and self-monitor his or her performance on real-life academic or social tasks.

Another challenge of assessment in this domain stems from the fact that executive functioning may not be highly stable across tasks and developmental stages (Bernstein & Waber, Chapter 3, this volume). For example, if an individual is strongly motivated to do well on a particular task and can muster up his energy and resources to optimize his functioning, he might do very well on a brief, isolated measure of executive functioning such as the Wisconsin Card Sort Test or the Trail Making Test. In contrast, in real-life academic or social situations, the same individual may have difficulty with such processes as planning, organizing, and self-monitoring, where the demands may be overwhelming due to their complexity (i.e., too much information to process), duration (e.g., a long-term project or a 2-hour discussion or play-date), and emotional valence. Moreover, since executive function processes encompass a broad range of disparate components from working memory to organization to self-regulation, it is difficult to identify a diversified yet comprehensive range of measures to assess this wide variety of skill sets. Therefore, the results of traditional neuropsychological or psychoeducational evaluations of executive function processes may be limited in their generalizability because of issues with reliability (i.e., variability) and validity (breadth and depth of measures). In other words, when conclusions regarding an individual's executive function are drawn primarily from performance on standardized measures such as the Wisconsin Card Sort Test, the Tower Test, the Trail Making Test, and the Stroop Color Word Test, these findings may not be representative of the individual's functioning in real-life situations. Alternative measures such as self-report questionnaires and rating scales provide a broader view of an individual's functioning in real-life situations; however, they are more subjective and highly dependent on the perceptions of the reporter.

These general assessment challenges in the realm of executive function are magnified when evaluating individuals with nonverbal learning disabilities. First and foremost, students with nonverbal learning disabilities are often more anxious when entering novel situations and performing new tasks. While performance on all assessment measures may be compromised by anxiety, executive function processes are among the most vulnerable to interference in the face of emotional disturbance (Airaksinen, Larsson, & Forsell, 2005; Ottowitz, Tondo, Dougherty, & Savage, 2002). Therefore, measures of executive function may be skewed depending on the comfort level and emotional well-being of the student.

In addition, children with nonverbal learning disabilities function quite differently depending on the structure of the tasks presented to them and the environment in which they are asked to perform. In an academic setting, for example, the performance of these students improves significantly when assignments are clearly explained, highly structured, and task-specific. A writing assignment based on an open-ended prompt such as "Why is math important in your life?" will elicit a very different response than a highly specific, well-defined prompt on the same topic, such as "Describe how math affects your daily life, including examples of how you use measurement, time, money, mathematical operations, fractions, and percentages." Similarly, in the testing situation, the evaluator must consider the nature of the tasks (e.g., open-ended vs. closed procedures), the explicitness of the instructions, and the level of inference, organization, and integration required by the student to complete the task. In many cases, students with nonverbal learning disabilities will perform well on tasks designed to measure executive function processes such as the Stroop Color Word Test and Trail Making Test because these measures are well defined, highly structured, and time limited. On the other hand, when given more open-ended tasks like the Design Fluency task (Delis–Kaplan Executive Function System; Delis et al., 2001) or the Category Shift task (Survey of Problem-Solving Skills; Meltzer, 1987), this group of children will likely have more difficulty. Therefore, the interpretation of test results must take into consideration the inherent structure and explicit nature of the tasks presented. Moreover, examiners need to be cautious about generalizing the results gleaned from a highly structured setting to a less organized, more ambiguous context such as the classroom or the playground.

Furthermore, these children often function at their best when interacting with adults. In the testing environment, these students are more likely to marshal their cognitive resources and perform optimally, especially given the supportive nature of most examiners. In addition, these children may perform tasks that tap executive function processes with greater proficiency because of the support and supervision available from the evaluator (i.e., repeated directions, explanations of the task, opportunities for practice, encouragement, and immediate feedback). In contrast, when these children are required to function independently in the classroom or at home when doing homework, they are more likely to flounder. Their executive function capacities may be further compromised when they are asked to work with a peer group. In this context, their heightened anxiety and poor interpersonal skills confound their ability to utilize their executive function processes in an effective manner. With respect to assessment, then, conclusions about executive function capacities based on adult–child interactions may have limited utility in the classroom or in social situations where peer-to-peer interactions dominate.

Diagnosticians who are mindful of these additional challenges when assessing students who present with difficulties characteristic of individuals with nonverbal learning disabilities will be in a position to provide more reliable and comprehensive information about students. Allowing ample time to develop rapport with these students, presenting both structured and open-ended complex tasks, and including a broad range of executive function measures (i.e., observer rating scales, process measures, and tasks that tap working memory, planning, prioritizing, organizing, flexibility, inhibition, and self-monitoring) are essential components of effective evaluations.

HOW DO WE ASSESS EXECUTIVE FUNCTION PROCESSES WITHIN THE SOCIAL REALM IN CHILDREN WITH NONVERBAL LEARNING DISABILITIES?

Assessment of executive function processes related to social competence involves similar challenges to the evaluation of other components of executive function. When evaluating children's social success, evaluators must measure a broad range of skills and abilities, including social perception, pragmatic language, social understanding and judgment, problem solving, emotional regulation, and behavioral control. Again, finding measures that are reliable and ecologically valid as well as practical is problematic. Without directly observing an individual's behavior in a social context, it is difficult to judge his or her social competence based on the data gathered in the testing environment. In order to optimize the assessment of executive function processes within the social realm, diagnosticians would benefit from using a variety of measures that could include the following:

Social Skills Observation Checklist

This measure is a standardized method for recording findings from a naturalistic observation and is described in detail in Michelson, Sugai, Wood, and Kazdin (1983). A social setting such as the classroom or playground is chosen, and one or more observers use a checklist to indicate the occurrence or absence of specific receptive and expressive social skills in a particular child, including (1) expressing and responding to positive statements, (2) expressing and responding to negative statements, (3) giving and following instructions and/or requests, (4) initiating and maintaining conversations and listening to others during conversation, and (5) expressing and responding to feelings. With respect to executive function processes, observers would want to pay particular attention to the child's ability to think about his or her response before speaking, to observe and utilize nonverbal and verbal feedback constructively, and to change his or her behavior as needed. One obvious advantage of utilizing this instrument is its inherently strong external validity and its direct connection to developing appropriate interventions to address the particular social difficulties that an individual may have. Disadvantages of using naturalistic observation include its time-consuming nature and its limited sampling of behaviors unless multiple observations occur.

Social Skills Role-Play Test

This instrument assesses the same receptive and expressive social skills as the Social Skills Observation Checklist, but the data is collected by observing individuals in contrived social situations. In other words, situations are presented to the child and several peers or adults, and they role-play the interactions that are dictated by written scripts. Examples of role plays that were developed by Bornstein, Bellak, and Hersen (1977) are described in Michelson and colleagues (1983). Again, in relation to executive function, observers could note how often the child is able to self-monitor her behavior and change it appropriately when verbal or nonverbal feedback is provided. In addition, the evaluator may want to ask the child to generate several possible responses in order to assess her ability to plan out her responses as well as to be flexible in her approach.

Children's Assertive Behavior Scale: Self-Report

This measure consists of 27 items in which a variety of situations and possible responses are presented, and the child is asked to select which response most accurately reflects his or her usual one to the particular social situation. A detailed discussion of the psychometrics of this scale is available in Michelson and Wood (1982). A corresponding questionnaire for parents and teachers is also available (Children's Assertive Behavior Scale: Informant's Report). With respect to executive function processes, none of the items directly assesses planning, cognitive flexibility, self-monitoring, or self-regulation; however, an analysis of the pattern of behavioral responses reported might provide some information about the child's level of functioning in this arena.

Other widely used informant and self-report questionnaires that assess social competence include the Peterson–Quay Behavior Problem Checklist (Quay & Peterson, 1967), the Achenbach Behavioral Checklist (Achenbach, 1991) and the Behavioral Assessment System for Children (BASC) (Reynolds & Kamphaus, 1992). These measures all present a list of problem behaviors that are rated according to the frequency or intensity of their occurrence. While these behavioral checklists are designed to assess a broad range of behaviors associated with emotional concerns (e.g., aggression, depression, anxiety), they all include a social competence/social skills scale. Reliability and other psychometric properties of each scale are available in the test manuals.

The variety of available social skills assessment tools is helpful for the clinician when trying to evaluate a child's social functioning and determine the presence or absence of a pervasive nonverbal learning disability. None of these measures is designed specifically to parcel out the executive function deficits that may be contributing to a child's social difficulties, but by using a variety of measures, one might be able to infer the level of planning, organization, and thoughtfulness that the child exhibited in his or her social interactions. For example, one might make the assumption that if a child exhibits overly passive or aggressive behaviors across many situations, then it is likely that difficulties in the executive function domain such as self-monitoring or self-regulation underlie this pattern of response.

HOW DO WE PROVIDE EFFECTIVE INTERVENTION AND INSTRUCTION?

Several chapters in this book address various aspects of intervention with students who have weak executive function processes, including in general classroom management, study skill strategies, math, and written expression (see Meltzer & Krishnan, Chapter 5, this volume; Meltzer, Pollica, & Barzillai, Chapter 8; Roditi & Steinberg, Chapter 11; Graham, Harris, & Olinghouse, Chapter 10). The following discussion focuses on the specific educational needs of students who meet the criteria for the diagnosis of a nonverbal learning disability. The major principles that guide intervention and specific strategy instruction are discussed, with particular emphasis on reading comprehension in order to round out the intervention discussions presented throughout this book.

Given the difficulties that these students experience with executive function processes such as anticipating events, planning, prioritizing, time management, and written output, they benefit from general classroom accommodations such as the following (Tanguay, 2002; Telzrow & Bonar, 2002; Thompson, 1997):

- Predictable schedules and routines
- Assigned seating that does not vary
- Advanced notice of syllabi, as well as test and exam schedules (for older students)
- Homework assigned for the week so the pattern is clearly evident
- Step-wise guides to long-term projects with phased timelines
- Access to models of finished products so the goal is clear
- Use of explicit linear, written rubrics so expectations are clear
- Access to software and appropriate templates (e.g., graph paper) to bypass visuospatial and fine-motor difficulties
- Balanced homework assignments that limit the number of visuospatial tasks
- Pairing visuals (e.g., complex maps, diagrams) with verbal explanations
- Alternatives to drawing or construction projects
- Extended time on tests and written tasks to offset motor and organizational weaknesses.

The level of support needed by a student clearly depends on the severity of his or her difficulties. Students with significant nonverbal learning disabilities often require very small, highly structured, and predictable learning environments. In some cases, these students continue to need this high level of support through the middle and high school years. The majority of students with nonverbal learning disabilities can be successful in mainstream educational settings. Nevertheless, in the absence of the appropriate kind of support, these students can quickly develop anxiety, a high level of frustration, depleted self-esteem, and, eventually, depression if their needs are not met (Thompson, 1997).

Students with nonverbal learning disabilities benefit from direct, systematic, structured instruction, as do all students with uneven learning profiles and processing difficulties. Within this general framework, there are specific principals that apply to the teaching of these particular students (Johnson & Myklebust, 1967).

Establishing the Gestalt

Students with nonverbal learning difficulties often struggle to integrate and synthesize details. This difficulty is why they need models and rubrics to help them conceptualize and visualize the "whole" or the final goal of a lesson or assignment. With respect to instruction within individual academic domains, students with nonverbal learning disabilities benefit greatly from a "whole-to-part-to-whole" progression in the curriculum, methods, and materials. This progression allows them to understand the connections among the parts and to conceptualize the whole as a sum of the parts (Johnson & Myklebust, 1967).

For instance, many students at the middle school level study a variety of ancient and medieval empires in social studies. Teachers expect them to abstract the characteristics of empires from these various examples and from classroom discussions. Often seventh- and eighth-graders are asked to write essays on whether there are modern empires or whether the United States meets the definition of "empire." This can be a very difficult and frustrating process for students with nonverbal learning disability profiles who struggle to synthesize diverse details to arrive at a single over-arching concept of empire. They benefit from a more direct approach to the concept, where a teacher begins by defining "empire" and laying out all the characteristics of empires in a systematic manner. With this schema, or organizational framework, before them, students can study various empires and systematically work at comparing and contrasting their characteristics. The foundational framework gives them "slots" into which they can insert specific details, so that they can analyze each empire they study in a systematic manner. A table, where they can tally the features of each topic, would provide a very simple but effective way to organize the information. When the discussion and curriculum proceed in this way, students feel a sense of security with respect to the information, which promotes learning and integration of the content.

An important component of establishing the whole or the gestalt for these students is the presence of a meaningful context. Teaching new material within a familiar context—that is, making the link between the new and the known very explicit—is essential. At all times, students with nonverbal learning disabilities benefit from establishing a personal connection to the skills or content they are learning.

Segmenting and Controlling Task Difficulty

Difficulties with executive function processes such as the sorting and prioritizing of details, organization, and cognitive flexibility can be circumvented by presenting tasks in small chunks. Once the main idea has been established, as described above, it is important to present the task or assignment in manageable, small steps. The added advantage of this approach is that it helps diminish and control the performance anxiety that many students with nonverbal learning disabilities experience, while ensuring that they experience incremental successes. This principle can easily be applied when teaching the writing process. When students with nonverbal learning disabilities are introduced to the concept of writing three-paragraph essays, for example, they benefit greatly from first looking at several examples of well-organized essays. Once this is done, they need to practice the individual skills involved in writing an essay systematically and in a step-wise fashion (e.g., how to write main idea sentences, how to select and group details, how to introduce a topic, how to conclude the essay).

Another way to control task difficulty is to reframe assignments and tasks so that they help students rely on their strengths while bypassing weaknesses. Programs that require students to remain at a particular level until they achieve mastery can be very frustrating to those who have nonverbal learning disabilities, and those students may choose to quit or avoid these tasks entirely. A common instance of this dilemma is the requirement in many math programs for timed math fact tests where students are required to achieve mastery at a particular level before they move on. This approach can be exasperating for students with nonverbal learning disabilities who often struggle with slower rates of processing than their peers, weak executive function skills, and anxiety. As long as they have reliable strategies for accessing math facts, they should be encouraged to move forward.

Sequencing

Many students with nonverbal learning disabilities are sequential learners. In other words, it is difficult for them to process large volumes of information simultaneously. Scanning complex visual information quickly (e.g., diagrams, illustrations, social situations) in order to extract the essential information is challenging for these students. They process sequential information more easily when the content is absorbed in small chunks. Whenever possible, they also benefit from using linear, verbal strategies that help them sequence more amorphous, or nonlinear, information that may appear to lack an internal structure. It is always important to ensure that the links from one step to the next are made explicit for these students so they can continuously update their formulation of the gestalt. For instance, in social studies or literature, when they are studying a long series of cause-and-effect relationships, students benefit from understanding the broad arc of the content (gestalt) and from addressing each specific event in turn, chronologically. At each step, it is important to summarize the information known thus far so that there is a feedback loop and a cumulative review that continuously relates each individual cause–effect outcome to the broad theme.

A Note about Segmenting and Sequencing Tasks

As Harris and Graham (1996) point out, lessons are usually taught with a strong focus on skill development, particularly at the elementary level. Often, teachers have been handed instructional guides and workbooks with specific instructions on the page numbers to be covered during a particular time span. This is not the type of systematic, step-wise instruction that benefits students with nonverbal learning disabilities. In fact, these traditional approaches to teaching often include a forced pace (everyone works on the same page at the same time) and a highly decontextualized skills-based approach that would be at loggerheads with the profiles of students who have weak spatial organization and motor skills and a deep need for a meaningful context for their learning. Instead, instruction for students with nonverbal learning disabilities must be linked to prior knowledge, embedded in a familiar context, and presented within a reasonable time frame.

Modeling and Providing Verbal Mediation

Teacher-modeled problem solving is essential for teaching students with learning disabilities, particularly those with nonverbal learning disabilities. This method is sometimes called cognitive apprenticeship and is modeled on the apprenticeship, where a novice can observe the process while an expert is working (Collins, Brown, & Hollum, 1991; Brown, & Newman, 1989). When the internal process of the expert is revealed through verbal mediation, or "think out loud," this approach becomes a cognitive apprenticeship. Students with nonverbal learning disabilities benefit greatly from "think-out-loud" formats that allow teachers to make their own problem-solving processes transparent and explicit. By systematically transferring these scripts to students, teachers can help them develop verbal mediation strategies that can be highly effective in limiting the impact of weaknesses in organization, sequencing, spatial processing, and strategy use. One of the most well-known scripts is contained in the format of reciprocal teaching methods developed by Palincsar and Brown (1984), where the teacher repeatedly models the essential subprocesses in reading comprehension: questioning, paraphrasing, summarizing, and predicting. In this format, teachers and students alternate roles, with teachers modeling the desired scripts and behaviors and students being asked explicitly to copy the teachers. This verbally mediated strategy has been highly effective and proven for teaching reading comprehension skills even with students as young as first-graders (Lysynchuk, Pressley, & Vye, 1990; Rosenshine & Meister, 1994). Think-out-loud protocols and verbal mediation are also highly effective in teaching metacognitive strategies for self-checking and self-correcting (Bereiter & Bird, 1985; Chan, Burtis, Scardamalia, & Bereiter, 1992; Fisher, 2002). In addition, teaching methods that integrate spatial and verbal processes, such as Visualizing and Verbalizing (Bell, 1986) are highly effective in helping students integrate their verbal strengths with their areas of weakness in order to develop more effective ways to learn, remember, and integrate information. Studies have shown marked gains for poor comprehenders when they are taught systematic strategies for integrating and synthesizing information across visual and verbal domains irrespective of their primary deficits (Bell, 1991; Johnson-Glenberg, 2000; Pressley et al., 1994).

Explicit and Direct Instruction

Students with nonverbal learning disabilities struggle to learn within constructivist models, of which one of the best-known applications is whole language. Students with nonverbal learning disabilities are typically detail-oriented, concrete thinkers who struggle to connect the dots, read between the lines, and draw inferences (Humphries, Cardy, Working, & Peets, 2004). They function best in settings where direct and explicit instruction is the norm. It is important to note that both the form and the content of the curriculum must be explicit. For example, when teaching these students to write responses to literature, they need a formula for the form (e.g., "Use part of the question in the first sentence of your answer") as well as the content (e.g., "Say where and when the events happened, including the season, time of day, and location of the characters during this event"). Once this has been learned, they need the consistency of using this structure for the format and content each and every time they answer that particular type of question. This kind of repetitive, highly routinized instruction is often counterintuitive to most teachers, who work hard to provide exciting, creative lessons. As described previously, however, any deviation from an established routine can be extremely frustrating and anxiety provoking for students with nonverbal learning disabilities. As Harris and Graham (1996) caution, students with learning disabilities also need sequential instruction in discrete skills to be integrated into a larger context. Failure to do so can result in a lack of meaningful learning, boredom, frustration, and even anxiety in students with nonverbal learning disability profiles.

Providing Drill and Practice

As is the case with all students who have learning difficulties, students with nonverbal learning disabilities need more practice than their typically achieving peers, but they often have fewer opportunities for practice because their slow processing speed, motor difficulties, and organizational skills can get in the way. Through consistent practice and drill, these students can accrue sufficient control over content to understand concepts at a more abstract level in a part-to-whole progression (Bargh & Chatrand, 1999; Hook & Jones, 2002). Thus, it is particularly important for these students to overlearn foundational educational skills and procedures. Once again, it is essential to help students understand how these discrete skills relate to a broader context.

Teaching Strategies Systematically

Several authors in this volume have stressed the importance of strategy instruction for students with weak executive function processes (see chapters by Meltzer, Sales Pollica, and Barzillai; Gaskins and Pressley; Roditi and Steinberg; Graham, Harris, and Olinghouse). Students with nonverbal learning disabilities are no exception. Through explicit and systematic cognitive strategy instruction, they can learn to compensate for a wide range of processing difficulties in the spatial, motor, and organizational domains. It is essential for these students to compile strategies that they have used successfully in a notebook, allowing them to refer to their strategies whenever they need to use them and promoting the integration and generalization of those strategies. One caveat that applies to students with nonverbal learning disabilities relates to their reliance on formulas. It is often the case that, given the type of sequential, step-wise strategies they need, many of these students adapt to their difficulties by becoming highly formulaic in their responses. It is as if they internalize a flowchart and follow it through to its end each time. Helping these students develop cognitive flexibility is particularly challenging both in the social realm and for higher-order academic tasks such as reading comprehension and written expression.

WHAT GUIDELINES SHOULD BE USED FOR TEACHING COMPLEX ACADEMIC SKILLS SUCH AS READING COMPREHENSION STRATEGIES?

The principles discussed above apply to other academic domains that require students to integrate and coordinate multiple subskills and strategies by using the necessary executive function processes. Reading comprehension instruction provides one context to understand some of these fundamental principles. Meltzer and Krishnan (Chapter 5, this volume) discuss the impact of weak executive function processes on a variety of academic areas, including reading comprehension. Reading comprehension requires students to decode the text while attending to the meaning of the material. At the same time, they need to monitor their performance with respect to tracking the text correctly, decoding words accurately, and synthesizing the content in order to build meaning. In order to construct meaning successfully, students need to draw on prior knowledge, to shift flexibly from main ideas to details, to attend to and interpret print, and to integrate known information with new content. Flexibility of thinking is continuously called into play when students interpret ambiguous words or language, draw inferences and conclusions, and process redundant information, all of which are features inherent to most written texts. Students need to prioritize and re-prioritize information in an effort to make the text useful for their particular purpose. Each time students are asked to respond to questions such as "What was the most important event in this book?" or "What were the key factors that contributed to World War I?" they are being asked to prioritize and synthesize information. In summary, executive function processes such as self-monitoring, flexible thinking, organizing, prioritizing, and self-checking play a critical role in a broad array of reading processes.

As discussed above, the presence of a nonverbal learning disability results in processing inefficiencies at multiple levels, including a more concrete interpretation of language and content, as well as difficulty with multiple interpretations (Rourke, 2000). These students also often struggle to understand the whole-to-part connection of main ideas to details and vice versa. In addition, the decoding efficiency of students with nonverbal learning disabilities is dependent on the efficiency and fluidity of their visual processing, including visual scanning and visuo-spatial discrimination.

The schema theory provides a useful framework for addressing the multiple challenges students with nonverbal learning disabilities encounter with respect to reading comprehension. Although the notion of schema as generic knowledge structures for complex phenomena has been understood since the 1930s (Bartlett, 1932), it was re-introduced in the 1970s to the cognitive science literature by Minsky (1975), Rumelhart and Ortony (1977), and Shank and Abelson (1977). Schema theory states that all knowledge is organized into units, or schemata, and that information is stored within these units. Thus, a schema is a generalized description or a conceptual system for understanding information—it is how knowledge is represented, stored, retrieved, and used. Though the system is called by different names (frames, schemata, and scripts), the common assumption is that new, incoming information actiates, or stimulates, these higher-order structures of relevant prior knowledge. The new information can then be encoded in terms of the information already present, thus facilitating integration. Scripts are a specific type of schema, which can be thought of as generic knowledge structures for frequently occurring sequences of events, such as a visit to a restaurant (Shank & Abelson, 1977). In the context of reading comprehension, a variety of scripts or schema can be invoked to help students with nonverbal learning disabilities. These include scripts that

- Establish the reasons for reading and activate background knowledge
- Activate the necessary language (style, dialect, essential vocabulary)
- Activate the necessary text structures (e.g., narrative, descriptive, persuasive)
- Acclimate the student to the format of the lesson.

Establishing the Reasons for Reading

Teachers could adopt a variety of approaches to clarify the purpose of reading. For younger students, it is often productive to predict events in the story by examining the title and cover illustration. Asking questions that serve to activate background knowledge and helping students formulate questions about the content they anticipate in the book also are very helpful in establishing a foundation for approaching new texts. Older students may benefit from anticipation guides (Buehl, 2001; Herber & Herber, 1993), which motivate them to read closely for specific information that will support their predictions. This can be done by asking students to respond to a series of statements that support or challenge their beliefs and experiences about the topic being studied. The *problematic situation* (Vacca & Vacca, 1993) is also a helpful technique. A problematic situation is identified and defined by the teacher so as to engage students' interest and require them to gather specific information that can be used to support their argument. This challenges students to draw upon prior knowledge, motivates them to read, and provides a clear focus for their reading. In the case of students with nonverbal learning disabilities, these activities must occur in the context of direct teaching, which seeks to make connections between ideas explicit. Prereading organizers should be completed with students with teacher-guided verbal mediation and modeling. The same prereading formats and templates must be used repeatedly, with a systematic procedure for helping students internalize these structures. Then, students must be cued and supported when accessing these templates strategically and independently.

Activating the Necessary Language

Students with nonverbal learning disabilities often have difficulty with the flexible interpretation of language (e.g., multiple meanings, connotative and denotative meanings of words, interpretation of idioms and metaphors). These difficulties sometimes play out in the social context and include weaknesses in social and linguistic pragmatics. When students with nonverbal learning disabilities read literature, they often have difficulty shifting their mindset to understand, accept, and interpret text that may be written in different dialects. The writings of Mark Twain, for example, present a typical challenge to students who may have trouble "switching codes" in the receptive domain. Thus, a student with a nonverbal learning disability may have difficulty empathizing with key characters in the literature he or she reads, understanding the substance of dialogues between characters, and appreciating literary elements such as the author's style. Teachers can alleviate some of these difficulties by laying appropriate groundwork prior to the reading in an explicit and direct manner that allows students to be open to alternate dialects and linguistic codes in the text. Students may also benefit from a broader framework (e.g., maps, history) creating a time and space that is comprehensible to them within which they can place the novel and characters. Providing information about the author, the reasons why he or she chose to write this type of book, and the political context, if applicable, are all extremely helpful ways to activate the necessary schema for students. Students may also benefit from watching well-produced film or stage adaptations of the books they are reading and from reading dialogue reciprocally so that they can better access the more nonverbal, or suprasegmental, features of the language such as rhythm, intonation, pitch, and stress, all of which contribute greatly to meaning.

Making Text Structures Explicit

The underlying organizational framework of written text can be explicitly taught using linear graphic organizers and flowcharts. The goal in teaching text structures and templates is to make the structure of information explicit and transparent for students. Thus, strategies, teaching materials, and methods that help students understand the *link* between the content of text and its form (language and format) are essential for students with nonverbal learning disabilities. Once again, these organizers and flowcharts need to be paired with organized, systematic, think-out-loud protocols that help students create an internal, contextualizing monologue, or verbal mediation. One of the challenges in teaching and practicing strategies for analyzing text structures is to choose material that is presented in a consistent format. Because students with nonverbal learning disabilities are often inflexible and unable to adapt easily to situations that may differ even in superficial attributes it becomes essential to have a consistent format that these students can use to practice their strategies. This raises many issues, particularly for older students who are included in mainstream classes. Literature, by definition, is a creative pursuit. As such, both the form and content vary considerably from one example to the next. Part of the study of literature is gaining an appreciation of the unique voices of different authors who may all be writing on the same topic (e.g., the human condition, nature, biography). How can we make this study accessible and relevant to students with nonverbal learning disabilities? What part of the experience of literature is essential for these students to have received a full and meaningful education? These are philosophical questions that need to be resolved on a case-by-case basis.

Acclimating Students to the Format of the Lesson

Throughout this chapter, we have emphasized the need for consistent structures and routines for students with nonverbal learning disabilities and weak executive function processes. One of the reasons why consistency is so important is the length of time and the number of opportunities for practice these students need in order to internalize and implement sequential procedures. Based on the purpose of the lesson, teachers may use varying formats in the course of teaching literature or language arts. It is always essential to ensure that students in the class who may have weak executive processes and nonverbal learning disabilities understand the format of the day's lesson. Students find it extremely helpful when the plan for the day is clearly outlined or bulleted in a prominent place (chalkboard, overhead projector slide, Power-Point presentation) so that they can anchor themselves within this framework. One may assume that, having experienced numerous similar lessons, a student will understand what is expected; however, students with weak nonverbal and executive function processes can be highly inconsistent and vulnerable to minute changes in their environment. Providing an outline for the day's lesson and showing how the lesson is progressing vis-à-vis the plan is an important way of supporting these students.

Higher-order language and cognitive processes that are involved in reading comprehension include drawing inferences, understanding alternate/multiple points of view, and interpreting complex, potentially ambiguous information. These are areas that can pose significant challenges to students with nonverbal learning disabilities. The complexity of these processes and the unique strengths and weaknesses of these students can appear to be diametrically opposed, but methodical, step-wise teaching, analytical approaches to methods and materials, and a close adherence to the principles laid out in this chapter can prove effective. For instance, when teaching students to draw inferences, a step-by-step approach can be used to show how discrete details can line up to suggest a particular interpretation. This type of structured, explicit instruction using highly controlled texts and materials can be supplemented with a more constructivist method such as reciprocal reading, which provides the student with guided practice in applying discrete skills within a broader context. When all of this occurs within a framework that activates the necessary schemata for understanding written text (schema for purpose, content, language, and style, as well as task), we can help students with nonverbal learning disabilities succeed in the classroom.

HOW DO WE ADDRESS THE SOCIAL DIFFICULTIES OF CHILDREN WITH NONVERBAL LEARNING DISABILITIES?

While the specifics of an effective intervention program for improving the social skills of children with nonverbal learning disabilities are beyond the scope of this chapter, general principles for addressing these needs will be discussed.

At the individual and small-group intervention level, a multitude of programs is available to address the social skills deficits that many children with nonverbal learning disabilities experience. Unfortunately, few social skills programs have been evaluated scientifically, and those that have been investigated have produced mixed results (Forness & Kavale, 1996). Nevertheless, researchers and clinicians have identified the critical components of social skills training for this group of children: nonverbal communication skills that involve understanding and using appropriate facial expressions, postures, touch, voice tone and prosody, and interpersonal distance (Duke, Nowicki, & Martin, 1996; Elksnin & Elksnin, 2006); emotional literacy (e.g., labeling emotions, empathic understanding, emotional control) (Elksnin & Elksnin, 2006); and problem-solving skills (Hazel, Schumaker, Sherman, & Sheldon, 1982; Kendall & Braswell, 1993; Michelson et al., 1983). Direct, explicit instruction that identifies each component of effective communication, models each skill and subskill, and provides opportunities for ample practice in contrived and real social situations enables students with nonverbal learning disabilities to overcome many of their social difficulties.

In most cases, the social success of children with nonverbal learning disabilities depends on interventions at the classroom level as well as at the individual and/or small-group level. Consistent with the approach to teaching general executive skills (e.g., planning, organizing, self-monitoring), classroom teachers need to take an active role in helping these students with executive function processes within the social realm. It is critical for teachers to provide the structure, support, and cues for children who are learning to initiate social interactions appropriately, to control their emotional and behavioral responses to others, and to problem-solve effectively in social situations. Equally important, teachers and administrators must establish a socially supportive and accepting environment in the classroom and on the playground and structure social activities that optimize the opportunities for these students to experience success. This type of school-wide support has been found to be effective in many forms. Whether establishing a "You Can't Say You Can't Play" policy on the playground so that all peers must be included in play activities (Paley, 1993), providing structured recess activities such as scavenger hunts, cooperative games, and opinion surveys that are conducted by children with nonverbal learning disabilities (www.ildlex.org), or implementing a schoolwide anti-bullying or social–emotional learning curriculum (www.connectforkids.org; www.open-circle.org), schools can provide a safe, supportive environment to foster positive interactions between children with social problems and their peers. In addition, teachers can directly and positively enhance children's social status and acceptance by providing recognition of a targeted child's talents and abilities, pairing the child with a popular and supportive peer for academic and social activities, and delegating valued roles and responsibilities to him or her (Lavoie, 1994). In this way, students with nonverbal learning disabilities will have more opportunities for initiating and practicing appropriate social interactions.

CONCLUSION

Students with nonverbal learning disabilities are characteristically strong with respect to their verbal reasoning abilities, vocabulary development, factual knowledge, auditory and automatic memory, receptive and expressive language, and reading skills. At the same time, these students may exhibit a broad range of deficits in the areas of tactile and visual perception, nonverbal reasoning, spatial orientation, integration and organization of information, inferential reasoning, adaptation to novelty, processing speed, mathematical problem solving, and production of written work. In addition, children with nonverbal learning disabilities experience significant difficulties in the area of executive function. Specifically, the executive function processes of planning, prioritizing, organizing, self-monitoring, and self-regulation are often problematic for these students. The combination of their nonverbal processing weaknesses and their executive function deficits contributes to their notable social difficulties.

Evaluating students with nonverbal learning disabilities poses a number of challenges to the diagnostician. Given the particular sensitivities and behavioral characteristics of this group of students, evaluators will need to provide ample time to develop rapport, present both structured and open-ended complex tasks, and include a broad range of executive function and social competence measures in order to gather the most accurate and comprehensive information.

With respect to effective intervention, students with nonverbal learning disabilities benefit from structured, systematic methods and materials, as do all students with uneven learning profiles and processing difficulties. Special considerations to keep in mind when working with students who have nonverbal learning disabilities include the following:

- Progression from whole-to-part-to-whole
- Making links between individual processes or concepts explicit
- Making explicit the links between individual processes and the gestalt

- Building in strong verbal mediation strategies to foster metacognition, integration, and synthesis and to enhance memory
- Using technology to bypass processing weaknesses in the visual–motor and fine-motor domains.

Finally, the success of children with nonverbal learning disabilities often depends on their ability to learn appropriate social behaviors and to develop close relationships with their peers. Interventions designed to help these children develop more effective social skills are often required at the individual level (e.g., individual and small-group instruction), in the classroom (e.g., teacher coaching, cueing, and ample structure), and in the school (e.g., providing a safe and supportive environment, recognizing students' strengths, and fostering positive interactions among all students).

REFERENCES

Achenbach, T. M. (1991). *Manual for the Child Behavior Checklist.* Burlington, VT: University of Vermont, Department of Psychiatry.

Airaksinen, E., Larsson, M., & Forsell, Y. (2005). Neuropsychological functions in anxiety disorders in population-based samples: Evidence of episodic memory dysfunction. *Journal of Psychiatric Research, 39*(2), 207–214.

Bargh, J. A., & Chatrand, T. L. (1999). The unbearable automaticity of being. *American Psychologist, 54*(7), 462–279.

Bartlett, F. C. (1932). *Remembering.* Cambridge, UK: Cambridge University Press.

Bell, N. (1991). *Visualizing and verbalizing: For language comprehension and thinking, second edition.* Paso Robles, CA: Nancibell, Inc.

Bell, N. (1991). Gestalt imagery: A critical factor in language comprehension. *Annals of Dyslexia, 41*, 246–260.

Bereiter, C., & Bird, M. (1985). Use of thinking aloud in identification and teaching of reading comprehension strategies. *Cognition and Instruction, 2*(2), 131–156.

Bornstein, M. R., Bellak, A. S., & Hersen, M. (1977). Social-skills training for unassertive children: A multiple-baseline analysis. *Journal of Applied Behavior Analysis, 10*, 183–195.

Buehl, D. (2001). *Classroom strategies for interactive learning* (2nd ed.). Madison, WI: International Reading Association.

Chan, C. K. K., Burtis, P. J., Scardamalia, M., & Bereiter, C. (1992). Constructive activity in learning from text. *American Educational Research Journal, 29*(1), 97–118.

Collins, A., Brown, J. S., & Hollum, A. (1991). Cognitive apprenticeship: Making thinking visible. *American Educator, 6*(11), 38–46.

Collins, A., Brown, J. S., & Newman S. E. (1989). Teaching the crafts of reading, writing, and mathematics. In L. B. Resnick (Ed.), *Knowing, learning, and instruction: Essays in honor of Robert Glaser* (pp. 453–493). Hillsdale, NJ: Erlbaum.

Cornoldi, C., Rigoni, F., Tressoldi, P. E., & Vio, C. (1999). Imagery deficits in nonverbal learning disabilities. *Journal of Learning Disabilities, 32*(1), 48–57.

Delis, D. C., Kaplan, E., & Kramer, J. H. (2001). *Delis–Kaplan Executive Function System Manual.* San Antonio, TX: Psychological Corporation.

Drummond, C. R., Ahmad, S. A., & Rourke, B. P. (2005). Rules for the classification of younger children with nonverbal learning disabilities and basic phonological processing disabilities. *Archives of Clinical Neuropsychology, 20*(2), 171–182.

Duke, M. P., Nowicki, S., & Martin, E. A. (1996). *Teaching your child the language of social success.* Atlanta, GA: Peachtree.

Elksnin, L., & Elksnin, N. (2006). *Teaching social–emotional skills at school and at home.* Denver, CO: Love Publishing.

Fisher, R. (2002). Shared thinking: Metacognitive modeling in the literacy hour. *Reading, 36*(2), 65–67.

Forness, S. R., & Kavale, K. A. (1996). Treating social skill deficits in children with learning disabilities: A meta-analysis of the research. *Learning Disability Quarterly, 19*(1), 2–13.

Gioia, G. A., Isquith, P. K., Guy, S. C., & Kenworthy, L. (1996). *Behavior Rating Inventory of Executive Function: Professional manual.* Lutz, FL: Psychological Assessment Resources, Inc.

Harris, K. R., & Graham, S. (1996). Constructivism and students with special needs: Issues in the classroom. *Learning Disabilities Research and Practice, 11*(3), 134–137.

Hazel, J. S., Schumaker, J. B., Sherman, J. A., & Sheldon, J. (1982). Application of a group training program in social skills and problem solving to learning disabled and non-learning disabled youth. *Learning Disability Quarterly, 5*(4), 398–408.

Heaton, R. K. (1981). *Wisconsin Card Sorting Test* (WCST). Odessa, FL: Psychological Assessment Resources.

Herber H. L., & Herber J. N. (1993). *Teaching in content areas with reading, writing and reasoning.* Boston: Allyn & Bacon.

Hook, P. E., & Jones, S. D. (2002). The importance of automaticity and fluency for efficient reading comprehension. *Perspectives (International Dyslexia Association Quarterly Newsletter), 28*(1), 9–14.

Humphries, T., Cardy, J. O., Working, D. E., & Peets, K. (2004). Narrative comprehension and retelling abilities of children with nonverbal learning disabilities. *Brain and Cognition, 56*(1), 77–88.

Jing, J., Wang, Q. X., Yang, B. R., & Chen, X. B. (2004). Neuropsychological characteristics of selective attention in children with nonverbal learning disabilities. *Chinese Medical Journal, 117*(12), 1834–1837.

Johnson, D. J., & Myklebust, H. R. (1967). *Learning disabilities: Educational principles and practices.* New York: Grune & Stratton.

Johnson-Glenberg, M. C. (2000). Training reading comprehension in adequate decoders/poor comprehenders: Verbal versus visual strategies. *Journal of Educational Psychology, 92*(4), 772–782.

Kendall, P., & Braswell, L. (1993). *Cognitive-behavioral therapy for impulsive children* (2nd ed.). New York: Guilford Press.

Lavoie, R. (1994). *Do's and don'ts for fostering social competence; Teacher's guide for Last One Picked, First One Picked on: Learning disabilities and social skills*. www.ldonline.org

Little, L. (1999). The misunderstood child: The child with a nonverbal learning disorder. *Journal of the Society of Pediatric Nurses, 4*(3), 113–121.

Lysynchuk, L. M., Pressley, M., & Vye, N. J. (1990). Reciprocal teaching improves standardized reading comprehension performance in poor comprehenders. *Elementary School Journal, 90*(5), 469–484.

Meltzer, L. (1987). *Surveys of problem-solving and educational skills: Manual.* Cambridge, MA: Educators Publishing Service, Inc.

Michelson, L., Sugai, D. P., Wood, R., & Kazdin, A. E. (1983). *Social skills assessment and training with children.* New York: Plenum Press.

Michelson, L., & Wood, R. (1982). Development and psychometric properties of the Children's Assertive Behavior Scale. *Journal of Behavioral Assessment, 4*, 3–14.

Minsky, M. (1975). A framework for representing knowledge. In P. H. Winston (Ed.), *The psychology of computer vision* (pp. 211–277). New York: McGraw-Hill.

Ottowitz, W. E., Tondo, L., Dougherty, D. D., & Savage, C. R. (2002). The neural network basis for abnormalities of attention and executive function in major depressive disorder: Implications for application of the medical disease model to psychiatric disorders. *Harvard Review of Psychiatry, 10*(2), 86–99.

Paley, V. G. (1993). *You can't say you can't play.* Cambridge, MA: Harvard University Press.

Palincsar, A. S., & Brown, A. L. (1984). Reciprocal teaching of comprehension-fostering and comprehension-monitoring activities. *Cognition and Instruction, 1*(2), 117–175.

Pelletier, P. M. (2001). Nonverbal learning disabilities and BPPD: Rules for classification and a comparison of psychosocial subtypes. *Dissertation Abstracts International: Section B: The Sciences and Engineering, 61*(9-B), 5030.

Pressley, M., Almasi, J., Shuder, T., Bergman, J., Hite, S., El-Dinary, P. B., et al. (1994). Transactional instruction of comprehension strategies: The Montgomery County, Maryland, SAIL Program. *Reading and Writing Quarterly: Overcoming Learning Difficulties, 10*, 5–19.

Quay, H. C., & Peterson, D. R. (1967). *Manual for the Problem Behavior Checklist.* Unpublished manuscript, University of Miami.

Reitan, R. M., & Wolfson, D. (1993). *The Halstead–Reitan Neuropsychological Test Battery: Theory and clinical interpretation* (2nd ed.). South Tucson, AZ: Neuropsychology Press.

Reynolds, C. R., & Kamphaus, R. W. (1992). *Behavioral Assessment System for Children manual.* Circle Pines, MN: American Guidance Service, Inc.

Rosenshine, B., & Meister, C. (1994). Reciprocal teaching: A Review of the research. *Review of Educational Research*, 64(4), 479–530.

Rourke, B. P. (1989). *Nonverbal learning disabilities: The syndrome and the model.* New York: Guilford Press.

Rourke, B. P. (1995). *Syndrome of nonverbal learning disabilities: Neuro-developmental manifestations.* New York: Guilford Press.

Rourke, B. P. (2000). Neuropsychological and psychosocial subtyping: A review of investigations within the University of Winsor Laboratory. *Canadian Psychology*, 41(1), 34–51.

Rumelhart, D. E., & Ortony, A. (1977). The representation of knowledge in memory. In R. C. Anderson & R. J. Spiro (Eds.), *Schooling and the acquisition of knowledge* (pp. 99–135). Hillsdale, NJ: Erlbaum.

Shank, R. C., & Abelson, R. P. (1977). *Scripts, plans, goals and understanding.* Hillsdale, NJ: Erlbaum.

Tanguay, P. B. (2002). *Nonverbal learning disabilities at school.* London: Jessica Kingsley Publishers.

Telzrow, C. F., & Bonar, A. M. (2002). Responding to students with nonverbal learning disabilities. *Teaching Exceptional Children*, 8, 13.

Thompson, S. (1997). *The source for nonverbal learning disorders.* East Moline, IL: LinguiSystems.

Vacca, R. T., & Vacca, J. L. (1993). *Content area reading.* New York: HarperCollins.

CHAPTER 7

Executive Dysfunction in Autism Spectrum Disorders

From Research to Practice

SALLY OZONOFF
PATRICIA L. SCHETTER

This chapter examines the executive function (EF) difficulties that have been widely reported in children with autism spectrum disorders. We first review the empirical research that has been done, highlighting central findings and important themes to emerge from this work. We then extend the research findings to the clinical realm through discussions of assessment and intervention applications. The vast majority of the work that has been done on EF in autism has focused on individuals who are verbal and function intellectually above the range of mental retardation. Such individuals usually fall into the categories of high-functioning autism and Asperger disorder, and this paper concentrates on those conditions. We begin with background information about these diagnoses.

CLINICAL MANIFESTATIONS AND SYMPTOMS

Autism involves impairments in social interaction, communication, and behaviors and interests. In the social domain, symptoms may include impaired use of nonverbal behaviors (e.g., eye contact, facial expression, gestures) to regulate social interaction, failure to develop age-appropriate peer relationships, little seeking to share enjoyment or interests with others, and limited social–emotional reciprocity. Communication deficits include delay in or absence of spoken language, difficulty with conversational reciprocity, idiosyncratic or repetitive language, and imitation and pretend play deficits. In the behaviors and interests domain, there are often encompassing, unusual interests, inflexible adherence to nonfunctional routines, stereotyped body movements, and preoccupation with parts or sensory qualities of objects (American Psychiatric Association, 2000). In order to meet DSM-IV-TR criteria for autistic disorder, an individual must demonstrate at least six of these 12 symptoms, with at least two coming from the social domain and one each from the communication and restricted behaviors/interests categories, and symptoms or delays must be present before 3 years of age. Some individuals who meet criteria for autistic disorder function intellectually in the average or better range; this subgroup is typically referred to as having "high-functioning autism," or HFA.

The second diagnosis relevant to this chapter is Asperger disorder. This condition shares the social deficits and restricted, repetitive behaviors of autism, but language abilities are well developed and intellectual functioning is average or better. Its symptoms are identical to those just listed for autistic disorder except that there is no requirement that the child demonstrate any difficulties in communication. The main point of differentiation from autistic disorder, especially HFA, is that those with Asperger disorder do not exhibit significant delays in the onset or early course of language development. This is defined as communicative use of single words by age 2 and use of meaningful phrase speech by age 3. Autistic disorder and Asperger disorder are the focus of this chapter; hereafter, they will be referred to collectively as autism spectrum disorders (ASDs).

Individuals with ASDs have long been noted to display behaviors thought to be indicative of executive problems and possibly mediated by underlying frontal dysfunction (Damasio & Maurer, 1978; Rumsey, 1985; Russell, 1995). Their singular focus on special topics, their difficulty transitioning between activities or relinquishing favored objects, resistance to change, repetitive language and motor behavior, and tendency to perseverate in ways of doing things are all signs of executive dysfunction. As discussed in more detail later, executive impairments can cause a host of difficulties in the classroom setting that may go unrecognized or misinterpreted.

REVIEW OF EF RESEARCH IN ASDs

Executive dysfunction has been found in both individuals with ASD and their family members, across many ages and functioning levels, on many different instruments purported to measure EF. This section summarizes the still growing literature. The first report of executive impairments in individuals with autism was published two decades ago, using the Wisconsin Card Sorting Test with normal-IQ adults with mild symptoms of ASD (Rumsey, 1985). The findings of this study stimulated a great deal of research on EF in ASD; within a decade, 14 studies had been published on EF deficits in autism, demonstrating significant group differences between children and adults with ASD and both typically developing and clinical samples (Ozonoff, Pennington, & Rogers, 1991; Szatmari, Tuff, Finlayson, & Bartolucci, 1990). In a review of this literature, Pennington and Ozonoff (1996) reported that impaired performance was found on at least one EF task in 90% of these studies, including 25 of the 32 executive tasks reported. The magnitude of group differences tended to be quite large, with an average effect size (Cohen's d; Cohen, 1988) across all studies of .98, marked by especially large effect sizes for the Tower of Hanoi ($d = 2.07$) and the Wisconsin Card Sorting Test ($d = 1.04$).

In the following decade, the field began to divide the multidimensional category of EF into dissociable component skills to examine the breadth of impairment. The consensus emerging from this more recent work is that ASD involves significant difficulties in both planning and flexibility (including shifting of attention and conceptual set) but not in inhibitory functions, such as stopping motor responses, inhibiting the processing of irrelevant material or distracters, or suppressing prepotent but incorrect responses (Brian, Tipper, Weaver, & Bryson, 2003; Hughes, Russell, & Robbins, 1994; Kleinhans, Akshoomoff, & Delis, 2005; Ozonoff et al., 2004; Ozonoff & Jensen, 1999; Ozonoff & Strayer, 1997). Deficits in flexibility are apparent at both the conceptual level (e.g., shifting set from one category or topic to another) and the attentional level (e.g., disengaging and moving attention among spatial locations; Courchesne, Akshoomoff, & Cieselski, 1990; Landry & Bryson, 2004; Wainwright-Sharp & Bryson, 1993).

A number of interesting issues have emerged from the EF literature in recent years. The research reported above was conducted with school-age children, adolescents, and adults with ASD, largely because of the relative difficulty of testing younger participants and the need to adapt existing experimental paradigms for them. More recently, using very simple executive tasks originally developed for nonhuman primates and human infants, several studies have failed to find group differences between preschool-aged children with autism and mental-age-matched typical and developmentally delayed controls (Dawson et al., 2002; Griffith, Pennington, Wehner, & Rogers, 1999; McEvoy, Rogers, & Pennington, 1993). This deals a blow to the hypothesis that underlying executive impairments lead to the specific symptoms of the autism spectrum and suggests that EF problems may be secondary to other, earlier-appearing core impairments. In a similar vein, it has been suggested that EF deficits directly give rise to the repetitive behaviors that are so characteristic of ASD (Turner, 1997), but predicted relationships between performance on EF tests and everyday repetitive behavior have not been found (Lopez, Lincoln, Ozonoff, & Lai, 2005; South, Ozonoff, & McMahon, 2005). Finally, as amply demonstrated in this volume, it has become clear in the last decade that ASDs are by no means the only conditions that involve executive dysfunction. In summary, with new studies have come new questions, most still unanswered, regarding the developmental course of executive dysfunction and its relationship to other symptoms of autism and other neurodevelopmental disorders. These emerging issues notwithstanding, 20 years of research documents that people with autism spectrum conditions experience significant impairments in executive processes. In the remainder of this chapter, we discuss practical implications of this empirical research, specifically assessment and intervention applications.

EVALUATION OF EF IN INDIVIDUALS WITH ASDs

A number of tests thought to tap the executive system exist. Here we will concentrate on those that have reliably demonstrated impairments in individuals with ASD, relative to control groups, in empirical research.

Wisconsin Card Sorting Test

The Wisconsin Card Sorting Test (WCST) has been the gold standard test of executive processes used in numerous studies of individuals with autism (summarized in Pennington & Ozonoff, 1996). It measures flexibility by requiring subjects to shift from a prepotent, previously reinforced cognitive set to a new sorting concept that the individual must generate (Grant & Berg, 1948; Heaton, 1981). Several investigations have demonstrated that individuals with frontal damage perform poorly on this test (e.g., Grafman, Jonas, & Salazar, 1990; Robinson, Heaton, Lehman, & Stilson, 1980). The task is appropriate for both children and adults (Chelune & Baer, 1986; Welsh, Pennington, & Groisser, 1991), with normative data available from ages 6 to 90 (Heaton, Chelune, Talley, Kay, & Curtiss, 1993).

Several computer programs for administering and scoring the WCST have been developed (Beaumont, 1981; Beaumont & French, 1987; Harris, 1990; Loong, 1990), which are appealing because they are less time consuming to administer and score and provide greater accuracy in data collection. Persons with ASDs often perform better on computer versions of the test (Ozonoff, 1995). If the WCST is being given to document deficits for the purposes of service eligibility, it may be best to use the examiner-administration format. If, however, the examiner wants to evaluate best possible performance under scaffolded conditions, then the computer-administration format may be preferable. Computer administration is also more time and cost efficient, so when evaluators face practical constraints like third-party reimbursement rates or limited time with patients (Groth-Marnat, 1999), it may be an acceptable choice.

Tower Tasks

The Tower of Hanoi and related Tower of London are the next most widely used tests in empirical research on autism. They are thought to be primary measures of planning (Shallice, 1982) and are appropriate for use with both children and adults (Levin et al., 1991; Welsh et al., 1991). Both consist of three pegs and three discs or rings of different color or size. Subjects must move the discs from an initial starting position to a specified goal state in the fewest moves possible. This places substantial demands on planning and organizational capacities. To complete the task successfully, subjects must plan a number of moves ahead, anticipate intermediate ring configurations, and determine the most efficient order of moves to achieve the goal state. Deficits in planning have been demonstrated in frontal-damaged adults (Shallice, 1982) and individuals with ASDs (summarized in Pennington & Ozonoff, 1996). Previous research used experimental versions of Tower tests, but more recently, administration and scoring procedures have been standardized and normative data provided through the inclusion of Tower tasks in two recently published neuropsychological batteries, reviewed next.

Developmental Neuropsychological Assessment (NEPSY)

The NEPSY (Korkman, Kirk, & Kemp, 1998) is a comprehensive battery that includes several measures of EF, such as a Tower subtest, a design fluency subtest, and two subtests measuring inhibitory control. It can be given to children ages 3 to 12 and has been used with children with autism (Joseph, McGrath, & Tager-Flusberg, 2005), demonstrating group differences consistent with the literature reviewed above.

Delis–Kaplan Executive Function System (D-KEFS)

The D-KEFS (Delis, Kaplan, & Kramer, 2001) provides a battery of tests that assess cognitive flexibility, concept formation, planning, impulse control, and inhibition in children and adults. It was standardized on a sample of more than 1,700 children and adults aged 8 to 89. Most of its nine subtests are adaptations of traditional research measures of EF that have been refined to examine skills more precisely, with fewer confounding variables. These subtests are Trail Making, Verbal Fluency, Design Fluency, Color-Word Interference (similar to a Stroop test), Sorting (similar to the WCST), Twenty Questions, Tower (similar to the Towers of Hanoi or London), Word Context, and Proverbs. Two recently published studies have reported significant group differences on various D-KEFS subtests between samples with autism and matched controls (Kleinhans et al., 2005; Lopez et al., 2005), suggesting it is a sensitive and valid measure of EF in individuals with ASDs. Consistent with previous literature, impairments have been found on subtests measuring cognitive flexibility and attention shifting, whereas performance on subtests measuring inhibitory processes is intact (Kleinhans et al., 2005; Lopez et al., 2005).

Behavior Rating Inventory of Executive Function (BRIEF)

The BRIEF (Gioia, Isquith, Guy, & Kenworthy, 2000) is a parent- or teacher-rated questionnaire for children ages 5 to 18 years that has 86 questions and takes about 10 minutes to complete. Clinical scales measure inhibition, cognitive flexibility, organization, planning, metacognition, emotional control, and initiation. Specific items tap everyday behaviors indicative of executive dysfunction that may not be captured by performance measures, such as organization of the school locker or home closet, monitoring of homework for mistakes, or trouble initiating leisure activities. Thus, this measure may have more ecological validity than other EF tests. It can be especially useful for documenting the impact of executive deficits on the child's real-world functioning and for planning treatment and educational accommodations. Some children who perform adequately on directly administered measures of EF, such as those just reviewed, when tested in a structured, quiet, one-on-one setting will still demonstrate profound EF deficits by parent report on the BRIEF. Correlational analyses between the BRIEF and EF tests provide evidence of convergent validity (Gioia et al., 2000). It has been used empirically with samples of students with autism (Gilotty, Kenworthy, Sirian, Black, & Wagner, 2002).

EF INTERVENTIONS FOR STUDENTS WITH ASDs

Individuals with ASDs often exhibit maladaptive patterns of behavior in the classroom that are directly related to executive dysfunction. Many times it is the occurrence of problematic behaviors in school that first leads educators to refer a student for diagnostic assessment. Since students with ASDs are verbal and function intellectually above the range of mental retardation, their deficits are often unrecognized early in their educational careers. It is typical for concerns to be raised around third grade, when curriculum and expectations of students make a significant shift, requiring more conceptual knowledge, prediction/abstraction, and self-initiated organization and learning. As students with ASDs struggle with these new challenges, they often begin to act out to gain support or attention or to express frustration. Some typical problematic behaviors observed in the classroom include noncompliance, prompt dependence, off-task behaviors, disorganization, socially inappropriate behavior, inappropriate verbalizations, defiance, and emotional "meltdowns" or aggression.

It is critical for teachers, care providers, and parents to realize that people with ASDs do not engage in inappropriate behaviors intentionally to be malicious or manipulative. Problematic behaviors are associated with skill deficits. Individuals with ASDs and executive dysfunction have not successfully learned better ways to function or the skills necessary for creating effective action plans and coping strategies. These students are engaging in maladaptive behaviors because they have not been effectively taught or sufficiently rewarded for doing things in a more acceptable way. A common misconception is that they are capable of learning to behave differently but are just lazy or unmotivated. Students with ASDs and other neurodevelopmental disorders (such as attention-deficit/hyperactivity disorder, obsessive–compulsive disorder, etc.) have documented structural and functional brain differences that affect learning (Hendren, De Backer, & Pandina, 2000). They cannot learn different ways of behaving without interventions that are specifically geared to their learning strengths and styles. It is the responsibility of parents and educators working with these students to address their specific deficits and find effective methods for teaching and reinforcing more appropriate and adaptive behaviors. There are two equally important components to intervention: (1) teaching students to work around deficits (e.g., accommodations, modifications, and compensatory strategies), and (2) directly training weak or missing skills. We describe each in turn after commenting on some specific features of the cognitive profile of ASD that are critical to effective teaching.

Typical Learning Profiles of Students with ASDs

It is critical for educators to understand the learning strengths and weaknesses of individuals with ASDs (Table 7.1) when designing educational programs and determining strategies for teaching. Without this understanding, well-meaning educators may contribute to the frustration these students feel in the learning process, exacerbating maladaptive behaviors. Areas of strength can and should be utilized when addressing executive problems. For students with ASDs, one of the most common areas of strength is visual–spatial processing; another is memory. As illustrated in the rest of this chapter, visual and memory strengths can be utilized to develop effective accommodation and compensation strategies, as well as directly to teach missing executive skills.

TABLE 7.1. Typical Learning Strengths and Weaknesses in ASD

Learning area	Spared	Impaired
Language/ communication	Phonology/syntax	Pragmatics
Math	Calculations	Concepts
Reading	Decoding	Comprehension
EF	Inhibition	Flexibility Organization skills Planning Self-monitoring
Perceptual skills	Visual	Auditory
Attention	Focused/sustained	Divided/shifting
Memory	Memorization	Working memory Memory strategies and organization
Generalization		Stimulus generation Response generalization
Motivation	Immediate Direct	Delayed Indirect Social
Sensory–motor	Fine motor	Sensory registration Sensory modulation Motor planning

Working Around Executive Dysfunction

An accommodation is a change in a course, standard, or test (e.g., preparation, location, timing, scheduling, expectations, response) that allows a student with a disability to participate without fundamentally altering or lowering the standard or expectation. Simply put, accommodations are physical or environmental changes around the student that assist him or her in accessing the standard curriculum. A modification, on the other hand, is a change in a course, standard, or test that does alter or lower the standard or expectation. Modifications involve structural, cognitive changes in the level of the material or curriculum. The goal of accommodations in education is to allow the student to access the core curriculum in the least restrictive environment, without having to modify (lower) the curriculum standards. Since students with ASDs have intelligence within normal limits and are capable of learning skills at or close to grade level, inclusive education in the general education curriculum is an appropriate consideration. Accommodations are typically necessary and effective for assisting students with ASDs to be fully included, but modifications are also sometimes necessary and appropriate. Table 7.2 explains and helps differentiate among some common accommodations and modifications used for students with ASDs in inclusive education.

Compensatory skills are skills that a student needs to access independently and utilize successfully the accommodations provided. Just because necessary accommodations have been identified and developed by an individualized education plan (IEP) team does not mean that a student can make use of them without some instruction. Often, the student must be explicitly taught the skills necessary to be independent and effective with the accommodations provided. For example, the IEP team may determine that the student needs to have assignments written on the board (rather than dictated by the teacher). The accommodation is provided, but the student still will need to learn to locate the assignment on the board, copy it into a planner, and then use the planner to gather materials and complete the work on time. Thus, IEP teams should carefully identify any compensatory skills that the student must be taught effectively to utilize the accommodations provided. Table 7.3 outlines compensatory skills students may need to learn in order to utilize accommodations successfully.

There are several programs for children with ASDs that focus on accommodations and compensatory skills and assist with executive impairments. The TEACCH program, for example, teaches students to follow visual schedules, provides highly structured and predictable routines, organizes environment and task demands using visual cues to promote independent performance, and uses work systems to clarify task

TABLE 7.2. Accommodations and Modifications Typically Used for Students with ASD

Accommodations

Pacing: extending/adjusting time; allowing frequent breaks; varying activity often; omitting assignments that require timed situations.

Environment: leaving class for academic assistance; preferential seating; altering physical room arrangement; defining limits (physical/behavioral); reducing/minimizing distractions (visual, auditory, both); cooling-off period; interpreter.

Presentation of material: emphasizing teaching approach (visual, tactile, multimodal); individual/small-group instruction; taping lectures for replay; demonstrating/modeling; using manipulative hands-on activities; preteaching vocabulary; utilizing organizers; providing visual cues.

Materials and equipment/assistive technology: taping texts; highlighting material; supplementing material/laminating material; note-taking assistance/copies from others; access to lecture outlines; typing teacher's material rather than writing on board; color overlays; using calculator, computer, word processor; having access to any special equipment.

Assignments: giving directions in small, distinct steps; allowing copying from paper/book; using written back-up for oral directions; adjusting length of assignment; changing format of assignment (matching, multiple choice, fill-in-the-blank, etc.); breaking assignment into series of smaller assignments; reducing paper/pencil tasks; reading directions/assignments to students; giving oral/visual cues or prompts; allowing recording/dictated/typed answers; maintaining assignment notebook; avoiding penalizing for spelling errors on every paper.

Reinforcement and follow-through: using positive reinforcement; using concrete reinforcement; checking often for understanding/review; providing peer tutoring; requesting parent reinforcement; having student repeat/explain the directions; making/using vocabulary files; teaching study skills; using study sheets/guides; reinforcing long-term assignment timelines; repeating review/drill; using behavioral contracts/check cards; giving weekly progress reports; providing tutoring before and/or after school; conferring with student (daily, 2 times/week, weekly, etc.).

Testing adaptations: reading test verbatim to student (in person or recorded); shortening length of test; changing test format (essay vs. fill-in-the-blank vs. multiple choice, etc.); adjusting time for test completion; permitting oral answers; writing test answers for student; permitting open-book/notes exams; permitting testing in isolated/different location.

Modifications

Presentation of subject matter: utilizing specialized curriculum written at a lower level of understanding.

Materials and equipment/assistive technology: adapting or simplifying texts for lower level of understanding; modifying content areas by simplifying vocabulary, concepts, and principles.

Grading: modifying weight of examinations.

Assignments: lowering reading level of assignment; adapting worksheets with simplified vocabulary.

Testing adaptations: lowering reading level of test.

TABLE 7.3. Common Accommodations and Compensatory Skills Needed to Utilize Them

Accommodation	Compensatory skill
Providing checklists for task steps and materials needed.	Student must learn to use the checklist by looking, doing, and crossing off items in the sequential order they are presented.
Utilize written schedule or other time-management systems.	Student must learn to identify needed information, plug it into the system, and then actively use the system by looking at, doing, and crossing off items in the sequential order in which they are presented.
Post written rules.	Student must learn the rules or the behaviors identified, recall them in the appropriate context, and engage in the specified behaviors to obtain the desired outcomes.
Set time limits utilizing a visual timer.	Student must learn to start and/or stop when the timer indicates. (Student may also learn to set timer for himself.)
Visual presentation of content or information (e.g., providing written notes, graphic organizers, highlighted material).	Student must attend to the correct cues or visual information provided.
Working individually on assignments rather than in groups.	Student must independently complete the steps of the assignment (often this accommodation is paired with checklists or other types of visual instruction).
Providing reinforcement and follow-through.	Student must learn to complete the behaviors indicated in the reinforcement system or behavior contract within the time specified. A self-management program may be taught.
Allowing frequent breaks as needed.	Student must learn what to do during the breaks to meet personal needs. Student may also need to learn to ask for a break when needed.

expectations and workload. Data from the TEACCH program indicate that these strategies do result in a greater level of independence and greater productivity for individuals with ASDs (Mesibov, 1997). These protocols can be easily implemented in a variety of settings, including the general education classroom, community, and home.

Once a student is able to utilize accommodations and compensatory skills independently, the focus should shift to self-advocacy, with the student learning to identify and request needed accommodations for him- or herself. Self-advocacy is often formally addressed as part of the educational plan when the student transitions to high school, as mandated by the Individuals with Disabilities Education Act (IDEA). This is an important time to consider how well an individual can advocate for him- or herself. IEP teams are responsible for determining and implementing appropriate accommodations during a student's education, but the responsibility shifts to the student following graduation from high school (Shore, 2004). The student must have the awareness to determine his or her needs and possess the skills to access the supports and assistance required for success in the adult world. Many critical self-advocacy skills can and should be identified and acquired much earlier in the student's educational career. These early self-advocacy skills can include learning about strengths, areas of challenge, and the nature of the student's learning differences, as well as asking for assistance from others when needed. Table 7.4 outlines some critical self-advocacy skills and strategies for addressing them.

Teaching Specific Executive Skills

While it is always critical to identify and develop compensatory skills and accommodation plans as part of an IEP, it is equally necessary to develop goals and objectives that directly build the underlying deficits in specific executive functions. Building one set of skills often does not build the other set. For example, an IEP goal might state, "To assist Johnny with homework completion skills, when the assignments are written on the board, Johnny will copy them into the appropriate location in his student planner with 80% accuracy as measured by teacher observation." The intention of the goal—to build a specific compensatory skill (i.e., writing the assignment in a planner) that makes use of a given accommodation (i.e., the assignments are written on the board)— is good. If left at this level of intervention, however, Johnny will not become independent with the entire process of homework completion nor will he have the skills to function when the accommodation is not provided for him. In fact, the underlying executive skill deficits are not being identified or directly taught at all.

TABLE 7.4. Self-Advocacy Skills and Methods for Addressing Them

Self-advocacy skill	Method/strategy for addressing
Self-awareness/ disability awareness	The student should learn and understand the nature of his or her disability and how it affects he or she across all areas (social, academic, motor, cognition, sensory). This can be done through counseling and self-awareness programs (Faherty, 2000).
Asking for help	The student should learn how to request additional help or information when it is needed. This can be done by teaching help-seeking routines and providing visual cues such as a "HELP" card with the steps for help seeking in bullet points.
Asking for a break or an appropriate sensory activity	A student may need to exit a situation temporarily to regain self-control or obtain input that will help him or her focus and sustain attention to task. The student should be taught to identify these indicators and learn ways to access a break appropriately.
Asking for clarity	The student should be taught how to ask for the necessary visual supports and cues he or she needs to be successful. He or she may be taught how to ask for visual instructions, checklists, timers, or time limits.
Asking for environmental supports and modifications	The student should be taught how to identify the necessary environmental supports he or she needs, identify those things that are distracting or creating barriers to success, and communicate these needs to others.

To learn independent completion of any complex task, the student must be taught the process of task analysis: how to break tasks down, prioritize and order steps, and plan for their completion. Few programs specifically address these underlying cognitive skills. Educators and parents alike find it challenging to write goals about a *process* rather than a *product*. It is even more challenging to write a goal about a process that is supposed to occur internally (as a private thinking event) and can only be inferred after observing a successful outcome.

Many interventions focus on teaching students with ASDs how to complete actions through rote compliance and rule following (e.g., "If _____ happens, then do _____"). Because students with ASDs have excellent memorization skills and are able to follow explicitly stated rules, they are able to execute such if-then action plans, many times independently. There are problems, however, with generalization to new situations and if-then rules that have not been explicitly taught. Furthermore, students with ASDs often become rigid with the rules they have been taught because they do not truly understand *why* an action plan was chosen or necessary and lack the flexibility to modify the rule.

Cognitive remediation is a systematic approach for overcoming cognitive deficits that arise from brain dysfunction. Specific neuropsychological deficits, such as executive, attention, and memory problems, are identified, and specific cognitive activities are designed to improve areas of weakness. Typically, cognitive remediation is only part of a more comprehensive program that also includes accommodations, modifications, compensatory strategies, and other treatment modalities, such as psychotherapy and organized social activities (Butler & Copeland, 2002). Cognitive remediation programs have been developed and shown to be effective for adults with acquired brain injury and schizophrenia (Gianutsos, 1991; Kurtz, Moberg, Gur, & Gur, 2001; Pilling et al., 2002). One of the more widely utilized approaches is Attention Process Training (Sohlberg & Mateer, 1987), which contains activities designed to improve focused, sustained, alternating, and divided attention. Recently, several papers have described cognitive remediation programs that are appropriate for children, targeting attention and executive functions such as planning, shifting set, and inhibiting prepotent but incorrect responses. Such programs have been used with both typically developing children (Rueda, Rothbart, Davis-Stober, & Posner, 2005) and those with attention-deficit/hyperactivity disorder (Kerns, Eso, & Thomson, 1999; Klingberg, Forssberg, & Westerberg, 2002). In each of these studies, training resulted in improvements on nontrained cognitive tests, including attention, EF, and abstract reasoning.

There are not yet any published efficacy studies of cognitive remediation programs for children with autism, but a controlled trial of Posner and colleagues' computer-based Attention Training Program (Rueda et al., 2005) is currently underway in our laboratory. This program was not specifically developed for children with ASDs but works well for this population because it is highly visual and takes advantage of the children's interest in computers. Through repetition and massed trials, it contains many opportunities to practice specific executive functions, such as planning, shifting attention, and inhibiting prepotent responses.

Any program to remediate executive dysfunction in individuals with ASDs should capitalize on their visual–spatial strengths. A heavy emphasis on generalization must also be applied. Students first need to learn to use particular visual strategies and then be provided with ample opportunities for practice and feedback using real-life, meaningful situations in context. A cognitive remediation program that was developed explicitly for children with ASDs, called "Learning the R.O.P.E.S. for Improved Executive Function" (Schetter, 2004), is described next. This program relies heavily on graphic organizers, which are visual representations of knowledge that organize information for later functional use (see Figure 7.1). They can be used as a form of input (i.e., the way in which information is presented to the student), which is a common accommodation strategy. Of even greater importance, graphic organizers are used in the R.O.P.E.S. program as a form of output (i.e., the way in which the student demonstrates understanding and knowledge). When students are taught to select, create, and develop their own graphic organizers, they are being taught several specific executive skills. We give examples below from the R.O.P.E.S. program.

Sequential Thinking and Evaluation

The ability to think sequentially and see relationships among situations, actions, and outcomes is a critical skill to teach children with ASDs. The use of a simple graphic organizer can provide the student with a visual thinking tool or mental construct for sequential thinking (see Figure 7.1). In the initial teaching of this process, the instructor provides prompting through directed questions to assist the student in completing the graphic organizer. Reinforcement is provided for progressively more independent responding and eventually only for independent completion of the graphic organizer on a given topic or situation. Once this basic process for sequential thinking is learned and the student is able independently to fill in the graphic organizer demonstrating the sequential

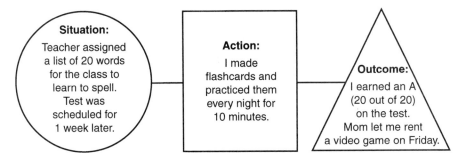

FIGURE 7.1. A graphic organizer illustrating the relationships between behaviors and consequences.

process for a variety of situations, more complex sequential thinking processes and social problem solving can be taught with graphic organizers (see Figures 7.2–7.4).

Task Analysis

Another critical process to teach students with ASDs is how to break large tasks into smaller, more functional chunks. This requires a graphic organizer that helps them see the parts or components of a larger whole, such as a simple cluster or web organizer, illustrated in Figure 7.5. The initial teaching of this process is conducted using real-life activities that the student is highly proficient at completing. Through prompting and guided questions, the instructor assists the student in completing the cluster organizer for a specific task, systematically breaking the task down into components. This practice is repeated with several activities or routines until the student is able independently to break down diverse

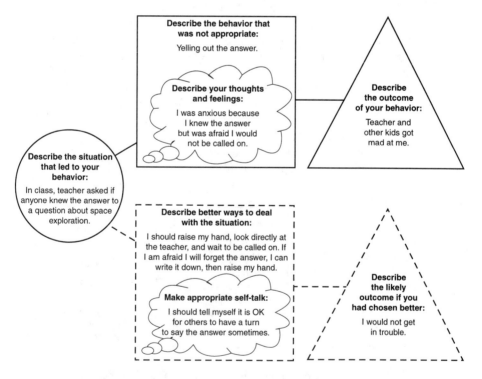

FIGURE 7.2. A graphic organizer to teach appropriate behavior.

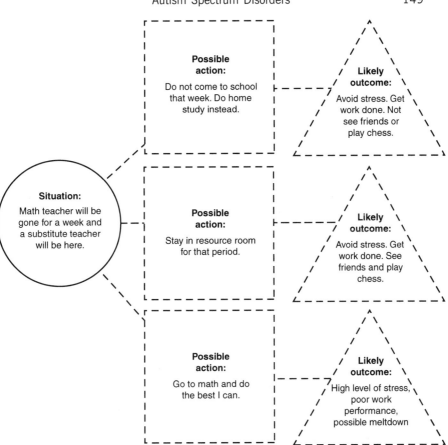

FIGURE 7.3. A graphic organizer to teach a student to predict potential outcomes and select appropriate action plans.

tasks using the cluster organizer without prompting or input. The final teaching phase involves sequencing the steps or chunks. The student is taught to order the chunks in a first-to-last sequence, ultimately creating a checklist that can then be used to assist him or her with task completion as a compensatory strategy. One subskill that deserves particular attention in the task analysis process is identification of the materials and resources necessary to complete a specific activity or assignment. This skill is imperative to teach, as gathering materials for task completion is often a trigger for off-task behavior and inefficient use of time. A simple extension of the cluster or web organizer can be used for this process (refer to Figure 7.6).

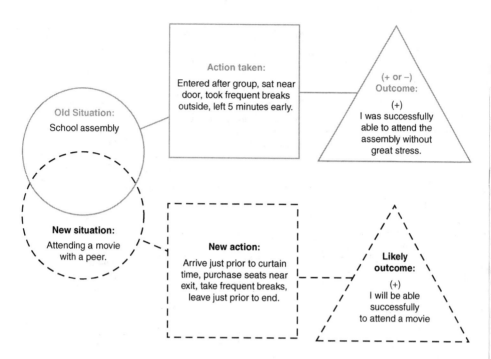

FIGURE 7.4. A graphic organizer to teach a student to evaluate a novel situation.

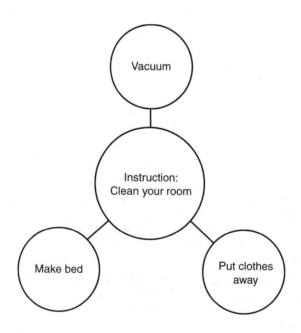

FIGURE 7.5. A graphic organizer to teach task analysis.

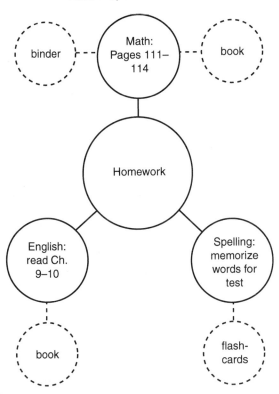

FIGURE 7.6. A graphic organizer to teach a student to identify needed materials for task completion.

Prioritization

The ability to prioritize items, demands, and activities significantly influences functional and adaptive skills. The student with executive impairments needs to be taught how to compare activities and their outcomes and order them in terms of importance. The critical variables to consider when prioritizing are due dates/deadlines and potential bonus/penalty outcomes. A graphic thinking tool such as a decision matrix can assist the student in conceptualizing and learning this comparative process. See Figure 7.7 for an example. Initially, the student is taught to plug items from a list of generated goals or assignments into the decision matrix with prompting and feedback from the instructor. The prompting and feedback are gradually decreased as the student is more independent in the process. Additional skills, such as time management and planning, must ultimately be addressed once this critical prerequisite skill is established.

	Heavy bonus or penalty outcome	No or light bonus or penalty outcome
Urgent deadline	**High priority** • **Book report** • **Study for calculus test (50 points)**	**Moderate priority** • **Spelling test (10 points)** • **Math homework (10 points)** • **Soccer practice and games**
No deadline or distant deadline	**Moderate priority** • **History term paper (250 points)**	**Low priority** • **Play video game and beat brother's score** • **Chat with friends online** • **Extra soccer practice**

FIGURE 7.7. A decision matrix to teach prioritization.

Promoting Acquisition, Generalization, and Maintenance of Executive Skills

The compensatory strategies and methods of direct cognitive remediation just discussed must be addressed across settings and within functional, real-life routines. These settings and routines should not be limited to the school day. Parents should be taught and encouraged to work with their children on these skills in home and community settings. Varying the instructors, settings, and situations will make the student more likely to generalize the skills and apply them to a broader class of behaviors.

The Role of Instructional Aides

Students with ASDs often require additional support or supplementary instruction to be successful in inclusive settings with the core curriculum. For this reason, educators and parents often feel it is necessary for an instructional aide to be assigned to a student. More important than *who* will be providing the additional support is *how* and *what type* of support should be provided. The ultimate goal of the support should be independence in the learning process. Often, however, the aide becomes a secretary for the student, taking on all of the organizational and planning components of the learning process. The aide breaks the tasks down for the student, provides step-by-step instructions, gathers the necessary materials for task completion, reminds the student of potential outcomes, and provides consequences for performance. The aide, in effect, has taken over the student's EF needs. Often the only thing the student is required to do is produce the answer or *product*, without having to participate in the *process*. Because executive skills are a core cognitive deficit for children with ASDs, these are the exact skills that the students should be actively learning. By providing an aide to perform these functions, the learning of necessary executive skills may actually be impeded and the student may become even more prompt dependent. A more productive use of aide support is to *coach* the student as he or she uses the accommodations provided and *train* the student in the cognitive remediation strategies discussed above. Aides can be used to teach the identified executive and compensatory skills and provide positive reinforcement and corrective feedback until the skills are firmly in the student's repertoire.

Self-Management Procedures

Once students can independently perform the executive skills reviewed above, self-management and maintenance of skills should become the focus of intervention. Self-management is a technique that facilitates independence by systematically fading reliance on external controls (e.g., instructions, feedback, praise) through shifting control to the child (Smith & Fowler, 1984). Self-management has been defined as "the personal and systematic application of behavior change strategies that result in the desired modification of one's own behavior" (Cooper, Heron, & Heward, 1987, p. 517). Multiple studies have shown that self-management techniques can be taught to children with ASDs, even those with significant intellectual limitations and those who are nonverbal (reviewed in Quinn, Swaggart, & Myles, 1994). Research has shown that when self-management of specific target behaviors is taught, there may also be a decrease in other maladaptive behaviors that were not specifically targeted for intervention (Koegel, Koegel, Hurley, & Frea, 1992). Research has also shown that changes in behaviors achieved through self-management training are maintained over periods of time and across instructional settings, including settings in which there are no trained service providers (Gardner, Berry, Cole, & Nowinski, 1983).

There are many components to a comprehensive self-management program. Self-monitoring (also referred to as self-recording, self-observation, or self-assessment) involves the individual observing and recording the occurrence or nonoccurrence of the target behavior. It is necessary for a person to accurately measure his or her own behavior in order to determine if that behavior is changing in the desired direction. In fact, the mere act of recording or monitoring one's behavior can have the effect of changing that behavior in the desired direction (see, for example, Broden, Hall, & Mitts, 1971). To self-monitor effectively, the student must be able to define an occurrence and nonoccurrence of the targeted behavior and must have a method for measuring the behavior and a process for determining reliability. Reliable self-monitoring is typically defined as 80% or better agreement with a designated instructor or care provider.

Another component of self-management is self-reinforcement. Having the student identify and self-administer his or her own reinforcers (and/or punishers) can have profound effects on behavior (Cooper et al., 1987). For students with ASDs, an important part of this process is to recognize the naturally occurring consequences of their actions. The ability to evaluate the outcomes of behavior, discussed in a previous section, is critical to successful self-management and maintenance of learned behaviors. Teaching students to determine natural consequences can be done with a graphic organizer much like those discussed earlier, as illustrated in Figure 7.8.

The Role of Parents

All efficacious treatments for children with ASDs involve parents in some role (Lord & McGee, 2001; Rogers, 1998), so, as with other intervention programs for children with ASD, inclusion of parents is critical

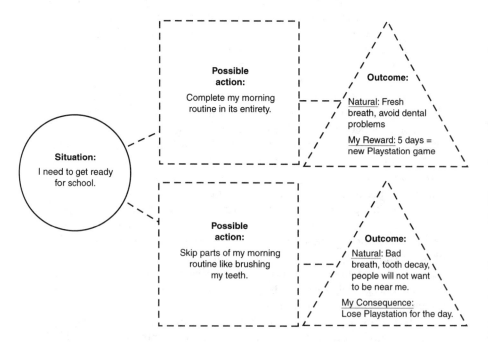

FIGURE 7.8. A graphic organizer to identify natural consequences of action choices.

for successful acquisition and generalization of executive skills. It is important that educators and professionals work with parents until parents feel confident in their understanding of executive impairments and abilities to address these complex cognitive deficits. They should understand how to accommodate these differences in the home and community; they should be assisted with identifying and teaching compensatory skills; and, when possible, they should be taught how to provide cognitive remediation.

Students learn faster and acquire more skills when they are provided with multiple contextual teaching opportunities. This requires practice outside the classroom, ideally supported by parents. It requires ongoing parent training, communication, and collaboration between home and school. Parent training can come in the form of in-services or workshops, lending libraries, shared resources, and hands-on coaching and demonstration. Ongoing communication can be in the form of conferencing, phone calls, communication logs, or other correspondence. Collaboration, which requires trust and commitment, is often the most challenging aspect for parents and professionals to achieve. Although the ability of families to be involved in their child's education will vary, educators must solicit parent input and involvement to foster collaboration. If educators and parents put forth this effort, the students will ultimately gain more educational benefit.

CONCLUSION

We began this chapter with a summary of the large research literature on executive dysfunction in autism. Over the last two decades, it has become clear that people with autism suffer from executive impairments at a high rate. Executive function is important to school success (Clark, Prior, & Kinsella, 2002), predicts response to treatment (Berger, Aerts, van Spaendonck, Cools, & Teunisse, 2003) and long-term outcome (Szatmari, Bartolucci, Bremner, Bond, & Rich, 1989), and is associated with real-world adaptive skills (Clark et al., 2002; Gilotty et al., 2002). Despite knowledge of the importance of EF to autism, practical applications have been slow to come. There are no commercially available programs to treat executive dysfunction in people with ASDs, nor are there any published studies of efficacy. At the end of this chapter, we described some important components in the remediation of executive problems and how to make the interventions maximally appropriate for people with autism. It is critical that researchers and service providers collaborate, as we have done in this chapter, to better meet the needs of people with autism.

REFERENCES

American Psychiatric Association. (2000). *Diagnostic and statistical manual of mental disorders* (4th ed., text revision). Washington, DC: Author.

Beaumont, J. G. (1981). A PASCAL program to administer a digit span test. *Current Psychological Reviews, 1,* 115–117.

Beaumont, J. G., & French, C. C. (1987). A clinical field study of eight automated psychometric procedures: The Leicester/DHSS project. *International Journal of Man Machine Studies, 26,* 661–682.

Berger, H. J. C., Aerts, F. H. T. M., van Spaendonck, K. P. M., Cools, A. R., & Teunisse, J. P. (2003). Central coherence and cognitive shifting in relation to social improvement in high-functioning young adults with autism. *Journal of Clinical and Experimental Neuropsychology, 25,* 502–511.

Brian, J. A., Tipper, S. P., Weaver, B., & Bryson, S. E. (2003). Inhibitory mechanisms in autism spectrum disorders: Typical selective inhibition of location versus facilitated perceptual processing. *Journal of Child Psychology and Psychiatry, 44,* 552–560.

Broden, M., Hall, R., & Mitts, B., (1971). The effect of self-recording on the classroom behavior of two eighth-grade students. *Journal of Applied Behavior Analysis, 4,* 191–199.

Butler, R. W., & Copeland, D. R. (2002). Attentional processes and their remediation in children treated for cancer: A literature review and the development of a therapeutic approach. *Journal of the International Neuropsychological Society, 8,* 115–124.

Chelune, G. A., & Baer, R. A. (1986). Developmental norms for the Wisconsin Card Sorting Test. *Journal of Clinical and Experimental Neuropsychology, 8,* 219–228.

Clark, C., Prior, M., & Kinsella, G. (2002). The relationship between executive function abilities, adaptive behavior, and academic achievement in children with externalizing behavior problems. *Journal of Child Psychology and Psychiatry, 43,* 785–796.

Cohen, J. (1988). *Statistical power analysis for the behavioral sciences* (2nd ed.). Hillsdale, NJ: Erlbaum.

Cooper, J. O., Heron, T. E., & Heward, W. L. (1987). *Applied behavior analysis.* New York: Macmillan Publishing.

Courchesne, E., Akshoomoff, N. A., & Ciesielski, K. (1990). Shifting attention abnormalities in autism: ERP and performance evidence. *Journal of Clinical and Experimental Neuropsychology, 12,* 77.

Damasio, A. R., & Maurer, R. G. (1978). A neurological model for childhood autism. *Archives of Neurology, 35,* 777–786.

Dawson, G., Munson, J., Estes, A., Osterling, J., McPartland, J., Toth, K., et al. (2002). Neurocognitive function and joint attention ability in young children with autism spectrum disorder versus developmental delay. *Child Development, 73,* 345–358.

Delis, D. C., Kaplan, E., & Kramer, J. H. (2001). *Delis–Kaplan Executive Function System (D-KEFS).* San Antonio, TX: Psychological Corporation.

Faherty, C. (2000). *Aspergers . . . What does it mean to me?* Arlington, TX: Future Horizons.

Gardner, W., Berry, D., Cole, C., & Nowinski, J. (1983). Reduction in disruptive behaviors in mentally retarded adults: A self-management approach. *Behavior Modification, 7,* 76–96.

Gianutsos, R. (1991). Cognitive rehabilitation: A neuropsychological specialty comes of age. *Brain Injury, 5,* 353–368.

Gioia, G. A., Isquith, P. K., Guy, S. C., & Kenworthy, L. (2000). *Behavior Rating Inventory of Executive Function.* Odessa, FL: Psychological Assessment Resources.

Gilotty, L., Kenworthy, L., Sirian, L., Black, D. O., & Wagner, A. E. (2002). Adaptive skills and executive function in autism spectrum disorders. *Child Neuropsychology, 8,* 241–248.

Grafman, J., Jonas, B., & Salazar, A. (1990). Wisconsin Card Sorting Test performance based on location and size of neuroanatomical lesion in Vietnam veterans with penetrating head injury. *Perceptual and Motor Skills, 71,* 1120–1122.

Grant, D. A., & Berg, E. A. (1948). A behavioral analysis of degree of reinforcement and ease of shifting to new responses in a Weigle-type card-sorting problem. *Journal of Experimental Psychology, 32,* 404–411.

Griffith, E. M., Pennington, B. F., Wehner, E. A., & Rogers, S. I. (1999). Executive functions in young children with autism. *Child Development, 70,* 817–832.

Groth-Marnat, G. (1999). Financial efficacy of clinical assessment: Rational guidelines and issues for future research. *Journal of Clinical Psychology, 55,* 813–824.

Harris, M. E. (1990). *Wisconsin Card Sorting Test: Computer version, research edition.* Odessa, FL: Psychological Assessment Resources.

Heaton, R. F. (1981). *Wisconsin Card Sorting Test manual.* Odessa, FL: Psychological Assessment Resources.

Heaton, R. F., Chelune, G. J., Talley, J. L., Kay, G. G., & Curtiss, G. (1993). *Wisconsin Card Sorting Test manual: Revised and expanded.* Odessa, FL: Psychological Assessment Resources.

Hendren, R. L., De Backer, I., & Pandina, G. J. (2000). Review of neuroimaging studies of child and adolescent psychiatric disorders from the past 10 years. *Journal of the American Academy of Child and Adolescent Psychiatry, 39,* 815–828.

Hughes, C., Russell, J., & Robbins, T. W. (1994). Evidence for executive dysfunction in autism. *Neuropsychologia, 32,* 477–492.

Joseph, R. M., McGrath, L. M., & Tager-Flusberg, H. (2005). Executive dysfunction and its relation to language ability in verbal school-age children with autism. *Developmental Neuropsychology, 27,* 361–378.

Kerns, K. A., Eso, K., & Thomson, J. (1999). Investigation of a direct intervention for improving attention in young children with ADHD. *Developmental Neuropsychology, 16,* 273–295.

Kleinhans, N., Akshoomoff, N., & Delis, D. C. (2005). Executive functions in autism and Asperger's disorder: Flexibility, fluency, and inhibition. *Developmental and Neuropsychology, 27,* 379–401.

Klingberg, T., Forssberg, H., & Westerberg, H. (2002). Training of working memory in children with ADHD. *Journal of Clinical and Experimental Neuropsychology, 24,* 781–791.

Koegel, L., Koegel, R., Hurley, C., & Frea, W. (1992). Improving social skills and disruptive behavior in children with autism through self-management. *Journal of Applied Behavior Analysis, 25,* 341–353.

Korkman, M., Kirk, U., & Kemp, S. L. (1998). *NEPSY Developmental Neuropsychological Assessment manual.* San Antonio, TX: Psychological Corporation.

Kurtz, M. M., Moberg, P. J., Gur, R. C., & Gur, R. E. (2001). Approaches to cognitive remediation of neuropsychological deficits in schizophrenia: A review and meta-analysis. *Neuropsychology Review, 11,* 197–210.

Landry, R., & Bryson, S. E. (2004). Impaired disengagement of attention in young children with autism. *Journal of Child Psychology and Psychiatry, 45,* 1115–1122.

Levin, H. S., Culhane, F. A., Hartmann, J., Evankovich, F., Mattson, A. J., Harward, H., et al. (1991). Developmental changes in performance on tests of purported frontal lobe functioning. Special issue: Developmental consequences of early frontal lobe damage. *Developmental Neuropsychology, 7,* 377–395.

Loong, J. W. K. (1990). *Wisconsin Card Sorting Test: IBM version.* San Luis Obispo, CA: Wang Neuropsychological Laboratory.

Lopez, B. R., Lincoln, A. J., Ozonoff, S., & Lai, Z. (2005). Examining the relationship between executive functions and restricted, repetitive symptoms of autistic disorder. *Journal of Autism and Developmental Disorders, 35,* 445–460.

Lord, C., & McGee, J. P. (2001). *Educating children with autism.* Washington, DC: National Academy Press.

McEvoy, R. E., Rogers, S. J., & Pennington, B. F. (1993). Executive function and social communication deficits in young autistic children. *Journal of Child Psychology and Psychiatry, 34,* 563–578.

Mesibov, G. B. (1997). Formal and informal measures on the effectiveness of the TEACCH programme. *Autism, 1,* 25–35.

Ozonoff, S. (1995). Reliability and validity of the Wisconsin Card Sorting Test in studies of autism. *Neuropsychology, 9,* 491–500.

Ozonoff, S., Cook, I., Coon, H., Dawson, G., Joseph, R., Klin, A., et al. (2004). Performance on subtests sensitive to frontal lobe function in people with autistic disorder: Evidence from the CPEA network. *Journal of Autism and Developmental Disorders, 34,* 139–150.

Ozonoff, S., & Jensen, J. (1999). Specific executive function profiles in three disorders. *Journal of Autism and Developmental Disorders, 29,* 171–177.

Ozonoff, S., Pennington, B. F., & Rogers, S. J. (1991). Executive function deficits in high-functioning autistic individuals: Relationship to theory of mind. *Journal of Child Psychology and Psychiatry, 32,* 1081–1105.

Ozonoff, S., & Strayer, D. L. (1997). Inhibitory function in nonretarded children with autism. *Journal of Autism and Developmental Disorders, 27,* 59–77.

Pennington, B. F., & Ozonoff, S. (1996). Executive functions and developmental. *Journal of Child Psychology and Psychiatry, 37,* 51–87.

Pilling, S., Bebbington, P., Kuipers, E., Garety, P., Geddes, J., Martindale, B., et al. (2002). Psychological treatments in schizophrenia: II. Meta-analyses of randomized controlled trails of social skills training and cognitive re-mediation. *Psychological Medicine, 32,* 783–791.

Quinn, C., Swaggart, B. L., & Myles, B. S. (1994). Implementing cognitive behavior management programs for persons with autism: Guidelines for practitioners. *Focus on Autistic Behavior, 9,* 1.

Robinson, A. L., Heaton, R. K., Lehman, R. A., & Stilson, D. W. (1980). The utility of the Wisconsin Card Sorting Test in detecting and localizing frontal lobe lesions. *Journal of Consulting and Clinical Psychology, 48,* 605–614.

Rogers, S. J. (1998). Empirically supported comprehensive treatments for young children with autism. *Journal of Clinical Child Psychology, 27,* 167–178.

Rueda, M. R., Rothbart, M. K., Davis-Stober, C. P., & Posner, M. I. (2005, April). *Development and training effects on children's executive attention.* Paper presentation at the Society for Research in Child Development, Atlanta, GA.

Rumsey, J. M. (1985). Conceptual problem solving in highly verbal, nonretarded autistic men. *Journal of Autism and Developmental Disorders, 15,* 23–36.

Russell, J. (1995). *Autism as an executive disorder.* New York: Oxford University Press.

Schetter, P. (2004). *Learning the R.O.P.E.S. for improved executive functioning: A cognitive-behavioral approach for children with high-functioning autism and other behavioral disorders.* Woodland, CA: Autism and Behavior Training Associates.

Shallice, T. (1982). Specific impairments in planning. In D. E. Broadbent & L. Weiskrantz (Eds.), *The neuropsychology of cognitive function* (pp. 199–209). London: Philosophical Transactions of the Royal Society of London.

Shore, S. (2004). Using the IEP to build skills in self-advocacy and disclosure. In S. Shore (Ed.), *Ask and tell: Self-advocacy and disclosure for people on the autism spectrum* (pp. 65–105). Shawnee Mission, KS: Autism Asperger Publishing Co.

Smith, L., & Fowler, S. (1984). Positive peer pressure: The effects of peer moni-toring on children's disruptive behavior. *Journal of Applied Behavior Analysis, 17,* 213–227.

Sohlberg, M. M., & Mateer, C. A. (1987). Effectiveness of an attention training program. *Journal of Clinical and Experimental Neuropsychology, 9,* 117–130.

South, M., Ozonoff, S., & McMahon, W. M. (2005). Repetitive behavior in the high-functioning autism spectrum: Phenotypic characterization and rela-tionship to cognitive functioning. *Journal of Autism and Developmental Disorders, 35,* 145–158.

Szatmari, P., Bartolucci, G., Bremner, R., Bond, S., & Rich, S. (1989). A follow-up study of high-functioning autistic children. *Journal of Autism and Developmental Disorders, 19,* 213–225.

Szatmari, P., Tuff, L., Finlayson, A. J., & Bartolucci, G. (1990). Asperger's syndrome and autism: Neurocognitive aspects. *Journal of the American Academy of Child and Adolescent Psychiatry, 29,* 130–136.

Turner, M. (1997). Towards an executive dysfunction account of repetitive behavior in autism. In J. Russell (Ed.), *Autism as an executive disorder* (pp. 57–100). New York: Oxford University Press.

Wainwright-Sharp, J. A., & Bryson, S. E. (1993). Visual orienting deficits in high-functioning people with autism. *Journal of Autism and Developmental Disorders, 23,* 1–13.

Welsh, M. C., Pennington, B. F., & Groisser, D. B. (1991). A normative-developmental study of executive function: A window on prefrontal function in children. *Developmental Neuropsychology, 7,* 131–149.

PART III

Interventions to Address Executive Function Processes

What they should learn first is not the subjects ordinarily taught,
however important they may be; they should be given lessons of will,
of attention, of discipline; before exercises in grammar, they need to
be exercised in mental orthopedics; in a word they must learn how
to learn.

—BINET AND SIMON (1916, p. 257)

Nearly 100 years after the publication of Alfred Binet's work, school
curricula still emphasize the three R's: reading, writing, and arithmetic.
Unfortunately, there is not yet widespread recognition of the importance
of providing all children with an education in the fourth critical literacy
skill, *reasoning*. Ideally, this should include the metacognitive strategies
students need to think about *how* they think and learn. This is particularly surprising in view of the fact that increased accessibility to vast
sources of information has highlighted the importance of embedding the
teaching of executive function processes into the classroom curriculum.
The six chapters in this section address the principles and practicalities
of teaching executive function processes both at the level of the classroom and as part of a broader schoolwide curriculum.

In Chapter 8, Meltzer, Sales Pollica, and Barzillai build on the definitions and theoretical paradigms of executive function processes discussed in the other two sections of this book and provide a rationale for systematic, classroom-based strategy instruction that addresses executive function processes explicitly. They emphasize approaches that teachers can use to create "strategic classrooms." Discussion focuses on practical classroom-based strategies for teaching executive function processes such as goal setting and planning, organizing, shifting approaches flexibly, and self-checking. The next three chapters address the teaching of executive function processes in relation to the specific academic domains of reading, writing, and math.

In Chapter 9, Gaskins, Satlow, and Pressley address approaches to teaching reading comprehension strategies using a systematic, goal-oriented approach and emphasize the importance of students using "smart effort." In Chapter 10, Graham, Harris, and Olinghouse discuss their self-regulated strategy development model (SRSD) for teaching students to use goal setting, self-monitoring, and self-reinforcement to regulate the use of writing strategies, the writing task, and their behaviors. Their model also addresses students' motivation by emphasizing the role of effort in learning and making the (positive) effects of instruction visible and concrete. In Chapter 11, Roditi and Steinberg focus on the impact of executive function processes in the math classroom. They discuss the importance of providing systematic strategy instruction in math to all students, particularly those with learning and attention problems, as well as students who lack the motivation, confidence, and resilience to succeed in math. They provide specific strategies for addressing automatic memory of math facts, prioritizing in math word problems, and checking answers. This focus on the classroom is broadened to an entire school curriculum in Chapter 12. Gaskins and Pressley describe the goals and instructional approaches they consider critical for an across-the-grades curriculum to develop metacognitive processes and enhance executive processes. They reiterate the principles emphasized in Chapter 8 by Meltzer, Sales Pollica, and Barzillai and the need for a curriculum where students know when, how, and why to use strategies and understand their learning styles. In Chapter 13, Rose and Rose argue that we need to address curriculum disabilities by using modern technologies and universal design to teach content. They propose that learning opportunities be designed to accommodate the diverse needs of all students, including those with executive function problems.

All chapters in this section underscore the importance of long-term, school-based research that identifies specific methods for teaching *all* students strategies for addressing executive function processes, so that students can show what they know in school and work settings and can perform at the level of their potential.

REFERENCE

Binet, A., & Simon, T. (1916). *The development of intelligence in children (the Binet–Simon scale)* (E. S. Kite, Trans.). Baltimore: Williams & Wilkins.

CHAPTER 8

Executive Function in the Classroom

Embedding Strategy Instruction
into Daily Teaching Practices

LYNN MELTZER
LAURA SALES POLLICA
MIRIT BARZILLAI

The strategies gave me a structure so that I could put boundaries and parameters around those whizzing little molecules in my mind and turn them into something that really made sense.
— BRANDON, COLLEGE GRADUATE

As we enter the 21st century, with its reliance on rapid communication, advanced technology, efficient media, and fast access to vast sources of information, the importance of teaching executive function processes such as planning, organizing, prioritizing, and self-editing has become more evident. Even in the elementary grades, teachers require students to complete long-term projects, lengthy writing assignments, and open-book tests that rely heavily on efficient executive function processes. Nevertheless, students are not taught these executive processes systematically, and classroom instruction tends to focus on the content or *what* of learning rather than the process or *how*, leaving many students over-whelmed and frustrated. The critical importance of addressing these executive processes through systematic strategy instruction has become increasingly evident over the past decade.

This chapter builds on current definitions and theoretical paradigms of executive function processes (see Chapters 1–4) and provides a rationale for teaching strategies that address executive function processes in the classroom. We focus on approaches that teachers can use to create strategic classrooms and discuss the importance of teaching strategies that enhance executive function processes such as goal setting, planning, organizing, prioritizing, shifting strategies flexibly, and self-checking.

TEACHING STRATEGIES THAT ADDRESS EXECUTIVE FUNCTION PROCESSES

So, if I had a history test I could think back to that note page and it all fitted into place—as opposed to remembering a liquefied gobble of notes that I had picked up here and there along the way.
                                        —BRANDON, COLLEGE GRADUATE

Reading comprehension, homework, note taking, long-term projects, studying, and test taking all require students to integrate and organize multiple subprocesses simultaneously and to shift approaches frequently. Academic success in all of these content areas is dependent on students' ability to plan their time, organize and prioritize information, separate main ideas from details, monitor their progress, and reflect on their work. These core executive function processes are the underpinning of most academic work from as early as the fourth grade, when the school curriculum increasingly emphasizes performance on tasks that require the coordination, integration, and synthesis of many of these executive function processes (see Figure 5.2 in Chapter 5).

Students with weaknesses in these important processes often understand complex concepts easily but struggle to show what they know, due to difficulties with planning, setting realistic goals, prioritizing, initiating tasks, and organizing materials and information. They may also have trouble shifting strategies flexibly, monitoring their progress and time, and checking and reflecting on their work. One of the most effective ways of addressing these executive function weaknesses is through strategy instruction. As is evident from Figure 8.1, effective strategy instruction focuses on helping students to become metacognitive learners by teaching them *how* to learn. As they gain an understanding of the learning process, students are able to recognize their personal strengths and

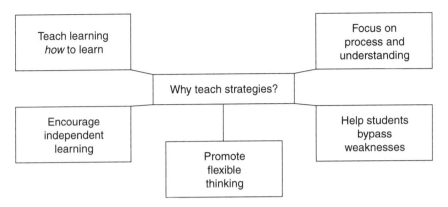

FIGURE 8.1. Purpose of teaching strategies that address executive function processes.

to realize the importance of these executive function processes for their academic success. Teaching these students strategies that address the core executive function processes allows them to become independent learners and flexible thinkers so that they can more easily bypass their weaknesses and use their strengths to learn efficiently and effectively (see Figure 8.1).

The impact of strategies on the learning process has been demonstrated in numerous studies that have shown that successful learners use effective strategies to process information (Brown & Campione, 1986; Harris & Graham, 1992; Meltzer, 1993; Palincsar, Winn, David, Snyder, & Stevens, 1993; Pressley, Goodchild, Fleet, Zajchowski, & Evans, 1989). This research has also indicated the importance of strategy instruction for enhancing students' conceptual understanding, transfer and creative use of knowledge, and ability to self-reflect about the learning process (Brown, 1997; Deshler, Schumaker, & Lenz, 1984; Pressley, Woloshyn, et al., 1995). In fact, findings have shown that explicit instruction can play a critical role in helping all students use metacognitive strategies to learn more efficiently and easily (Deshler et al., 2001; Ellis, 1997; Graham & Harris, 2003; Harris & Graham, 1996; Meltzer, Katzir, Miller, Reddy, & Roditi, 2004; Swanson, 1999a; Zimmerman & Schunk, 2001). These metacognitive strategies are beneficial for all students and are especially critical for students with learning disabilities. These students often show weaknesses in executive function processes such as planning, organizing large chunks of information, shifting mindsets, initiating new tasks, and self-monitoring (Meltzer & Montague, 2001; Meltzer, Reddy, Pollica, & Roditi, 2004; Meltzer,

Reddy, Pollica, et al., 2004). Nevertheless, there is still no clear consensus about the most effective methods for teaching students to use strategies independently and consistently.

Principles of Effective Strategy Instruction

How can strategies for enhancing executive function processes be taught effectively? Most studies have focused on evaluating the efficacy of strategy instruction for students with learning disabilities in one-on-one settings and small remedial groups rather than in general education classrooms (see Swanson & Hoskyn, 1998, for review). Recently, a few models of classroom-based strategy instruction have emerged, such as the Kansas intervention model (Deshler & Schumaker, 1988), the Benchmark model (Gaskins & Pressley, Chapter 12, this volume; Pressley & Woloshyn, 1995), and the *Drive to Thrive* approach (Meltzer, Reddy, Pollica, & Roditi, 2004). Comparisons of different interventions highlight several important principles of strategy instruction:

- Strategy instruction should be directly linked with the curriculum.
- Metacognitive strategies should be taught explicitly.
- Strategies should be taught in a structured, systematic way using scaffolding and modeling and providing time for practice.
- Students' motivation and self-understanding should be addressed to ensure generalized use of strategies.

These principles are discussed below in greater detail.

- *Strategies for teaching executive function processes should be directly linked with the curriculum.* In their meta-analysis of 51 study skills intervention studies, Hattie, Biggs, and Purdie (1996) showed that study skills programs that were separate from the curriculum "did not seem very effective." Rather, the most effective programs taught metacognitive strategies that were directly linked with the curriculum and used tasks that were perceived by students to be relevant to their classroom and homework assignments (Hattie et al., 1996). Further, embedding strategy instruction in the curriculum helped students learn and remember content material more easily and acquire efficient means of accessing information for lifelong learning (Deshler, Ellis, & Lenz, 1996; Ellis, 1993, 1994).

- *Metacognitive strategies should be taught explicitly.* While some students are able to use executive function processes independently, and even unconsciously, many need to be taught these processes explicitly. In fact, strategies are only effective learning tools if explicit instruction is provided about *how*, *when*, *where*, and *why* to use them (Carnes, Lindbeck, & Griffin, 1987; Merkley & Jeffries, 2001). Thus, in order to maximize the effectiveness of strategies, it is important to incorporate explicit instruction, including teacher modeling and extended practice (Boyle & Weishar, 1999; Idol & Croll, 1987; Scanlon, Deshler, & Schumaker, 1996). Furthermore, research findings have indicated that explicit and highly structured metacognitive instruction benefits all students and is essential for the academic progress of students with learning disabilities (Deshler et al., 1996; Deshler & Schumaker, 1988; Meltzer, Katzir, et al., 2004; Paris, 1986; Pearson & Dole, 1987; Rosenshine, 1997; Swanson, 2001; Swanson & Hoskyn, 1998, 2001). Thus, instead of assuming that students know how to use learning strategies, those strategies should be discussed clearly and their importance explicitly stated (e.g., "This strategy will help you to write longer, more interesting sentences"). When students recognize the importance of making the effort to use strategies, they value these strategies, and their academic performance improves.

• *Strategies should be taught in a structured, systematic way.* Strategy instruction presumes systematic modeling, guided practice, and frequent feedback, with instruction focused on helping students internalize and generalize the strategies that are taught (Deshler et al., 1996; Meltzer, Katzir, et al., 2004; Putnam, Deshler, & Schumaker, 1993). Further, research on strategy instruction has demonstrated that unless students are provided with numerous opportunities to practice a strategy, they will not use the strategy correctly or independently (Scanlon et al., 1996). Thus, students need opportunities to use strategies consistently and to receive constructive feedback so that they can learn to monitor and evaluate the effectiveness of the strategies they apply to their work. Specifically, each student needs to understand when, why, and how a given strategy will be effective because it matches his or her learning style. For instance, when students are required to use a specific strategy such as a graphic organizer or a linear outline each time they write a paragraph, and they find that this visual aid helps them to organize their writing and succeed, they eventually will use this strategy independently and will generalize it to different settings. Conversely, if the strategy is not a good fit for a particular student's learning profile, he or she needs to have the self-understanding to recognize what does or does not work in order to develop as an effective and flexible learner. The goal of strategy instruction should be to help each student develop fluent and automatic use of strategies that work best for him or her.

• *Strategy instruction should address students' motivation and effort.* Motivation plays a critical role in strategic learning, as students are more likely to use strategies if they are aware that these strategies will result in improved performance and higher grades. Students' motivation to use learning strategies is heavily dependent on their self-awareness and self-understanding (Deshler, Warner, Schumaker, & Alley, 1983; Deshler & Shumaker, 1986; Meltzer, 1996; Meltzer, Roditi, Houser, & Perlman, 1998; Paris & Winograd, 1990; Pressley et al., 1989). More specifically, students' awareness of their own strengths and weaknesses is an underlying component of effective strategic learning, as is their understanding of the impact that strategies can have on their performance (Meltzer, 1996; Meltzer, Katzir-Cohen, Miller, & Roditi, 2001; Meltzer, Katzir, et al., 2004). Furthermore, students' willingness to make the effort to use strategies is affected by their self-concept and self-confidence in the learning situation, particularly when they have experienced considerable frustration and failure in school as a result of learning and attention problems. Thus, as students become increasingly aware of the benefits of strategy use, they become independent learners and are more motivated to invest the effort to continue to use the strategies that work for them (Meltzer, Katzir, et al., 2004; Meltzer, Reddy, Pollica, & Roditi, 2004). Academic success results in positive academic self-concepts and shifts in self-perceptions so that students view themselves as capable learners with the potential to succeed in the classroom. *Drive to Thrive* is one model of an intervention program that is designed to train teachers to promote strategy use, focused effort, and positive academic self-concepts in their students (ResearchILD, 2005). This program is described in greater detail in a later section of this chapter.

CREATING STRATEGIC CLASSROOMS

Every grade level heralds changes in the curriculum, the setting, the expectations, and in each student's cognitive and social development. Students' learning profiles are not static but often change as a function of the match or mismatch between their specific strengths and weaknesses and the demands of the classroom, the teacher, and the curriculum (Meltzer, Roditi, Steinberg, et al., 2005). Critical transition times in the curriculum such as first grade, fourth grade, middle school, high school, and college can be particularly problematic for students. Each of these transitions corresponds with increased organizational demands and the introduction of tasks such as complex writing assignments, book reports, and multiple-choice tests that require the coordination and integration of multiple skills and strategies. Thus, learning metacognitive strategies in the context of the classroom curriculum becomes increasingly important and valuable, as these skills are crucial for all grade levels (Meltzer, Roditi, Steinberg, et al., 2005). For example, a strategy used to enhance reading comprehension of a novel in the fifth grade can also be used when reading books and articles at the college level. While the content changes from year to year, the process, or *how*, of learning is consistent and can be modified to address the changes in the curriculum and the task requirements. When classroom-based strategy instruction is implemented, the content becomes a springboard for teaching students how to learn and is not an end in itself. These strategies, if taught systematically and consistently, can begin to address many of the most important executive function processes, such as planning, organizing, prioritizing, accessing working memory efficiently, shifting, and checking. More specifically, these strategies can be used to teach students:

- How to plan and organize new concepts and material
- How to memorize (e.g., vocabulary, science terms, history facts)
- How to shift flexibly in order to process and learn new information efficiently and easily (e.g., active reading strategies)
- How to check and edit for errors in spelling, writing, and math.

The following section focuses on strategies for addressing each of these executive function processes.

Planning and Setting Goals

Planning, or the organization of information and details ahead of time, is an important executive function process that is not taught systematically in schools even though it is a prerequisite for reading, writing, and completing projects in content areas such as science and social studies. Students are not usually taught to set short- and long-term goals that guide their approach to homework, studying, and test taking. Many students with executive function difficulties may begin tasks impulsively with no plan of action. This often results in their "getting stuck" when the next step is unclear and in an end product that is disorganized and incoherent. The critical executive function processes of planning and goal setting help students understand the objective of a particular task, visualize the steps of the task, organize time effectively, and determine the resources needed to complete the task. Planning and goal setting are integral parts of many successful self-regulated learning interventions. When students set their own goals, they show greater commitment and are more motivated to attain these goals (Schunk, 2001; Winnie, 1996, 2001; Zimmerman, 2000; Zimmerman & Schunk, 2001). Goal setting has also been found to enhance self-efficacy, achievement, and motivation (Schunk, 2001).

Students can be taught effective planning and goal-setting strategies from the early grades. Teachers can model the planning process by making daily schedules, using calendars, and setting agendas for class meetings. Younger students can be taught strategies for planning their homework, long-term projects, study time, and classroom activities. These strategies are even more important in the middle and high school grades, when students are required to plan their study time, long-term projects, and papers. At these levels, time management is critically important, as students are required to juggle multiple deadlines for many different ongoing assignments and projects. They often underestimate the amount of work involved in major projects and open-ended tasks and need strategies for breaking down tasks into manageable parts. Time-management strategies help students schedule their homework and study time after school when time is less structured. Use of weekly and monthly calendars for tracking deadlines for long-term projects and assignments as well as self-pacing to complete assignments helps impose structure and self-monitoring. These executive function processes are critical for promoting independent learning as part of the homework process (Hughes, Ruhl, Schumaker, & Deshler, 2002; Sah & Borland, 1989). Figure 8.2 provides an example of a time management strategy for homework completion.

Organizing and Prioritizing

Organization, or the ability to systematize and sort information, is an executive function process that underlies most academic and life tasks. Strategy instruction needs to focus on teaching students systematic approaches for organizing their materials, information, and ideas and applying these strategies to their writing, note taking, studying, and test preparation. Each of these areas is discussed below (Meltzer, Roditi, Steinberg, et al., 2005).

Homework Time Sheet		
Assignment	**Estimated Time**	**Actual Time**
Social studies reading and note taking	30 min.	1 hour
Math problems	20 min.	25 min.
Spanish worksheet	20 min.	15 min.

FIGURE 8.2. Homework planning sheet.

Organization of Materials

Explicit systems and strategies are important for teaching organization of materials, such as color-coding strategies for teaching students how to organize their notebooks, binders, and assignment books. It is critical to teach students to allot a specific time period each week to organize their materials and folders in a systematic way.

Organization of Ideas and Information

At the middle and high school levels, students are presented with an enormous volume of detailed information in their curricula. How well they learn and remember this information depends on how effectively they use strategies for organizing and prioritizing concepts and details so that working memory is less cluttered (Hughes, 1996). While many students are able to participate in class lessons and to complete structured homework assignments accurately, they have more difficulty with independent, open-ended tasks. Reading and note-taking tasks, studying for tests, and completing writing assignments all require students to impose their own structure on the information. When strategies are taught that structure these open-ended tasks, students are more likely to achieve higher grades. Success results in increased motivation to use these strategies independently and to generalize across different contexts (Meltzer, 1996; Swanson, 1999b). Strategies for organizing and prioritizing information are critically important for writing, note taking, studying, and test preparation, all of which are discussed below in greater detail.

Organizational Strategies for Writing

From late elementary school on, the writing process can often be overwhelming for students who are required to complete lengthy writing assignments and essay tests that rely heavily on executive function processes. Writing requires the coordination and integration of many different cognitive processes and skills, including memory, planning, generating text, and editing (Flower et al., 1990; Flower, Wallace, Norris, & Burnett, 1994). While writing, students need to monitor multiple goals (Hayes, 1996) and to satisfy many constraints, such as those of topic and purpose. Therefore, students also need to switch flexibly among various writing processes, such as critical thinking (e.g., perspective, logic), rhetorical devices (e.g., description, persuasion), and writing conventions (e.g., tone, mechanics, spelling) (Bruning & Horn, 2000). Thus, writing requires the coordination and integration of a broad range of executive function processes. Students benefit from strategies that address these processes, such as planning, monitoring, evaluating, and revising their work (Bruning &

Horn, 2000; Kellogg, 1987; Ransdell & Levy, 1996; Scardamalia & Bereiter, 1986; Zimmerman & Risemberg, 1997).

Many students have particular difficulty when they are required to organize their ideas for writing and need the writing process to be broken down explicitly with organizers and templates that match both the goals of the assignment and the student's learning style. Writing templates and graphic organizers need to be well-structured so that students can easily translate their ideas into paragraph form. Such templates and organizers are helpful for many different genres of writing, including book reports, persuasive essays, descriptive paragraphs, news articles, summaries, reflections, and narratives (Schunk & Swartz, 1993).

Graphic organizers used in middle school for helping students plan and prioritize their ideas for essay writing can be extrapolated to more complex reports and papers at the high school and college levels (see Figure 8.3).

With consistency and feedback, teachers can help students internalize these strategies and organize their writing independently by prioritizing and breaking writing tasks into manageable parts. This allows students to monitor their progress and to experience success during the writing process (Bruning & Horn, 2000). In fact, research has shown that teacher guidance and feedback have a significant impact on students' willingness to use these strategies and also increase their self-confidence and writing performance (Pajares & Johnson, 1996; Skinner, Wellborn, & Connell, 1990). Further, when strategies that address executive function are successfully incorporated into the teaching of writing, they increase the likelihood of strategy use in the future (Graham & Harris, 2000, 2003; Harris & Graham, 1996; Scardamalia & Bereiter, 1985; Zimmerman & Risemberg, 1997). Rubrics such as the one in Figure 8.4), from the *Drive to Thrive* program (Meltzer, Steinberg, Button, et al., 2005) provide a structured approach that teachers can use for teaching and evaluating students' use of executive function processes when they write.

Organizational Strategies for Note Taking

The way my mind works with that liquefied gobble of dots, my notes would look scattered on a page. One of the most useful strategies I learned was multicolumn notes. With this system, I learned to make a hierarchy of notes and have it structure around itself and relate to things. This structure helped me to study and to write long papers.
—BRANDON, COLLEGE GRADUATE

Note taking from reading and lecture material is a common assignment given to students like Brandon, especially at the high school and college

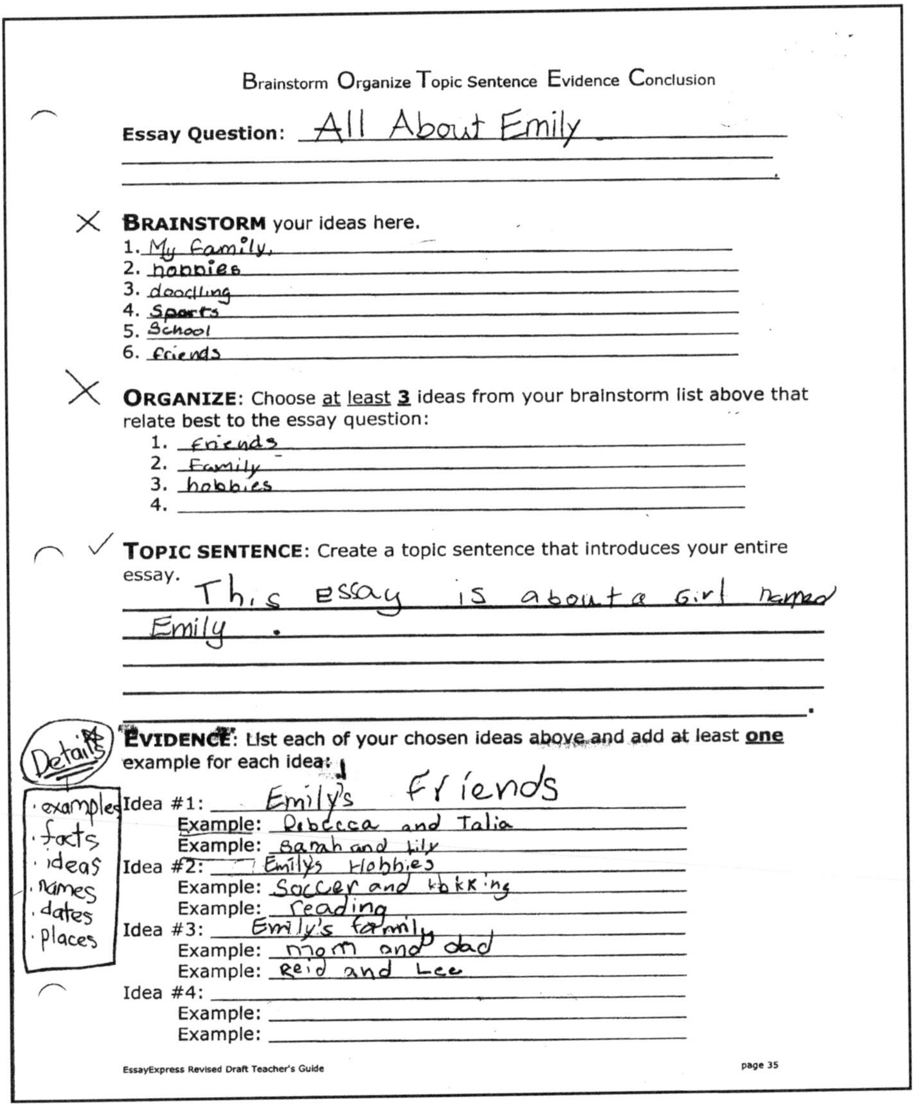

Brainstorm Organize Topic Sentence Evidence Conclusion

Essay Question: _All About Emily_

✗ **BRAINSTORM** your ideas here.
1. My family.
2. hobbies
3. doodling
4. Sports
5. School
6. friends

✗ **ORGANIZE:** Choose at <u>least</u> **3** ideas from your brainstorm list above that relate best to the essay question:
1. friends
2. Family
3. hobbies
4.

✓ **TOPIC SENTENCE:** Create a topic sentence that introduces your entire essay. This essay is about a Girl named Emily.

(Details)

EVIDENCE: List each of your chosen ideas above and add at least **one** example for each idea:

· examples
· facts
· ideas
· names
· dates
· places

Idea #1: _Emily's Friends_
   Example: Rebecca and Talia
   Example: Sarah and Lily
Idea #2: _Emily's Hobbies_
   Example: Soccer and Hokking
   Example: reading
Idea #3: _Emily's family_
   Example: mom and dad
   Example: Reid and Lee
Idea #4: _____
   Example: _____
   Example: _____

EssayExpress Revised Draft Teacher's Guide   page 35

FIGURE 8.3. A student's use of the BOTEC template (from Essay Express; Research Institute for Learning and Development & FableVision, 2005) to plan and organize her essay.

Objectives	Below Average	Needs Improvement	Proficient	Exemplary Performance	Earned Points
Planning	**1 point** Little or no evidence of planning.	**2 points** A planning sheet is included but it is incomplete.	**3 points** Student includes an outline or graphic organizer that is partially filled out. Planner is somewhat related to final essay.	**4 points** Student includes completely filled out outline or graphic organizer and final essay reflects its use.	
Organizing	**1 point** Student does not include a rough draft.	**2 points** Student includes a partially completed rough draft that does not follow an organizational plan.	**3 points** Student includes a rough draft that roughly follows his or her outline or graphic organizer.	**4 points** Student includes a rough draft that is well organized and follows the planning tool.	
Shifting	**1 point** Student shows no changes from the rough draft to the final draft.	**2 points** Only slight evidence of improvements is seen between the rough and final drafts.	**3 points** Student makes at least two changes beyond spelling and punctuation in the final draft.	**4 points** The student takes a different point of view in the final draft or makes at least three major improvements between the rough draft and the final draft.	
Prioritizing	**1 point** Essay includes no transition words to show sequence, contrast, or relative importance of ideas.	**2 points** Essay includes only transition words such as "and," "also," and "but."	**3 points** Essay includes two more sophisticated transition words that indicate sequence, importance, or contrast, such as "however," "on the other hand," "another example," etc.	**4 points** Essay includes more than two transition words to connect ideas or paragraphs.	
Checking	**1 point** Student does not submit a checklist with the writing project.	**2 points** Student checks for a few mistakes but not for others.	**3 points** Student checks off the checklist to indicate that he or she checked most of the items on the list.	**4 points** Student submits checklist indicating that he or she has checked for each item on the list. Student's writing reflects no errors that are listed on the checklist.	
	0 points	**0 points**	**0 points**	**0 points**	
				Score:	

FIGURE 8.4. Writing rubric from the *Drive to Thrive* program.

levels (Putnam et al., 1993). Independent note taking has been found to increase class participation and improve the recall of material (Ruhl & Suritsky, 1995), and many teachers assume that students know how to take notes that will be used for homework, studying, or other assignments. The note-taking process is complex, however, and requires the coordination and integration of multiple processes including listening, differentiating main ideas from details, and writing (Kiewra et al., 1991). As a result, many students have difficulties transcribing their notes, as well as discerning which information should be recorded (Hughes, 1991; Hughes & Suritsky, 1994; Suritsky, 1992). In fact, many students read their textbooks and articles without taking notes or take notes using a format that is not very helpful to them. Teaching and requiring organizational strategies for note taking ensures that students are interacting with text as they read instead of reviewing the information passively (Deshler et al., 1996; Hughes & Suritsky, 1994). Further, by providing note-taking templates and teaching students how to use these, teachers create a structure for students to organize information and to differentiate major themes from details, which results in improved performance (Boyle, 1996, 2001; Boyle & Weishaar, 1999; Katamaya & Robinson, 2000; Lazarus, 1991).

These templates, thinking maps, and graphic organizers can be particularly effective for helping students bypass their difficulties when they are required to recall and organize verbal information (Kim, Vaughn, Wanzeki, & Shangjin, 2004). In fact, findings have shown that graphic organizers provide frames that help students learn material in a clear, logical format and relate new information to known information (Ausubel, 1963; Mayer, 1984). Graphic organizers are also effective for improving student performance across a wide range of subject areas, including reading, science, social studies, language arts, and math (Bos & Anders, 1992; Bulgren, Schumaker, & Deshler, 1988; Darch, Carnine, & Kame'enui, 1986; Herl, O'Neil, Chung, & Schacter, 1999; Ritchie & Vokl, 2000), and across multiple grade levels from elementary school through high school (Alverman & Boothby, 1986; Horton, Lovitt, & Bergerud, 1990; Ritchie & Volkl, 2000; Scanlon, Duran, Reyes, & Gallego, 1992; Willerman & Mac Harg, 1991). Templates such as the one shown in Figure 8.5 help students take notes more efficiently and access the most important information.

Similarly, taking two-column notes instead of using a traditional note-taking format helps students to ask themselves active questions about the text they are reading. This format encourages them to find the main ideas, "chunk" information into manageable parts, and predict test questions (see Figure 8.6).

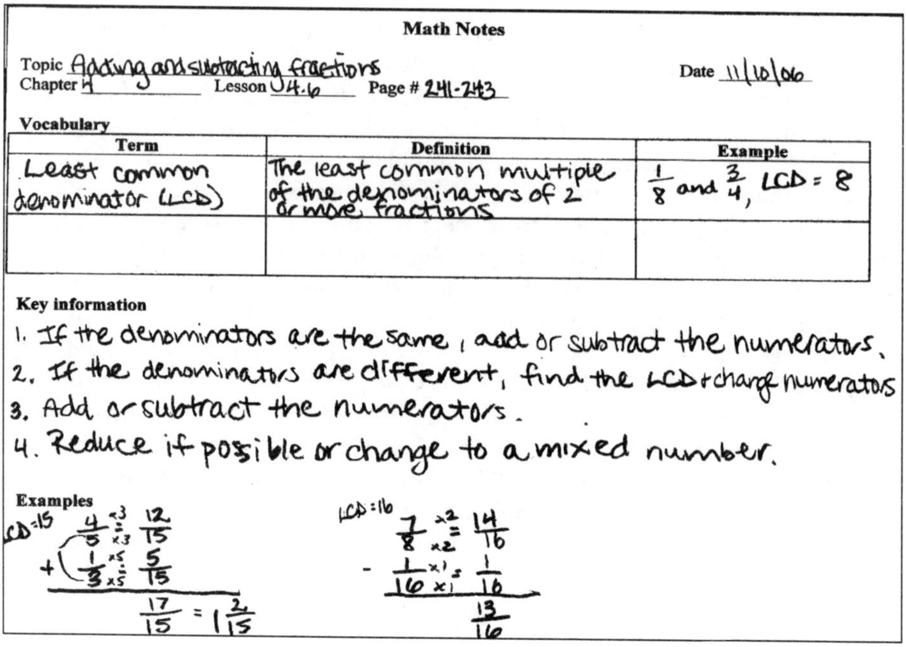

Math Notes

Topic Adding and subtracting fractions   Date 11/10/06

Chapter 4   Lesson 4.6   Page # 241-243

Vocabulary

Term	Definition	Example
Least common denominator (LCD)	The least common multiple of the denominators of 2 or more fractions	$\frac{1}{8}$ and $\frac{3}{4}$, LCD = 8

Key information

1. If the denominators are the same, add or subtract the numerators.
2. If the denominators are different, find the LCD + change numerators
3. Add or subtract the numerators.
4. Reduce if possible or change to a mixed number.

Examples

LCD=15
$$\frac{4}{5} \times 3 = \frac{12}{15}$$
$$+\frac{1}{3} \times 5 = \frac{5}{15}$$
$$\frac{17}{15} = 1\frac{2}{15}$$

LCD=16
$$\frac{7}{8} \times 2 = \frac{14}{16}$$
$$-\frac{1}{16} \times 1 = \frac{1}{16}$$
$$\frac{13}{16}$$

FIGURE 8.5. Note-taking template for math.

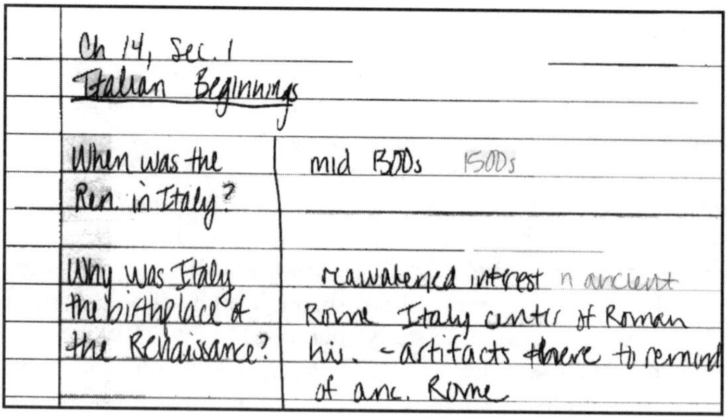

Ch 14, Sec. 1
Italian Beginnings

When was the Ren. in Italy?	mid 1300s 1500s
Why was Italy the birthplace of the Renaissance?	reawakened interest n ancient Rome Italy center of Roman his. —artifacts there to remind of anc. Rome

FIGURE 8.6. Example of a student's use of the two-column note-taking template.

Organizational Strategies for Studying and Test Preparation

Test results are the gateway to school success, graduation, college entry, and job advancement. Study and test-taking strategies are critically important in view of the demanding curriculum standards and the pressure on all students to perform optimally in test situations. Many students, especially those with learning and attention problems, often lack "test-wiseness," or facility with test-taking strategies, and their grades on tests do not reflect their understanding, the extent of their preparation, or their level of ability (Meltzer, Roditi, & Stein, 2002; Meltzer, Roditi, Steinberg, et al., 2005). They need systematic instruction in study strategies that help them organize their materials when they study and complete homework, prioritize and figure out what is most important to study, shift flexibly among different strategies, analyze questions on tests and work assignments, and check their answers in their written work. When strategies are taught systematically in each of these cognitive areas, students improve their efficiency and accuracy before, during, and after tests (see Figure 8.7). One

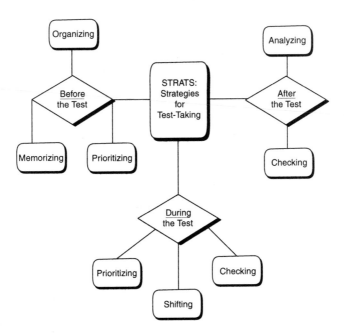

FIGURE 8.7. STRATS paradigm of addressing test-taking strategies before, during, and after a test.

example of an easy-to-use, systematic approach for teaching students strategies that address these executive function processes is represented in BrainCogs (Research Institute for Learning and Development & FableVision, 2002). BrainCogs is a computer program that is designed to help students develop strategies for learning, studying, and successful test taking and apply strategies that match their learning profiles. Approaches like this are important for helping students learn *how* to organize, prioritize, integrate, and retrieve information while simultaneously learning the required content. Students also learn *when* to use *which* strategies in *which* contexts.

The BrainCogs Triple Note Tote strategy (Figure 8.8) helps students organize and memorize information simultaneously. As is evident from Figure 8.8, the student writes the vocabulary term in the first column, the definition in the second column, and a memory strategy in the third.

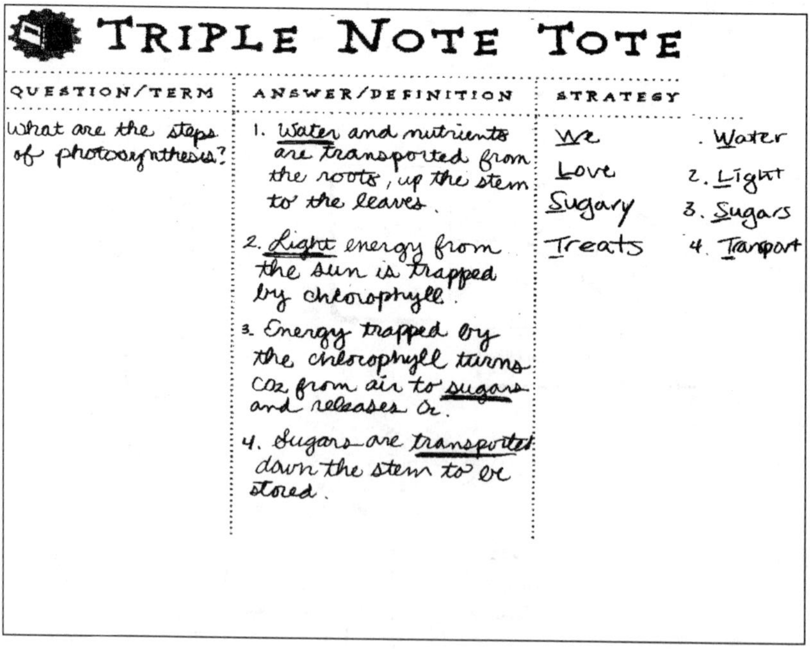

FIGURE 8.8. A student's use of the Triple Note Tote template (BrainCogs; Research Institute for Learning and Development & FableVision, 2002) to organize information.

Shifting Flexibly

Cognitive flexibility, or the ability to shift mindsets, is often extremely challenging for students, especially those with learning and attention difficulties (Meltzer, 1993; Meltzer, Soloman, Fenton, & Levine, 1989). Shifting requires students to interpret information in more than one way, change their approach when needed, and choose a new strategy when the first one is not working (Westman & Kamoo, 1990). Bereiter and Scardamalia (1985) have argued that instruction must include opportunities for students to use their acquired knowledge flexibly. Similarly, Bransford, Vye, and Adams (1989) have emphasized the importance of providing students with opportunities to solve problems from a variety of perspectives to teach cognitive flexibility.

In the classroom setting, cognitive flexibility is essential for effective reading, writing, math problem solving, and test taking. To read novels with complex or figurative language, students must shift between the concrete and the abstract, between the literal and the symbolic, and between major themes and extraneous details. Similarly, when writing, students must shift between their own perspective and that of the reader and between the main ideas and supporting details. When taking tests, students are required to shift among multiple topics or problem types and are often faced with information that is presented differently from the way in which they learned or studied it. Similarly, when students read words or phrases that have multiple meanings, they have to shift their mindsets or perspectives. Students can practice identifying multiple meanings in newspaper headlines, jokes, and riddles. Students can also be provided with sets of questions at their desks, in their binders or folders, on bookmarks, or posted in the classroom to help them shift more efficiently. When students come across words or sentences that do not make sense to them, they can stop reading and ask themselves the following questions:

- Does the word have more than one meaning?
- Can the word be used as both a noun and a verb?
- Can I emphasize a different syllable of the word to give it a different meaning?
- Can I emphasize different parts of the sentence to change its meaning?
- Does the passage contain any figurative language, such as metaphors or expressions that may be confusing?

Similar shifting strategies can be applied to writing. Students can be required to shift roles when they edit their writing (e.g., pretending they are space aliens or the teacher and switching pens while editing their writing). By playing different roles, students are more likely to find mistakes and identify areas that need improvement. This helps them shift perspectives to check whether they have explained information clearly and have supported their arguments with enough details.

In the area of math, shifting is essential for working efficiently and accurately. Students often get stuck trying to solve a problem in one way when there may be an easier or more efficient way to find a solution. Similarly, students may have seen problems presented in a particular format while in class or completing homework but may have trouble recognizing similar problems when these are presented differently on tests. Furthermore, while students can often solve problems of the same type that are grouped together for homework practice, they often have difficulty shifting among multiple problem types in a test situation. Cognitive flexibility can be enhanced when students use strategies like asking themselves the following questions while completing math homework or while taking math tests:

- Do I know more than one way to solve the problem?
- Does this look similar to anything I have seen before?
- Is this problem the same or different from the problem before it?

Teachers can also help students recognize that specific problems require them to shift from one operation (e.g., addition) to another (e.g., subtraction). Teachers can also help students solve certain types of math problems, and recognize and differentiate different problem types from one another.

Self-Monitoring and Self-Checking

Self-checking, or the ability to reflect on one's performance and identify errors, is an executive function process that is often extremely challenging for students. While students are often told to check their work, many students do not know *how* to check or *what* to check for. The most effective checking involves learning what types of errors to check for, how to check for these errors, and how to self-correct. Self-monitoring strategies are effective for improving the performance of students with learning disabilities (Harris, 1986; Reid, 1996; Reid & Harris, 1993; Shimabukuro, Prater, Jenkins, & Edelen-Smith, 1999; Webber, Scheuermann, McCall, & Coleman, 1993). Students need to know exactly what is expected from them on an assignment and how to check for their most common mistakes in order to be successful (Maccini & Hughes, 1997; Mastropieri & Scruggs, 1995).

Students often have difficulty with open-ended projects or assignments that involve multiple components. They may complete these quickly without checking for the details that teachers expect. Providing explicit checklists for particular assignments means students will know what to check for and make fewer errors. While general checklists work for many students, personalized checklists help students become aware of and search for *their own* most common errors (Dunlap & Dunlap, 1989). While one student may consistently make spelling errors but have no difficulty with organization, another may have the opposite profile. Students can make personalized checklists that include their most common mistakes and can develop their own acronyms to help them remember the details that need to be corrected. For example, the acronym STOPS (see Figure 8.9) was developed by a sixth-grader to help check his writing for errors he commonly made.

Students should be encouraged to make checklists for all content areas and to post these in the appropriate places such as folders, binders, bulletin boards, or even on the refrigerator. In addition to studying content, students should be encouraged to study their checklists. Personalized checklists are useful for all students, whether they complete their homework inaccurately, make careless errors on tests, or struggle with the mechanics of writing. Figure 8.10 is an example of a student-made personalized checklist.

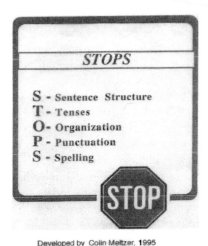

Developed by Colin Meltzer, 1995

FIGURE 8.9. Personalized acronym for self-checking.

```
┌─────────────────────────────────────────────────┐
│ MATH CHECKLIST                                    │
│ • READ DIRECTIONS CAREFULLY                       │
│ • REDUCE FRACTIONS                                │
│ • LABEL ANSWERS                                   │
│ • Ask "DOES MY ANSWER MAKE SENSE?"                │
└─────────────────────────────────────────────────┘
```

FIGURE 8.10. Personalized math checklist.

Creating a Culture of Strategy Use in the Classroom

While strategy instruction is critical for students with learning and attention problems, it is beneficial for all students in order to enhance their
use of executive function processes (Meltzer, Katzir, et al., 2004). While
some students automatically use strategies without being taught them
explicitly, most students need systematic strategy instruction. The classroom teacher plays a critical role in teaching students executive function
strategies that they can use throughout their lives. Research has shown
that strategy instruction works best when it is consistent and embedded
in the curriculum (Deshler et al., 2001; Hattie et al., 1996). Teachers can
create "strategic classrooms" by making strategy use a core component
of the classroom culture. The following are ways that a strategic classroom culture can be fostered.

- Explicit instruction and modeling can make strategies a part of
  the language of the classroom.
- Students can develop their own personalized strategy notebooks
  where they collect the strategies that work best for them.
- Students can participate in "strategy share" discussions, where
  they teach other students the personalized strategies that they
  have created.
- Strategies can be collected throughout the year and made into a
  "strategy book" for the classroom that can be used by other students.
- Teachers can make strategy use a required part of their curriculum by grading students based on the processes and strategies
  they have used to reach their goals, in addition to the end product. Each test or assignment can include a strategy reflection component at the end, where students record the strategies they have
  used to complete assignments or to study for tests (see Figure
  8.11).
- To motivate students to use strategies, teachers can help students
  keep track of their progress and strategy use through charts or

Strategy Reflection for Studying

Check off the strategies you used to study for this test.

____ Flash cards/Strategy cards	____ Two-column notes
____ Triple Note Tote (©BrainCogs)	____ Mapping/webbing
____ Acronyms	____ Discussing with a parent/friend
____ Crazy Phrases (©BrainCogs)	____ Other _____

© ResearchILD 2004

FIGURE 8.11. Strategy reflection card. Copyright 2004 by ResearchILD. Reprinted by permission.

graphs of their performance on homework, tests, projects, and writing assignments.

- To encourage strategy use, teachers can help their students access previous memories of success through leading questions, such as:
  - Do you remember another time you had trouble with a similar task? What did you do?
  - Have you learned a strategy to help you solve this problem?
  - Do you remember how easy the last vocabulary test was when you used a particular strategy? Why not try that again?
  - Do you remember the last time you made an outline before writing your essay? Wasn't it much easier to write when your ideas were organized?

The *Drive to Thrive* program, summarized below, is one example of a model program designed to integrate strategy instruction into the school curriculum to teach students the core executive function processes.

The Drive to Thrive Program

Studies of student motivation, effort, and strategy use indicate that students who understand the importance of applying strategies to their schoolwork begin to recognize that their academic struggles are not insurmountable and that they can achieve greater success when they use learning strategies (Meltzer, Reddy, Pollica, & Roditi, 2004, 2005b). Results from a 6-month, strategy-based classroom instruction intervention showed significant improvements for at-risk students with learning and attention problems (Meltzer et al., 2001; Meltzer, Katzir, et al.,

2004). Specifically, teachers reported that their students made academic gains, were academically more strategic, and invested more effort in their schoolwork. These at-risk students were more self-confident and viewed themselves as more successful in their academic performance on reading, writing, and spelling tasks. Most important, all students, including those with no immediate academic problems, benefited from learning a broad array of strategies to improve their performance on classwork and tests (Meltzer et al., 2001; Meltzer, Katzir, et al., 2004; Meltzer, Katzir-Cohen, & Roditi, 2000). These results indicated that successful strategy use mediates the relationship between students' self-reported levels of effort and their academic self-concepts (Meltzer, Katzir, et al., 2004; Meltzer, Reddy, Pollica, & Roditi, 2004). The *Drive to Thrive* program builds on these findings by emphasizing that teaching students how to implement strategies successfully can initiate a positive cycle in which students focus their effort and use strategies effectively, resulting in more efficient performance and improved academic performance. This, in turn, results in positive academic self-concept so that students are more willing to work hard and to use strategies again (see Figure 5.3 in Chapter 5).

The *Drive to Thrive* intervention program has been designed to address these interactions among effort, strategy use, academic self-concept, and classroom performance by teaching students strategies that strengthen the executive function processes. Teachers are trained to infuse strategy instruction that addresses executive function processes into the standards-based curriculum in their inclusive classrooms and to evaluate their students on the basis of their strategy use as well as their content knowledge (Meltzer, Roditi, Button, Pollica, Steinberg, Stein, et al., 2005b). The overall goal of the *Drive to Thrive* program is to create a school culture where general and special education teachers have a shared understanding of the importance of nurturing efficient strategy use, executive function processes, focused effort, and positive academic self-perceptions in their students.

CONCLUSIONS

As the demands of our school curricula increase, students are expected to use executive processes for more and more assignments in order to prepare for high school, college, and beyond. The primary goal for teachers has been to prepare students by teaching them the content and skills valued by our highly literate society, such as reading, writing, spelling, math, history, and science. While the end product of learning is important, it is evident that students do not retain all the content they are taught from year to year. Therefore, it is even more important to teach students the executive function processes that *will* carry over from elementary school to middle school, high school, college, and even into the real world.

REFERENCES

Alvermann, D. E., & Boothby, P. R. (1986). Children's transfer of graphic organizer instruction. *Reading Psychology*, 7(2), 87–100.

Ausubel, D. P. (1963). *The psychology of meaningful verbal learning.* New York: Grune & Stratton.

Bereiter, C., & Scardamalia, M. (1985). Cognitive coping strategies and the problem of "inert knowledge." In S. F. Chipman, J. W. Segal, & R. Glaser (Eds.), *Thinking and learning skills: Current research and open questions* (Vol. 2, pp. 65–80). Hillsdale, NJ: Erlbaum.

Bos, C. S., & Anders, P. L. (1992). Using interactive teaching and learning strategies to promote text comprehension and content learning for students with learning disabilities. *International Journal of Disability, Development, and Education*, 39, 225–238.

Boyle, J. (1996). Thinking while note taking: Teaching college students to use strategic note-taking during lectures. In B. G. Grown (Ed.), *Innovative learning strategies: Twelfth yearbook* (pp. 9–18). Newark, DE: International Reading Association.

Boyle, J. (2001). Enhancing the note-taking skills of students with mild disabilities. *Intervention in School and Clinic*, 36, 221.

Boyle, J., & Weishaar, M. (1999). Note-taking strategies for students with mild disabilities. *The Clearing House*, 72, 392–396.

Bransford, J. D., Vye, N. J., & Adams, L. T. (1989). Learning skills and the acquisition of knowledge. In A. Lesgold & R. Glaser (Eds.), *Foundations for a psychology of education* (pp. 199–249). Hillsdale, NJ: Erlbaum.

Brown, A. L. (1997). Transforming schools into communities of thinking and learning about serious matters. *American Psychologist*, 52(4), 399–413.

Brown, A. L., & Campione, J. C. (1986). Psychological theory and the study of learning disabilities. *American Psychologist*, 14, 1059–1068.

Bruning, R., & Horn, R. (2000). Developing motivation to write. *Educational Psychologist*, 35(1), 25–38.

Bulgren, J., Schumaker, J. B., & Deshler, D. D. (1988). Effectiveness of a concept teaching routine in enhancing the performance of LD students in secondary-level mainstream classes. *Learning Disability Quarterly*, 11(1), 3–17.

Carnes, E. R., Lindbeck, J. S., & Griffin, C. F. (1987). Effects of group size and advance organizers on learning parameters when using microcomputer tutorials in kinematics. *Journal of Research in Science Teaching*, 24(9), 781–789.

Darch, C. B., Carnine, D. W., & Kame'enui, E. J. (1986). The role of graphic organizers and social structure in content area instruction. *Journal of Reading Behavior, 18*(4), 275–295.

Deshler, D. D., Ellis, E. S., & Lenz, B. K. (Eds.). (1996). *Teaching adolescents with learning disabilities* (2nd ed.). Denver, CO: Love.

Deshler, D., & Shumaker, J. (1986). Learning strategies: An instructional alternative for low achieving adolescents. *Exceptional Children, 52*(6), 583–590.

Deshler, D., & Schumaker, J. B. (1988). An instructional model for teaching students how to learn. In J. L. Graden, J. E. Zins, & M. J. Curtis (Eds.), *Alternative educational delivery systems: Enhancing instructional options for all students* (pp. 391–411). Washington, DC: National Association of School Psychologists.

Deshler, D., Schumaker, J., & Lenz, B. (1984). Academic and cognitive interventions for LD adolescents: Part I. *Journal of Learning Disabilities, 17*, 108–117.

Deshler, D., Schumaker, J. B., Lenz, B. K., Bulgren, J. A., Hock, M. F., Knight, J., et al. (2001). Ensuring content-area learning by secondary students with learning disabilities. *Learning Disabilities Research and Practice, 16*(2), 96–108.

Deshler, D., Warner, M. M., Schumaker, J. B., & Alley, G. R. (1983). Learning strategies intervention model: Key components and current status. In J. D. McKinney & L. Feagans (Eds.), *Current topics in learning disabilities* (pp. 245–283). Norwood, NJ: Ablex.

Dunlap, L. K., & Dunlap, G. (1989). A self-monitoring package for teaching subtraction with regrouping to students with learning disabilities. *Journal of Applied Behavior Analysis, 22*(3), 309–314.

Ellis, E. S. (1993). Teaching strategy sameness using integrated formats. *Journal of Learning Disabilities, 26*, 448–482.

Ellis, E. S. (1994). Integrating content with writing strategy instruction: Part 2—Writing processes. *Intervention in School and Clinic, 29*, 219–228.

Ellis, E. S. (1997). Watering up the curriculum for adolescents with learning disabilities: Goals of the knowledge dimension. *Remedial and Special Education, 18*, 326–346.

Flower, L., Stein, V., Ackerman, J., Kantz, M. J., McCormick, K., & Peck, W. C. (1990). *Reading-to-write: Exploring a cognitive and social process.* New York: Oxford University Press.

Flower, L., Wallace, D. L., Norris, L., & Burnett, R. A. (1994). *Making thinking visible: Writing, collaborative planning, and classroom inquiry.* Urbana, IL: National Council of Teachers of English.

Graham, S., & Harris, K. R. (2000). The role of self-regulation and transcription skills in writing and writing development. *Educational Psychologist, 35*, 3–12.

Graham, S., & Harris, K. R. (2003). Students with learning disabilities and the process of writing. In H. L. Swanson, K. R. Harris, & S. Graham (Eds.), *Handbook of research on learning disabilities* (pp. 383–402). New York: Guilford Press.

Harris, K. (1986). Self-monitoring of attentional behavior versus self-monitoring of productivity: Effects on on-task behavior and academic response rates among learning disabled children. *Journal of Applied Behavior Analysis*, 19(4), 417–423.

Harris, K., & Graham, S. (1992). *Helping young writers master the craft: Strategy instruction and self regulation in the writing process*. Cambridge, MA: Brookline Books.

Harris, K., & Graham, S. (1996). *Making the writing process work: Strategies for composition and self-regulation*. Cambridge, MA: Brookline Books.

Hattie, J., Biggs, J., & Purdie, N. (1996). Effects of learning skills interventions on student learning: A meta-analysis. *Review of Educational Research*, 66(2), 99–136.

Hayes, J. R. (1996). *The science of writing*. Mahwah, NJ: Erlbaum.

Herl, H. E., O'Neil, H. F., Jr., Chung, G. K. W. K., & Schacter, J. (1999). Reliability and validity of a computer-based knowledge mapping system to measure content understanding. *Computers and Human Behavior, 15*, 315–333.

Horton, S. V., Lovitt, T. C., & Bergerud, D. (1990). The effectiveness of graphic organizers for three classifications of secondary students in content area classes. *Journal of Learning Disabilities, 23*, 12–22.

Hughes, C. A. (1991). Studying for and taking tests: Self-reported difficulties and strategies of university students with learning disabilities. *Learning Disability Quarterly, 13*, 66–79.

Hughes, C. (1996). Memory and test-taking strategies. In D. Deshler, E. Ellis, & B. Lenz (Eds.), *Teaching adolescents with learning disabilities: Strategies and methods* (2nd ed., pp. 209–266). Denver, CO: Love.

Hughes, C. A., Ruhl, K. L., Schumaker, J. B., & Deshler, D. D. (2002) Effects of instruction in an assignment completion strategy on the homework performance of students with learning disabilities in general education classes. *Learning Disabilities Research and Practice, 17*(1), 1–18.

Hughes, C. A., & Suritsky, S. K. (1994). Note-taking skills of university students with and without learning disabilities. *Journal of Learning Disabilities, 27*, 20–24.

Idol, L., & Croll, V. J. (1987). Story-mapping training as a means of improving reading comprehension. *Learning Disability Quarterly, 10*(3), 214–229.

Katamaya, A. D., & Robinson, D. H. (2000). Getting students "partially" involved in note-taking using graphic organizers. *Journal of Experimental Education, 68*, 119–134.

Kellogg, R. T. (1987). Effects of topic knowledge on the allocation of processing time and cognitive effort to writing processes. *Memory and Cognition, 15*(3), 256–266.

Kiewra, K. A., DuBois, N. F., Christian, D., McShane, A., Meyerhoffer, M., & Roskelley, D. (1991). Note-taking functions and techniques. *Journal of Educational Psychology, 83*, 240–245.

Kim, A. H., Vaughn, S., Wanzek, J., & Shangjin W. J. (2004) Graphic organizers and their effects on the reading comprehension of students with LD: A synthesis of research. *Journal of Learning Disabilities, 37*(2), 105–119.

Lazarus, B. D. (1991). Guided notes, review and achievement of secondary students with learning disabilities in mainstream content courses. *Education and Treatment of Children, 14,* 112–127.

Maccini, P., & Hughes, C. A. (1997). Mathematics interventions for adolescents with learning disabilities. *Learning Disabilities Research and Practice, 12*(3), 168–176.

Mastropieri, M. A., & Scruggs, T. E. (1995). Teaching science to students with disabilities in general education settings. *Teaching Exceptional Children, 27,* 10–13.

Mayer, R. E. (1984). Aids to text comprehension. *Educational Psychologist, 19*(1), 30–42.

Meltzer, L. (1993). Strategy use in learning disabled students: The challenge of assessment. In L. Meltzer (Ed.), *Strategy assessment and instruction for students with learning disabilities: From theory to practice.* Austin, TX: Pro-Ed.

Meltzer, L. (1996). Strategic learning in students with learning disabilities: The role of self-awareness and self-perception. In T. E. Scruggs & M. Mastropieri (Eds.), *Advances in learning and behavioral disabilities* (Vol. 10b, pp. 181–199). Greenwich, CT: JAI Press.

Meltzer, L., Katzir, T., Miller, L., Reddy, R., & Roditi, B. (2004). Academic self-perceptions, effort, and strategy use in students with learning disabilities: Changes over time. *Learning Disabilities Research and Practice, 19*(2), 99–108.

Meltzer, L., Katzir-Cohen, T., Miller, L., & Roditi, B. (2001). The impact of effort and strategy use on academic performance: Student and teacher perceptions. *Learning Disabilities Quarterly, 24*(2), 85–98.

Meltzer, L. J., Katzir-Cohen, T., & Roditi, B. (2000). *Effort, strategy use, and academic performance: Student and teacher perspectives.* Paper presented at the International Academy for Research in Learning Disabilities, British Columbia, Canada.

Meltzer, L., & Montague, M. (2001). Strategic learning in students with learning disabilities: What have we learned? In B. Keogh & D. Hallahan (Eds.), *Intervention research and learning disabilities.* Hillsdale, NJ: Erlbaum.

Meltzer, L., Reddy, R., Pollica, L., & Roditi, B. (2004). Academic success in students with learning disabilities: The roles of self-understanding, strategy use, and effort. *Thalamus, 22*(1), 16–32.

Meltzer, L., Reddy, R., Pollica, L., Roditi, B., Sayer, J., & Theokas, C. (2004). Positive and negative self-perceptions: Is there a cyclical relationship between teacher's and students' perceptions of effort, strategy use, and academic performance? *Learning Disabilities Research and Practice, 19*(1), 33–44.

Meltzer, L., Roditi, B., Button, K. S., Steinberg, J., Pollica, L., Stein, J., et al. (2005b). *Drive to thrive.* Lexington, MA: Research Institute for Learning and Development.

Meltzer, L., Roditi, B., Houser, R. F., & Perlman, M. (1998). Perceptions of academic strategies and competence in students with learning disabilities. *Journal of Learning Disabilities, 31*(5), 437–451.

Meltzer, L., Roditi, B., & Stein, J. (2002). Preserving process learning in the era of high stakes testing: Research-based strategies for teaching test-taking. *MASCD Review* (January), pp. 10–12.

Meltzer, L., Roditi, B., Steinberg, J., Biddle, K. R., Taber, S., Caron, K. B., et al. (2005a). *Strategies for success: Classroom teaching techniques for students with learning differences* (2nd ed.). Austin, TX: Pro-Ed.

Meltzer, L., Soloman, B., Fenton, T., & Levine, M. D. (1989). A developmental study of problem-solving strategies in children with and without learning difficulties. *Journal of Applied Developmental Psychology, 10,* 171–193.

Merkley, D. M., & Jeffries, D. (2001) Guidelines for implementing a graphic organizer. *The Reading Teacher, 54*(4), 350–357.

Pajares, F., & Johnson, M. J. (1996). Self-efficacy beliefs and the writing performance of entering high school students. *Psychology in the Schools, 33,* 163–175.

Palincsar, A. S., Winn, J., David, Y., Snyder, B., & Stevens, D. (1993). Approaches to strategic reading instruction reflecting different assumptions regarding teaching and learning. In L. J. Meltzer (Ed.), *Strategy assessment and instruction for students with learning disabilities* (pp. 247–270). Austin, TX: Pro-Ed.

Paris, S. G. (1986). Teaching children to guide their reading and learning. In T. E. Raphael (Ed.), *The contexts of school-based literacy* (pp. 115–130). New York: Random House.

Paris, S. G., & Winograd, P. (1990). Promoting metacognition and motivation of exceptional children. *Remedial and Special Education, 11*(6), 7–15.

Pearson, P. D., & Dole, J. A. (1987). Explicit comprehension instruction: A review of research and new conceptualization of instruction. *Elementary School Journal, 88,* 151–165.

Pressley, M., Goodchild, F., Fleet, J., Zajchowski, R., & Evans, E. D. (1989). The challenges of classroom strategy instruction. *Elementary School Journal, 89,* 301–342.

Pressley, M., & Woloshyn, V. (1995). *Cognitive strategy instruction that really improves children's academic performance.* Cambridge, MA: Brookline Books.

Putnam, M. L., Deshler, D. D., & Schumaker, J. B. (1993). The investigation of setting demands: A missing link in learning strategies instruction. In L. J. Meltzer (Ed.), *Strategy assessment and instruction for students with learning disabilities: From theory to practice* (pp. 325–354). Austin, TX: Pro-Ed.

Ransdell, S., & Levy, C. M. (1996). Working memory constraints on writing quality and fluency. In C. M. Levy & S. Ransdell (Eds.), *The science of writing* (pp. 93–105). Mahwah, NJ: Erlbaum.

Reid, R. (1996). Research in self-monitoring with students with learning disabilities: The present, the prospects, the pitfalls. *Journal of Learning Disabilities, 29,* 317–331.

Reid, R., & Harris, K. R. (1993). Self-monitoring of attention versus self-monitoring of performance: Effects on attention and academic performance. *Exceptional Children, 60*(1), 29–40.

Research Institute for Learning and Development & FableVision. (2002). *BrainCogs: The personal interactive coach for learning and studying.* Watertown, MA: Author.

Research Institute for Learning and Development & FableVision. (2005). *Essay Express: Strategies for effective essay writing.* Watertown, MA: Author.

Ritchie, D., & Volkl, C. (2000). Effectiveness of two generative learning strategies in the science classroom. *School Science and Mathematics, 100*(2), 83–89.

Rosenshine, B. (1997). Advances in research on instruction. In J. W. Lloyd, E. J. Kame'enui, & D. Chard (Eds.), *Issues in educating students with disabilities* (pp. 197–221). Mahwah, NJ: Erlbaum.

Ruhl, K. L., & Suritsky, S. (1995). The pause procedure and/or an outline: Effect on immediate free recall and lecture notes taken by college students with learning disabilities. *Learning Disability Quarterly, 18,* 2–11.

Sah, A., & Borland, J. H. (1989) The effects of a structured home plan on the home and school behaviors of gifted learning-disabled students with deficits in organizational skills. *Roeper Review, 12*(1), 54–57.

Scanlon, D. J. Duran, G. Z., Reyes, E. I., & Gallego, M. A. (1992). Interactive semantic mapping: An interactive approach to enhancing LD students' content area comprehension. *Learning Disabilities Research and Practice, 7,* 142–146.

Scanlon, D., Deshler, D. D., & Schumaker, J. B. (1996). Can a strategy be taught and learned in secondary inclusive classrooms? *Learning Disabilities Research and Practice, 11*(1), 41–57.

Scardamalia, M., & Bereiter, C. (1985). Helping students become better writers. *School Administrator, 42*(4), 16–26.

Scardamalia, M., & Bereiter, C. (1986). Written composition. In M. Wittrock (Ed.), *Handbook of research on teaching* (3rd ed., pp. 778–803). New York: Macmillan.

Schunk, D. H. (2001). *Self-regulation through goal setting.* ERIC Digest. ERIC Clearinghouse on Counseling and Student Services: Greensboro, NC. (ERIC Document Reproduction Service No. ED 462 671)

Schunk, D. H., & Swartz, C. W. (1993) Goals and progress feedback: Effects on self-efficacy and writing achievement. *Contemporary Educational Psychology, 18*(3), 337–354.

Shimabukuro, S. M., Prater, M. A., Jenkins, A., & Edelen-Smith, P. (1999). The effects of self-monitoring of academic performance on students with learning disabilities and ADD/ADHD. *Education and Treatment of Children, 22*(4), 397–415.

Skinner, E. A., Wellborn, J. G., & Connell, J. P. (1990). What it takes to do well in school and whether I've got it: A process model of perceived control and children's engagement and achievement in school. *Journal of Educational Psychology, 82,* 22–32.

Suritsky, S. K. (1992). Note-taking approaches and specific areas of difficulty reported by university students with learning disabilities. *Journal of Postsecondary Education and Disability, 10,* 3–10.

Swanson, H. L. (1999). Instructional components that predict treatment outcomes for students with learning disabilities: Support for a combined strategy and direct instruction model. *Learning Disabilities Research and Practice, 14,* 129–140.

Swanson, H. L. (2001). Research on intervention for adolescents with learning disabilities: A meta-analysis of outcomes related to high-order processing. *The Elementary School Journal, 101,* 331–348.

Swanson, H. L., & Hoskyn, M. (1998). Experimental intervention research on students with learning disabilities: A meta-analysis of treatment outcomes. *Review of Educational Research, 68,* 277–321.

Swanson, H. L., & Hoskyn, M. (2001). Instructing adolescents with learning disabilities: A component and composite analysis. *Learning Disabilities Research and Practice, 16*(2), 109–119.

Webber, J., Scheuermann, B., McCall, C., & Coleman, M. (1993). Research on self-monitoring as a behavior management technique in special education classrooms: A descriptive review. *Remedial and Special Education, 14,* 38–56.

Westman, A. S., & Kamoo, R. L (1990). Relationship between using conceptual comprehension of academic material and thinking abstractly about global life issues. *Psychological Reports, 66*(2), 387–390.

Willerman, M., & MacHarg, R. A. (1991). The concept map as an advance organizer. *Journal of Research in Science Teaching, 28*(8), 705–712.

Winne, P. H. (1996). A metacognitive view of individual differences in self-regulated learning. *Learning and Individual Differences, 8*(4), 327–353.

Winne, P. H. (2001). Self-regulated learning viewed from models of information processing. In B. J. Zimmerman & D. H. Schunk (Eds.), *Self-regulated learning and academic achievement: Theoretical perspectives* (2nd ed., pp. 153–189). Mahwah, NJ: Erlbaum.

Zimmerman, B. J. (2000). Attaining self-regulation: A social cognitive perspective. In M. Boekaerts, P. R. Pintrich, & M. Zeidner (Eds.), *Handbook of self-regulation* (pp. 13–39). San Diego, CA: Academic Press.

Zimmerman, B. J., & Risemberg, R. (1997). Becoming a self-regulated writer: A social cognitive perspective. *Contemporary Educational Psychology, 22,* 73–101.

Zimmerman, B. J., & Schunk, D. H. (Eds.). (2001). *Self-regulated learning and academic achievement: Theoretical perspectives.* Mahwah, NJ: Erlbaum.

CHAPTER 9

Executive Control of Reading Comprehension in the Elementary School

IRENE WEST GASKINS
ERIC SATLOW
MICHAEL PRESSLEY

Few would dispute that the purpose of reading is to understand text nor would there be any dispute that understanding text necessitates reading words correctly, but reading words correctly is not what reading is about. By definition, reading is an interaction among the reader, the situation, the task, and the text that results in the construction of meaning (Gaskins, 2005; RAND Reading Study Group, 2002). To assure that comprehension is occurring, the reader taps into the power of executive control, a volitional process that enables him or her to monitor and take charge of the construction of meaning while reading. Executive control is one of the most important, if not the most important, student aptitudes related to reading comprehension (Wagner & Sternberg, 1987). It is a student's capacity to plan, monitor, and, if necessary, replan comprehension strategies in the service of understanding (Wang, Haertel, & Walberg, 1997).

As students advance through the elementary years, instruction in reading comprehension pushes readers beyond what is known and comfortable and increasingly requires them to take charge of active, effortful, resource-demanding thinking and problem solving, processes that result in understanding (Kintsch, 2004). Students who consistently demonstrate good comprehension tend to be those who, over time, expand and flexibly use their word recognition and comprehension strategies and monitor their progress (Joyce & Weil, with Calhoun, 2004). Executive control manages and directs these processes that enable students to demonstrate good comprehension.

This chapter explains the components of executive control, principles for understanding the relationship between reading comprehension and executive control, and factors affecting comprehension that may benefit from executive control. Three frequently cited factors affecting comprehension are word recognition, background knowledge, and comprehension strategies (Pressley, 2000). These factors are crucial to reading comprehension; however, in getting to the root of comprehension deficiencies, challenges in these areas may be only the tip of the iceberg. Therefore, additional factors must be considered, factors that interact with the acquisition of word recognition, background knowledge, and comprehension strategies (Gaskins, 2005). These interactive factors fall into four categories: person, situation, task, and text variables (RAND Reading Study Group, 2002). This chapter discusses these variables as well as how one uses executive control to take charge of them. The examples cited in this chapter are from Benchmark School, a grade 1–8 school for struggling readers in Media, Pennsylvania.

WHAT IS EXECUTIVE CONTROL OF COMPREHENSION?

Executive control processes for comprehending text deal with how individuals plan, direct, select, and orchestrate the various cognitive structures and processes available to them for attaining their comprehension goals. To accomplish these actions, individuals use knowledge of their own cognitive processes for controlling which cognitive activities are carried out at which time (Schumacher, 1987). Five of the often cited executive control processes include planning, prioritizing, organizing, shifting mindsets flexibly, and self-checking (Meltzer, 2004; Meltzer, Sales Pollica, & Barzillai, Chapter 8, this volume). A sixth executive control process is self-assessing (Gaskins, 2005).

The intelligent application of these processes is the primary job of executive control (Wagner & Sternberg, 1987). Ideally, before reading, the reader forms comprehension goals regarding the text being read and devises a plan of action to monitor and accomplish these goals and to take charge of specific challenges to them. The plan often includes prioritizing so that time and effort can be allocated appropriately to reach the comprehension goal (Wagner & Sternberg, 1987). Next, the reader selects and coordinates the strategies that are needed to implement the plan and organize the incoming information. As the reader proceeds through the text, he or she self-checks to determine whether the actions being taken are successful or unsuccessful relative to understanding what is being read and gathering the data needed to reach the comprehension goals that were set. When a reader determines that his or her comprehension goals are not being successfully reached, he or she employs further executive control and self-modifies (Costa & Kallick, 2004). For example, the reader may shift mindset, looking again at the goals, perhaps in a new way such as shifting from main ideas to details or approaching the same information from different viewpoints (Meltzer, 2004; Meltzer & Krishnan, Chapter 5, this volume). Finally, the reader self-assesses his or her achievement of the comprehension goals, often as related to a unit of instruction. The self-assessing reader can positively answer, with evidence, the questions "Do I really grasp what I have read?" and "Can I demonstrate my understanding?"

Basic to engaging successfully in executive control of reading comprehension are general principles about the relationship between reading comprehension and executive control. Effective teachers explicitly teach students these principles, which we discuss next. These principles are grounded in a theoretical and empirical understanding of reading comprehension and the role executive control plays in achieving comprehension goals. In teaching and reteaching these principles during grades 1–8, teachers guide students to note how each principle builds on the previous one.

PRINCIPLES UNDERLYING THE READING COMPREHENSION– EXECUTIVE CONTROL RELATIONSHIP

The vast majority of kindergarten and first-grade students expect that *what is read to them* will make sense. They probably even suspect that *what they read* should make sense. Those who struggle in learning to decode or in recalling words, however, are often unable to deal with both recognizing words and making sense of what they read, so comprehension is sacrificed. Some may even respond as a struggling first-grade reader did when I (Gaskins) was conducting an informal reading inventory. When Marissa (*pseudonyms are used throughout this chapter*) was unable to answer a question I posed about a short passage she had just read aloud to me, I asked her if the passage made sense to her. "No," she answered with a big smile. "What I read never makes sense. The teacher just gives us books so we can practice reading words—they don't have to make sense."

Reading Must Make Sense

Because of experiences like this one with Marissa, the first executive control principle that should be explicitly taught to beginning readers when they enter school is that reading must make sense. One teacher's explanation for this principle sounded something like this:

> "If the words you are reading do not make sense, you may have misread a word. Therefore, when what you are reading isn't making sense, you must stop and take action to see if you can figure out what went wrong. One thing you can do is to notice whether the sounds in the words you read match the letters you see in each word. Let me demonstrate what happened when I was reading the newspaper last night. I have put the sentence from the newspaper on a sentence strip on your desk so you can follow along, pointing to each word as I read."

(Teacher reads: "The burglar entered though the open window," but the sentence strip contains the word *through* instead of *though*.)

> "Everyone point to the word on your sentence strip that doesn't make sense in that sentence? [Students put their fingers on the word *through*.] I have a feeling that some of you know what word we need there so the sentence will make sense. Sometimes when you misread a word you can figure out from the sense of the sentence what the word is. Who thinks they know what the word is? [A student replies.] Yes, the word is *through*. Everyone put your finger on the letter in the word *through* that I missed."

(Students point to the letter *R*, and a student explains that the word in the sentence strip has the /r/ sound, but *though* does not.)

> "Great detective work, class! Let me read the sentence again as you point to each word. This time I will read the correct word that contains the /r/ sound. 'The burglar entered through the open window.' Does the sentence make sense now? What is the difference between the sounds you hear and the letters you see in *though* and *through*? [Students respond that they hear /r/ and see *r* in *through*.] Isn't it amazing that my ignoring just one letter in that whole sentence, caused what I read not to make sense? I know that I was actively

involved in making meaning when I read that sentence because I knew that it did not make sense and I took action to figure out how to make sense of it. That is what I want you to do when what you are reading does not make sense."

Understanding Is the Result of Planning to Understand

The second principle of executive control of reading comprehension expresses the importance of planning how the comprehension goal will be achieved. A plan for approaching a new text that effective teachers can explicitly teach is to survey, predict, and set a purpose. The survey portion can be a picture walk in which students access their background knowledge and talk about what they see happening in the pictures. An alternative to a picture walk is to ask students to survey the text for clues to what the story will be about by reading the title and any subheadings and by looking at the pictures. Based on their picture walk or survey, students are asked to predict what they will learn from reading the text. Next, the teacher guides students in shaping a purpose that will direct the reading of the text. Teachers explain to students that the survey–predict–set-a-purpose strategy is a plan for how to become actively involved in understanding what they read.

Once the survey–predict–set-a-purpose strategy has been practiced under the guidance of the teacher for about 6 weeks, the teacher adds another strategy to the plan. Students are taught that most fiction stories have four story elements: characters, setting, problem, and resolution. Teachers explicitly teach each element separately, and when each element is understood, they are combined and used to summarize or retell the important information in a story. If a reader's comprehension goal is to understand a story well enough to summarize the critical elements, the story-elements strategy would be part of the reader's plan, in combination with the survey–predict–set-a-purpose strategy. The reader would also plan to use the story-elements strategy as a way to monitor understanding.

The reader's action plan will eventually also include how to proceed through the text. For example, the plan may be to read several paragraphs at a time, then, at the conclusion of reading the paragraphs, to tell a partner a summary of what has been learned so far about the story elements. An alternative plan might be to read the entire piece of fiction, taking notes about the story elements, then, at the conclusion, to write a summary of the story telling about the characters, setting, problem, and resolution. Whatever the plan, the teacher explicitly teaches students the steps of the planning process and models how he or she would construct a plan to achieve a specific comprehension goal. A plan of action directs the processes to be used in reading the text and serves as a way to monitor whether the comprehension goal is being achieved. Children must be taught that they are the executives in charge of these processes.

By the time Benchmark's struggling readers are reading on a second-grade level, about half the guided reading they experience during language arts instruction takes place in nonfiction texts that are more dense than the fiction typically found in their literature readers. Comprehending what is read in these nonfiction texts calls for additional principles of executive control, discussed below.

Prioritizing Leads to Maximizing Time and Effort

A third principle of executive control of reading comprehension is the importance of prioritizing how much time and effort to allocate to various goals. For example, Bart arrives home from school frustrated that he does not understand the concept of photosynthesis that his fifth-grade class is studying. His science homework is to read two pages in a trade book about plants, then to write a sentence or two summarizing his understanding of photosynthesis. He also has math homework to complete and a chapter to read in an independent reading book his group will be discussing tomorrow. Bart's teacher explicitly teaches students how to analyze and prioritize the completion of homework. She also provides students with an estimate of how much time to devote to each task. For example, she told the class that the math and independent reading assignments combined should take no longer than 45 minutes to complete. In the past, Bart has had no difficulty completing these assignments in 45 minutes or less. Therefore, he decides that they can safely be left for completion after dinner. He decides that he had better begin immediately on his science assignment so that, in case he continues not to understand photosynthesis after reading and taking notes on the two assigned pages, he will still have time to call a classmate to discuss the science assignment before dinner. Bart has set his priority as understanding his science assignment, and he has allocated ample time to pursue the assistance he may need. He has implemented the executive control processes of establishing priorities and making a plan for reaching his comprehension goal. Both are processes that have been explicitly taught and that will continue to be revisited throughout Bart's school years.

Accessing Background Information Helps Organize New Information

A fourth principle of executive control of reading comprehension is that background information must be accessed before and during the reading process to help organize new information. The reader takes charge of calling to mind information and images that are already known about the topic or topics encountered while surveying and reading the text. The reader also constructs and organizes propositions while reading that will illuminate further understanding. Some topics will be very familiar, so connecting what is being read to background information will happen almost automatically: Other topics will be less familiar, and the reader will need to make sense of the text by accessing any relevant information, analogous situations, or images that will provide a means of organizing the text and fostering understanding. The processes of accessing background information and using it to organize new information are most likely to be employed by students if these strategies are explicitly explained and modeled for them.

As students advance beyond beginning texts, there will be occasions when they are unfamiliar with the topics in the text, particularly in content areas such as science and social studies. One way teachers can guide students to handle these texts is explicitly to point out to them the differences in the density and organization of ideas in the content-area texts as compared to literature basals or fiction trade books and, therefore, the need to read these texts differently than they read fiction. Teachers model their thought processes aloud as they read a content-area text to give students a sense of the amount of information that can be packed into a paragraph and the need to organize the incoming information based on what they already know. Topics in fiction can also be unfamiliar. Again, teachers think aloud, modeling how they proceed more slowly than usual in reading the text, relating the new information to known information, constructing meaningful propositions as reading is taking place, and crosschecking these constructions for sense as reading proceeds.

An additional way students can take charge of a paucity of background knowledge for understanding either fiction or nonfiction is to read a text below their instructional reading level on the topic with which they lack familiarity. Such texts usually provide a mental outline of the most important ideas about a topic. Then, as the student later reads more detailed information about the topic, that information can be fit into the mental outline of the important ideas gained from the easier text.

I (Gaskins) regularly share with students how lost I was in the early 1980s as I read books about China in preparation for my first visit there. I had no background knowledge. Comprehension of dynasties, China's geography, and effects of the Cultural Revolution were assumed by the books I read, but I had no schema into which I could integrate these concepts. My solution was to ask the librarian for the least dense book that would provide a main-idea outline of China into which I could integrate new information. Reading a children's book about China written at the third-grade level provided me with the background knowledge I needed to begin to understand travel books written about China. Over the years, teachers have shared the story of my needing to read easy children's books to understand adult books about China. The story of how an adult coped with lack of background knowledge needed to organize the new information she was reading seems to make it palatable for students to seek out easy books when they realize that they are missing background information on a specific topic. Reading easier texts is a strategy that should be taught explicitly and modeled by teachers. Actively thinking beyond the text to hook what is being read to information already organized in schemas and propositions is the role of executive control processes.

Self-Checking Enhances Goal Achievement

A fifth principle of executive control of reading comprehension is that the reader must be actively involved in self-checking comprehension to ascertain whether information is being understood and that the information is relevant to achieving his or her comprehension goal. Self-checking should occur before, during, and after reading. One way teachers suggest that students self-check their comprehension is to use the story-elements strategy. This strategy keeps students actively involved looking for important information in the text and provides a mental checklist to aid students in monitoring what they read. For example, students learn that characters and setting are usually introduced early in fiction, particularly fiction written at a beginning level. After reading several pages, if the reader is unable to recall the characters and tell the time and place of the story, it is a signal that comprehension is not taking place. Not being able to identify the characters or the time and place of the story alerts the student that he or she needs to reread or skim the text to identify these elements. If the student reads farther into the piece and finds that he or she cannot identify a problem that the characters are trying to resolve, this is another signal that a fix-up strategy such as rereading is needed. Throughout the reading, the student's goal of identifying story elements keeps him or her focused on important information and helps him or her monitor for understanding. The reader has engaged executive control.

An example with a more advanced reader may be setting goals to select and organize the main points of a topic and attach to those main points the most important and/or relevant supporting details. The strategy used might be skimming the chapter headings in boldface type to see if the text contains information relevant to the purpose for reading, then, if it does, reading selectively those sections, rather than the entire chapter. While reading, the reader self-checks by summarizing periodically what has been read to see if it meets his or her goal for reading. Self-checking may also require dealing with inconsistencies between background knowledge and information in the text. This situation calls for evaluating the accuracy of the text and possibly revising inconsistent prior knowledge. Other cognitive strategies that the reader may use to self-check and accomplish his or her goal include noting unfamiliar words and figuring out their meanings from context and, upon concluding the text, writing notes about or paraphrasing important ideas in the text to evaluate whether the goal has been achieved.

Having a Flexible Mindset Provides Opportunities for Increased Understanding

A sixth principle of executive control of reading comprehension is that, when the data call for it, the reader should be willing to change his or her mindset with respect to strategies and interpretation. As an example regarding strategies, a reader may prefer to read all of an assignment before reflecting on it or attempting to summarize it yet find that he or she does not remember much of what was read using this strategy. Readers with flexible mindsets would be willing to try a new strategy, such as taking notes as they read or filling in a story-elements outline. With respect to interpretation, a reader may approach a text with a hypothesis about how something works or about the happenings of an event in history only to find that his or her hypothesis is incorrect. In such cases, the reader would need to rethink his or her hypothesis and revise it in line with the data. Another occasion for employing a flexible mindset is when several interpretations of a text are set forth in a discussion. In such instances, students must learn not to hold on to interpretations that may seem plausible but are unsupported and to withhold judgment about an interpretation until it is supported with text. Effective teachers guide readers in developing the mindset that seeing another point of view, especially when the data support it, is usually an opportunity to learn.

Understanding Is Improved by Self-Assessing

A seventh principle of executive control of reading comprehension is the need to self-assess. Self-assessing differs from self-checking. As used in this chapter, self-checking is the monitoring of one's understanding as one reads and taking action to clear up confusion. Self-assessing is evaluating whether one's comprehension goal was achieved and, if not, what person, situation, task, or text variables are interfering and what action needs to be taken to correct the situation. This principle reminds students that one reads for understanding and that, if that goal has not been met, one has not read. The job of self-assessing is to ensure that the reader's comprehension goals are met.

An example of self-assessment includes taking action to check one's preparedness for a quiz, such as by designing and taking a practice quiz that evaluates whether one understands and can apply knowledge integrated from reading texts and participating in class discussions and other learning experiences. Self-assessment may also include writing a critique of what seemed to work and not work in completing a project to enhance understanding or in studying for and taking a quiz. At Benchmark School, this critique is often the required last step before handing in a project or quiz. Another act of self-assessment occurs after a project or quiz is returned with feedback. At that time, students are asked to discuss the ways their approach would be the same or different next time they completed a similar project or quiz. As part of this discussion, students are often asked to assess the effect of person, situation, task, or text variables on their understanding and how they could take control of these variables in the future. These variables will be discussed next.

WHAT AFFECTS COMPREHENSION AND HOW CAN EXECUTIVE CONTROL HELP?

In the preceding section, comprehension was discussed through the lens of principles governing executive control of comprehension. In this section, a broader lens is used—the lens of multiple variables affecting comprehension. It is well established that, in addition to reading processes, there are many nonreading variables that are crucial to comprehension (RAND Reading Study Group, 2002). This multivariable lens has traditionally been left out of discussions of executive control of comprehension, but we advocate that, when programming for students who struggle to comprehend, nonreading variables should be considered as carefully as reading processes. Both reading and nonreading variables can benefit tremendously from the power of executive control.

Nonreading variables include the affective processes of effort, motivation, self-concept, and persistence; volition to monitor and regulate thinking processes and to change strategies as necessary; and self-understanding regarding assumed constraints that arise from beliefs and lack of understanding about the nature of knowing and learning (Greeno, Collins, & Resnick, 1996). Nonreading variables also include beliefs about the locus of responsibility, degree of self-determination, and sense of agency in creating positive possibilities for self-development and self-regulation, often through realizing when there is a need for assistance and knowing how to acquire that assistance (McCombs, 2001). In the next four sections, person variables such as these, as well as situation, task, and text variables, are discussed as are executive control strategies for taking charge of these variables.

Person Variables

Person variables are the affective, conative, and cognitive factors that are characteristic of an individual. They include cognitive style, beliefs, interests, self-efficacy, background knowledge, and more. A few of these characteristics are discussed below, and they are discussed further (as is how to take control of them) in Chapter 12 in this volume.

Temperament and Emotion

Temperament and emotion are components of affect, a student's usual emotional tendency. Temperament is a fairly stable characteristic, the likelihood one will behave or react in a particular way, and includes such characteristics as activity level, adaptability, intensity, mood, persistence/attention span, and distractibility (Carey, 2005). Emotion, on the other hand, is a less stable characteristic and refers to a specific feeling at a specific time. Temperament and emotion can support or interfere with a student's ability to construct understanding, making it important that readers have the awareness, willingness, and ability to self-assess the status of these variables and to take charge of them to their advantage, a major challenge for some children.

Helpful suggestions for teaching students how to take charge of aspects of temperament and emotion that interfere with comprehension can be found in Meichenbaum's classic book *Cognitive-Behavior Modification: An Integrative Approach* (1977). The Benchmark School staff has implemented Meichenbaum's techniques successfully, especially with respect to adaptability, persistence, and reflectivity (Gaskins & Baron, 1985). An example of Benchmark's adaptation of Meichenbaum's techniques follows.

In the Benchmark program, students set a goal to take charge of some personal characteristic that is compromising comprehension, such as lack of adaptability. The teacher and student (Bill) meet together for a goal-setting conference in which the teacher guides Bill to realize that his reluctance to consider the ideas of others regarding events in or interpretations of a text is interfering with his comprehension. The teacher points out Bill's reluctance to reread to check his facts, which might be contributing to his difficulty understanding what he reads. Together, the teacher and Bill set the goal that when Bill's responses in discussion or in writing do not agree with others, or when he is confused about how to answer a discussion question, he will reread the text to find information that supports his point of view. The teacher writes on Bill's goal card, "During discussion or written response, I will find information in the text to support my answers." Each time Bill finds information in the text to support an answer, the teacher makes a check on his goal card. Students like to see a string of checks confirming that they are meeting their goal and, in earning the checks, they are learning executive control.

Motivation and Volition

Motivation and volition are components of conation, a "crescendo of commitment" that runs "from wishing to wanting to intending to acting" (Cronbach, 2002, p. 87).

> Motivation is incentive or desire (the affective part) directed toward a particular action, whereas volition is the act of making a conscious choice or decision to take action (the cognitive part). Volition is the will or drive to achieve what one desires. *Interests* affect motivation, whereas volition is related to *cognitive style* and plays an important role in a person's realization of *purposes and goals*. (Gaskins, 2005, p. 36, italics in original)

Motivation is about needs and goals. Volition is about self-regulation and executive control, mindful effort investment, and self-monitoring that mediate the enactment of goals and intentions (Gaskins, 2005).

Explicitly teaching students about motivation and volition is an important part of our program, particularly in grades 4–8. The concept of volition is introduced using the word "control," sharing with students examples of how they are in control of telling their brains what to do and that talking to themselves about how to do things is a good way to take control. Some teachers also use the phrase "take charge" to remind students that they need to be exercising executive control (Gaskins, 2005). Teachers regularly model for students how they exercise executive control by using self-talk to accomplish a goal. For example, one teacher shared that she understands how her students feel when they have schoolwork to complete but would rather be doing something else. She shared that she has the same problem, so she talks to herself something like this:

"I've got two trimester reports to write and tomorrow's lessons to plan, but I would rather talk to Ms. Brown about our plans for the weekend. I know that I need to take charge and have a plan because, if I put off the reports and lessons, I'll end up staying up too late tonight to get them finished. I think I had better make a deal with myself. I will work on reports for 45 minutes, and then I will take a break to talk to Ms. Brown. After 15 minutes, I will come back to my desk and finish my work."

We also talk with our students about the ingredients of intelligent behavior—something each one of them cares about. This is another way to include explicit talk about executive control processes. We share that, to demonstrate intelligent behavior, students need three ingredients, and we put these ingredients on a poster that is displayed at the front of the classroom:

Intelligent Behavior = Knowledge + Motivation + Control

(Gaskins & Elliot, 1991). We talk about the different kinds of knowledge they need, particularly world knowledge and strategy knowledge, what it means to be motivated, and how they can take control of reaching their goals by having a plan, applying their strategies, checking their progress toward meeting the goal, and modifying their plan if it is not working. Teachers refer to the intelligent-behavior poster throughout the day. For example, if students are off task and not using their time well during small-group projects, the teacher might say:

"I'm not seeing what I consider intelligent behavior right now. What ingredient seems to be missing? What can we do about it?"

Thus, the intelligent-behavior phrase is another way to highlight the importance of executive control, particularly as it pertains to motivation and volition. The phrase further emphasizes that executive control is a primary goal for all students.

Knowledge of What, How, and When

Knowledge is a powerful factor that influences comprehension, but knowledge does not only mean information or facts. Researchers divide knowledge into several types, and each requires its own spotlight during instruction as teachers help students achieve executive control of reading comprehension. Further, comprehension requires understanding how the pieces of knowledge fit together (Mayer, 1987). Therefore, students must assess their knowledge prior to reading in order to facilitate three important control processes: (1) paying attention to incoming information from the text; (2) organizing the incoming information into a coherent structure; and (3) integrating the incoming information with existing knowledge structures.

Facts and information are a kind of *declarative knowledge*, the knowledge of *what*. This also includes "vocabulary knowledge, world/ domain knowledge, linguistic knowledge, discourse knowledge, beliefs, and so on" (Gaskins, 2005, p. 51). Knowledge of this sort is stored in mental structures known as schemas (Anderson & Pearson, 1984). Schemas represent world knowledge, such as events, and enable readers automatically to draw inferences about events in text. A second source of knowledge is built as readers process individual ideas in text, noticing as they read how the ideas are related to one another to construct networks of propositions and macropropositions that can be tapped when readers encounter ideas in the text related to knowledge encoded in these propositional networks (Pressley, 2000). Knowledge structures such as these have been shown to be potent predictors of comprehension (Alexander, 2005–2006). They direct students' understanding and can even override facts found in a text (Yekovich & Walker, 1987).

Readers benefit from being explicitly taught to consider consciously their declarative knowledge as it pertains to the text they are about to read. Prior to and during reading, the successful reader accesses his or her knowledge, considering the pertinent factual, world, and vocabulary knowledge he or she possesses relevant to the topic of the text. As described earlier, one way we teach students to do this is by surveying the text and accessing background knowledge that is related to the information gained from their survey.

In some cases, students do not have sufficient background knowledge to be able to read a text with understanding, and teachers prepare students to take charge of this eventuality. First, they explain to students the relationship between background knowledge and comprehension, then they model how students can cope when they discover they do not have the background knowledge assumed by the text. One way to cope that was discussed earlier is to read an easier text about the topic. Other ways are to watch a movie about the topic or to discuss the topic with a parent or other adult.

Students must also be taught how to be in charge of their comprehension during reading. For example, they are taught to "criss-cross the landscape" (Spiro, Vispoel, Schmitz, Samarapungavan, & Boerger,

1987)—that is, to reread several times a complicated portion of text, sometimes from several perspectives, making enough connections in the content of their reading to confirm their understanding and eliminate contradictions or misunderstandings. Researchers advocate that information that will need to be used in different ways needs to be experienced and represented in different ways, with the reader making connections across these ways (Spiro et al., 1987). One technique Benchmark teachers use to accomplish this in social studies with our fifth and sixth graders is to ask students to be prepared, when they complete an assigned reading (e.g., on California during the Gold Rush), to discuss the topic of the assignment from two or three points of view (e.g., values and beliefs, social factors, technology, economics, government, or geography) (Gaskins, 2005). We call these points of view "lenses." During discussions, the teacher may ask one student to explain the Gold Rush through the technology lens, another to explain it through the social lens, and still another through the economic lens. In the process of such discussions, students crisscross the Gold Rush landscape from six directions or more, experiencing and representing the information in many ways.

Procedural knowledge "includes knowledge of how to use cognitive and metacognitive strategies, how to read words fluently, how to integrate nonprint and text, how to use skills, as well as the how of countless tasks" (Gaskins, 2005, p. 51). Students are taught to consider their procedural knowledge prior to a reading task in order to match their reading goal with appropriate strategies. For example, teachers may ask beginning readers what they will do if the reading does not make sense or if they come to an unknown word, then review strategies for handling these situations. They also explicitly teach any new strategy that will be needed to achieve the comprehension goal successfully, such as how to determine the main idea of a section of content-area text or the theme of a novel.

A third and final type of knowledge is *conditional knowledge*. Conditional knowledge "deals with understanding *when, where*, and *for what reason*" background knowledge and knowledge of strategies should be brought into play (Alexander, 2006, p. 78). Conditional knowledge is closely aligned with executive control because it is the understanding of why specific background knowledge is appropriate or why one strategy is better than another for a particular comprehension task. In our experience, students who have been taught how the mind works with respect to principles of learning and comprehension are most adept at implementing the most appropriate strategy to understand a text.

When introducing strategies, it is a good idea for teachers to include the *when* and the *why* of a strategy. For example, a teacher might introduce a procedure for taking notes and explicitly explain to students why a note-taking strategy should be used instead of relying on memory. The teacher's explanation might sound like this:

> "We know that most of us can only hold five to seven new ideas in short-term memory before the newest pieces of information begin to push out some of the other information you just read. Therefore, it is a good idea to take notes when you anticipate a reading assignment will include more than five new pieces of information."

Throughout the course of the unit and later in the school year, the teacher will cue students to take notes, perhaps saying:

> "This section of text contains at least nine or ten new concepts that we will need to be familiar with to understand the entire unit. I would suggest that you take notes because we know that we probably only have room for five to seven new ideas in short-term memory."

Thus, students learn to orchestrate the implementation of these strategies—that is, to develop executive control.

Situation Variables

In the Benchmark model, situation or context variables include two groups of variables that affect reading comprehension: the cognitive group and the sociocultural group (Gaskins, 2005). Variables in the cognitive group include teacher knowledge, classroom culture, and instruction. Variables in the sociocultural group include friends and family demographics, language, values, and cultural expectations. Although not extensively discussed in this chapter due to the limited power of a student's executive control to modify many of them, situation variables must be considered by teachers and diagnosticians when assessing the etiology of reading comprehension problems.

Some of the situation variables over which students can exercise executive control are:

1. A time schedule that includes schoolwork and extracurricular activities
2. An appropriate space, free of disruptions and distractions, for completing school assignments

3. A plan for gathering all the materials and books necessary for completing school tasks
4. A plan for receiving any support needed to complete assignments.

In general, organization of time, space, materials, and support is difficult for many elementary and middle school students, but it is particularly challenging for struggling readers like those students we teach at Benchmark School. Therefore, from the first day a student attends Benchmark, teachers explicitly teach students executive control strategies for organizing time, space, materials, and support.

For example, teaching a group of young struggling readers how to pace the completion of a written response to reading within the time constraints of a classroom schedule might sound something like this:

"Learning how to make the best use of our time each day is an important skill for all of us to develop. One reason for learning to use our time well is that the number of words read and written each day is a good predictor of the progress you will make in reading and writing. Today, to make you aware of how you use your time, write the time on your response-to-reading sheet each time I tell you to do so. You will write the time at exactly the place where you last wrote a word. This will help us analyze how well you are using your time. This may sound confusing to you, so let me model how I would note the time on my response-to-reading sheet. [Teacher models.] For today, when I ask you to stop and write the time, I will circulate and help you mark the spot. After we have done this for about 15 minutes a day for a week or so, I will sit down with each one of you individually and we will analyze how many words you read and wrote correctly in a certain period of time. We will also talk about factors that helped and hindered your ability to use your time well and come up with a plan to deal with the factors that hinder your ability to use your time well."

No matter how old students are, teachers can guide them to take control of their use of time. For example, with older students, teachers can ask their students to fill in a weekly assignment sheet. On this sheet, based on a week-end conference students are required to have with a parent, students write all their extracurricular activities and outside appointments for the week. Based on this input, teachers can guide students in planning the completion of homework and long-term assignments.

Similar approaches are taken to helping students learn how executive control can help them manage their study space, materials, and support. Learning to take charge of time, space, materials, and support has proved to be a major factor in the success of our students.

Task Variables

The task in reading is to comprehend, but depending on the specific task, the levels of comprehension may vary from superficial to deep (Kintsch, 2004) and from literal to interpretative to application or critical analysis. To accomplish satisfactorily the task of comprehension, readers must engage in active problem solving, knowledge construction, self-explanation, and monitoring (Kintsch, 2004). In addition, they need tools to self-assess their comprehension, a skill many students lack.

The executive system determines how and where to apply one's reading resources to accomplish a specific comprehension task (Wagner & Sternberg, 1987) and to monitor the success of task performance, revising strategies to improve performance as necessary. The executive system also allocates resources of time, attention, and effort to task demands and determines what to read and how to read it via effective allocation of reading time and effective planning of task strategies.

The comprehension task can be as simple as locating a fact in a text or as complex as applying the understanding acquired from reading a chapter in a history book to a different time and place. To put students in control of accomplishing complex comprehension tasks, we teach students an executive control strategy we call ANOW. One purpose of ANOW is to provide students with a plan for answering essay questions. The letter A in ANOW stands for analyze. Before they answer a question, we ask students to analyze what the task involves, then to write a restatement of the task in their own words. The N stands for notes. Students are to jot down notes that result from brainstorming what they know about the question. The third letter, O, stands for organize. Students organize their notes by numbering them in the order they will use them in answering the question. Finally, W stands for write. Students write their essays following the outlines they have constructed.

Text Variables

Text variables are the elements of any printed or electronic materials that affect the reader's ability to process the information on a page. These include:

1. Level of the vocabulary
2. Proposed audience for the text
3. Characteristics of the text genre

4. Clarity of text structures
5. The nature of illustrations and graphics.

Just as with the previous variables that affect comprehension, students must be taught explicitly about the nature of text elements. This information is then available for executive monitoring and decision making. For example, at Benchmark even the youngest students are taught to assess the readability of a book before choosing it for nightly reading. Students are taught to open the books they are considering to a full page of text and to read the page to themselves, putting up a finger for each word they need to stop and decode. If they encounter more than one word per page that is not a sight word, the book may not be appropriate to read for fun. In addition, all of the books in the school library are color-coded. Students are guided to choose texts by the color that represents their independent level for reading. Students know which colors match their instructional and independent levels and tend to choose books for recreational reading that are at their independent level. With time, students develop the habit of exerting control over this aspect of the reading process, automatically checking that the books they choose for recreational reading are books they can comfortably read. They have learned from their teachers that the number of words they can read fluently correlates with progress in reading and reading books with too many hard words makes it difficult to comprehend what they read.

Another example of taking charge of text variables pertains to genre. Students are exposed to a variety of genres as they are instructed in reading and as teachers read aloud to them. Through this process, students can be explicitly taught some of the features of genres. Teachers can discuss with students differences between fiction and nonfiction texts as well as differences between realistic fiction, fanciful tales, science fiction, biographies, historical fiction, etc. Thus, when students approach a reading task, such as taking notes for a summary of a novel, they can identify the book's genre and know what form of note taking works best for it.

SUMMARY

Executive control processes enable readers to monitor what they read for sense and to be in charge of whether they understand what they read. Executive control processes for comprehending text include planning, directing, selecting, and orchestrating the various cognitive structures and processes available to them for attaining their comprehension goals.

To accomplish these actions, individuals use knowledge of their own cognitive processes for controlling which cognitive activities are carried out at which time. Executive control processes include planning, prioritizing, organizing, self-checking, shifting mindsets flexibly, and self-assessing. These processes tend to follow a developmental trajectory; thus, students should be able to demonstrate increased awareness and control with each passing year, especially if they have the benefit of specific, explicit instruction on how and why to implement these processes and if this instruction extends over 6–8 years of their schooling.

Seven principles for understanding the relationship between reading comprehension and executive control are:

1. Reading must make sense.
2. Understanding is the result of planning to understand.
3. Prioritizing leads to maximizing time and effort.
4. Accessing background information helps organize new information.
5. Self-checking enhances goal achievement.
6. Having a flexible mindset provides opportunities for increased understanding.
7. Understanding is improved by self-assessing.

Four categories of variables that interact to affect comprehension are person, situation, task, and text. Each affects whether comprehension will occur, and most are responsive to executive control. Exercising executive control instead of becoming discouraged by personal characteristics, situations, tasks, or texts that seem hostile to understanding is the hallmark of successful students. Not only are the cognitive benefits of taking control substantial, but so are the affective and conative benefits (e.g., feeling more confident, believing one can succeed, being more persistent).

Explicitly teaching students how to take control of understanding the texts they read is one of the greatest gifts a teacher can give. Students who have knowledge of and use executive control have the power to succeed in school and in life. Executive control is the aptitude that unlocks success.

ACKNOWLEDGMENTS

We appreciate the helpful suggestions of Helen Lawrence, Sandy Madison, Melinda Rahm, and Theresa Scott on earlier versions of this chapter.

REFERENCES

Alexander, P. A. (2006). *Psychology in learning and instruction.* Upper Saddle River, NJ: Pearson Education.

Alexander, P. A. (2005–2006). The path to competence: A lifespan developmental perspective on reading. *Journal of Literacy Research, 37,* 413–436.

Anderson, R. C., & Pearson, P. D. (1984). A schema-theoretic view of basic processes in reading comprehension. In P. D. Pearson (Ed.), *Handbook of reading research* (pp. 255–291). New York: Longman.

Carey, W. B. (2005). *Understanding your child's temperament* (rev. ed.). New York: Macmillan.

Costa, A. L., & Kallick, B. (2004). Launching self-directed learners. *Educational Leadership, 62,* 51–55.

Cronbach, L. (Ed.). (2002). *Remaking the concept of aptitude: Extending the legacy of Richard E. Snow.* Mahwah, NJ: Erlbaum.

Gaskins, I. W. (2005). *Success with struggling readers: The Benchmark School approach.* New York: Guilford Press.

Gaskins, I. W., & Baron, J. (1985). Teaching poor readers to cope with maladaptive cognitive styles: A training program. *Journal of Learning Disabilities, 18,* 390–394.

Gaskins, I. W., & Elliot, T. T. (1991). *Implementing cognitive strategy instruction across the school: The Benchmark manual for teachers.* Cambridge, MA: Brookline Books.

Greeno, J. G., Collins, A. M., & Resnick, L. (1996). Cognition and learning. In D. Berliner & R. Calfee (Eds.), *Handbook of educational psychology* (pp. 63–84). New York: Macmillan

Joyce, B., & Weil, M. (with Calhoun, E.). (2004). *Models of teaching* (7th ed.). Boston: Pearson Education.

Kintsch, W. (2004). The construction-integration model of text comprehension and its implications for instruction. In R. Ruddell & N. Unrau (Eds.), *Theoretical models and processes of reading* (5th ed., pp. 1270–1328). Newark, DE: International Reading Association.

Mayer, R. E. (1987). Instructional variables that influence cognitive processes during reading. In B. Britton & S. Glynn, *Executive control processes in reading* (pp. 201–216). Hillsdale, NJ: Erlbaum.

McCombs, B. L. (2001). Self-regulated learning and academic achievement: A phenomenological view. In B. Zimmerman & D. Schunk, *Self-regulated learning and academic achievement: Theoretical perspectives* (2nd ed., pp. 67–123). Mahwah, NJ: Erlbaum.

Meichenbaum, D. (1977). *Cognitive-behavior modification: An integrative approach.* New York: Plenum Press.

Meltzer, L. (2004, November). *Executive function in the classroom: Metacognitive strategies for fostering academic success and resilience.* Paper presented at the 20th annual Learning Differences Conference, Boston, MA.

Pressley, M. (2000). What should comprehension instruction be the instruction of? In M. Kamil, P. Mosenthal, P. Pearson, & R. Barr (Eds.), *Handbook of reading research* (Vol. 3, pp. 545–561). Mahwah, NJ: Erlbaum.

RAND Reading Study Group. (2002). *Reading for understanding: Toward an R and D program in reading comprehension*. Santa Monica, CA: RAND.

Schumacher, G. M. (1987). Executive control in studying. In B. Britton & S. Glynn (Eds.), *Executive control processes in reading* (pp. 107–144). Hillsdale, NJ: Erlbaum.

Spiro, R., Vispoel, W., Schmitz, J., Samarapungavan, A., & Boerger, A. (1987). Knowledge acquisition for application: Cognitive flexibility and transfer in complex content domains. In B. Britton & S. Glynn (Eds.), *Executive control processes in reading* (pp. 177–199). Hillsdale, NJ: Erlbaum.

Wagner, R. K., & Sternberg, R. J. (1987). Executive control in reading comprehension. In B. Britton & S. Glynn (Eds.), *Executive control processes in reading* (pp. 1–21). Hillsdale, NJ: Erlbaum.

Wang, M. C., Haertel, G. D., & Walberg, H. J. (1997). Learning influences. In H. Walberg & G. Haertel (Eds.), *Psychology and educational practice* (pp. 199–211). Berkeley, CA: McCuchan Pub.

Yekovich, F. R., & Walker, C. H. (1987). The activation and use of scripted knowledge in reading about routine activities. In B. Britton & S. Glynn (Eds.), *Executive control processes in reading* (pp. 145–176). Hillsdale, NJ: Erlbaum.

CHAPTER 10

Addressing Executive Function Problems in Writing

An Example from the Self-Regulated Strategy Development Model

STEVE GRAHAM
KAREN R. HARRIS
NATALIE OLINGHOUSE

Over the last 5,000 years, writing has evolved from a recording instrument for keeping track of goods and animals to a flexible and indispensable tool. Writing is now used as a means for communication, a vehicle for learning, and an instrument for artistic, political, spiritual, and self-expression (Graham, 2006a). Writing has become so important today that approximately 85% of the world's population now writes (Swedlow, 1999).

Those who do not learn to write or write well are at a considerable disadvantage. In school, writing is used to gather, remember, and share subject-matter knowledge as well as to explore, organize, and refine ideas about a topic (Durst & Newell, 1989). Thus, students who experience difficulty with writing cannot fully draw on its power to support and extend learning. Their grades are also likely to suffer, especially in classes where writing is the primary means for assessing progress (Graham, 1982).

The consequences of poor writing extend well beyond the school-house. Poor writers are also unlikely to realize their occupational or personal potential. For example, in a survey of 120 American corporations employing nearly 8 million people, writing was identified as a threshold skill for hiring and promoting salaried workers (National Commission on Writing, 2004). A subsequent survey found that writing is even more essential for the nearly 2.7 million state government employees (National Commission on Writing, 2005).

Unfortunately, many children have difficulty mastering this critical skill. Only about 25% of students in the most recent National Assessment of Educational Progress (Persky, Daane, & Jin, 2003) were classified as competent writers. While there are many possible reasons some children do not develop adequate writing skills (see, for example, Graham, in press a; Graham & Harris, 2000; MacArthur, Graham, & Fitzgerald, 2006), one factor that appears to influence writing development and contribute to writing difficulties is executive functioning. We define executive functioning as follows:

> Executive functioning involves the conscious, purposeful, and thoughtful activation, orchestration, monitoring, evaluation, and adaptation of strategic resources, knowledge, skills, and motivational states to achieve a desired goal. This involves analysis (e.g., sizing up the demands of the situation), decision making and planning (e.g., selecting or devising a plan of action), attentional control (focusing and maintaining attention as well as inhibiting interfering behaviors), coordination of cognitive resources, and flexible application (e.g., adjusting plans and goals to meet changing situations).

Skilled writing involves all of the processes that are included in our definition of executive functioning. For example, when Hayes and Flower (1980) asked adults to think aloud while composing, the resulting verbal protocols revealed that skilled writing is a self-directed activity, which is driven by the goals that writers set for what they want to do and say. To meet these goals, the writer must skillfully and flexibly (i.e., thoughtfully) apply and coordinate a variety of resources, including strategic processes (i.e., mental operations for planning, drafting, and revising), knowledge (e.g., about the topic, the intended audience), and skills (handwriting, spelling, sentence construction). The success of this enterprise rests on careful analysis (e.g., determining the demands of the writing task) as well as decision making and planning (e.g., determining a suitable approach to tackling the writing problem). The entire process places considerable demands on the writer's attention, as it requires simultaneously juggling or coordinating a number of constraints and processes. While motivation received little attention in the initial analyses of Hayes and Flower, this omission was corrected later, when Hayes (1996) emphasized that writers must also attend to affective factors such as goals, predispositions, beliefs, and attitudes when writing.

Even though executive functioning plays a central role in skilled writing, there is surprisingly little research on its function, development, or impact on children who are learning to write. In the next section, we examine a proposition that immature and struggling writers employ an approach to composing that minimizes the role of executive functioning skills in writing.

EXECUTIVE CONTROL AND ITS ROLE IN WRITING DEVELOPMENT AND DIFFICULTIES

The Knowledge-Telling Approach

One of the most important contributions of the work on skilled writing by Hayes and Flower (1980) was the recognition that composition did not necessarily proceed in a linear fashion from planning to drafting to revising. Instead, the skilled writers that they observed acted in a recursive manner, shifting among processes such as planning, drafting, and revising, nesting one within another.

Based upon their extensive observations of novice writers, Bereiter and Scardamalia (1987) indicated that developing or novice writers' approach to composing is much simpler. They primarily convert the writing task into telling what they know about the topic.

The architecture of Bereiter and Scardamalia's (1987) knowledge-telling model includes three components. One component, *mental representation of the assignment*, involves understanding the writing assignment by defining the topic and function of the text to be produced. A second component, *long-term memory*, includes two types of knowledge the writer can draw on to complete the assignment: content knowledge (what the writer knows about the topic) and discourse knowledge (linguistic knowledge and knowledge about the type of text to be produced). The third component, the *knowledge-telling process*, consists of a series of operations. The first two operations are constrained by the writer's mental representation of the assignment and involve making a decision on the topic and type of text to be produced. This serves to guide the writer's search and retrieval from long-term memory. The retrieved information is checked to determine if it matches the nature and topic decided on. If it is appropriate, this information is transcribed into written text. The text produced so far serves as a stimulus for conducting the next search of long-term memory.

For the most part, observations of how immature and struggling writers compose are generally consistent with the knowledge-telling model (e.g., Graham, 1990; Thomas, Englert, & Gregg, 1987). McCutchen (1988) has proposed that these writers adopt and continue to use the knowledge-telling approach because it serves an adaptive function. The process of translating ideas into text (e.g., handwriting, spelling) exerts considerable processing and attentional demands on young writers who have not fully mastered these skills. Executive functioning also requires considerable cognitive effort (Kellogg, 1987). The knowledge-telling approach minimizes (but does not eliminate) the use of executive functioning skills, such as planning and decision making, making writing a less demanding task—one that is less likely to overwhelm a developing writer. It also provides a reasonably successful approach to many of the types of writing tasks young children encounter (e.g., writing about personal experiences, telling what they know about a topic).

As children move from the primary grades to upper elementary school and beyond, writing tasks become more demanding and complicated, requiring a more thoughtful, planful, and reflective approach. In essence, executive functioning becomes more critical to writing success. Many children experience difficulty shedding an approach that requires less effort, especially when it has been relatively successful in the past, for one that requires considerably more. In our opinion, an important goal in writing instruction for developing and struggling writers is to help them upgrade the executive function skills they use when writing. Before presenting a specific approach for enhancing young writers' use of executive functioning skills in writing, we first examine evidence that supports the view that writing performance is influenced by executive functioning skills.

Evidence on the Impact of Executive Functioning on Writing Performance

One method for studying the role of executive functioning in writing is to examine the effects of providing external support in managing and coordinating the elements involved in writing (Graham, 2006a). Focusing on the skill of revising, Scardamalia and Bereiter (1983) provided such support to normally developing students in grades 4, 6, and 8. Students were prompted to use a routine for coordinating and managing the evaluative and tactical decisions involved when revising text. The routine was based on a model of revising involving three elements: compare (detecting a mismatch between what the author intended to say and what was written), diagnose (determining the cause of the mismatch), and operate (deciding on the type of change needed and carrying it out). This model was operationalized by having students read the first sentence in the first draft of their composition and select the one of a possible 11 evaluations (e.g., "This doesn't sound quite right") that best characterized the sentence (compare stage). Then, they were asked to explain orally how the evaluation applied (diagnose stage). Finally, students selected one of six operations (e.g., "I better say more") that they would carry out (operate stage). This routine ensured that the skills involved in revising occurred in a coordinated way. Providing this procedural support had a positive impact on the revising of the participating students, as they revised more and there was an improvement in the quality of their individual revisions. Similar results were found in a second study with normally achieving students in grades 6 and 12 using a more sophisticated executive control routine (Scardamalia & Bereiter, 1985). Graham and colleagues (De La Paz, Swanson, & Graham, 1998; Graham, 1997) also found that slightly modified versions of these executive control routines enhanced the revising performance of struggling writers with learning difficulties in grades 6 and 8.

These four studies provide support for the proposition that difficulties with executive functioning constrain the revising of normally developing and weaker writers, and there is considerable evidence that teaching executive control routines for planning has a positive and strong effect on the writing performance of these two groups of children. The average effect size for such instruction exceeds 0.80 (Graham, 2006b; Graham & Harris, 2003; Graham & Perrin, 2006). Furthermore, a study by Hooper, Swartz, Wakely, de Kruif, and Montgomery (2002) provides further support for the idea that executive functioning difficulties constrain writing development. They found that weaker writers were less adept than stronger writers on a broad array of executive functioning skills.

In our own intervention research, we made the facilitation and development of executive functioning a central element in how we teach students strategies for planning, drafting, and revising text (see Graham & Harris, 2003). We developed a specific instructional model for teaching these strategies, self-regulated strategy development (SRSD; Graham & Harris, 2005a, 2005b; Harris & Graham, 1996). With this model, students are explicitly and directly taught to apply the target writing strategies and how to use procedures such as goal setting, self-monitoring, self-instruction, and/or self-reinforcement to regulate their use of the writing strategies, the writing task, and their behavior. Content knowledge is increased by teaching students information they will need to use the selected writing strategies and self-regulation procedures effectively. Finally, the model is designed to enhance students' motivation for writing through a variety of procedures, including emphasizing the role of effort in learning, making the positive effects of instruction concrete and visible, and promoting a "can do" attitude.

We specifically designed the SRSD model so that it would support the following five aspects of executive functioning: analysis, decision making and planning, execution and coordination of mental and affective resources, attentional control, and flexible adaptation. Procedures to support the application and development of these processes are integrated throughout the model's six instructional stages (illustrated in the next section). The SRSD model has proven very effective. In an examination of the writing intervention literature in grades 4–12 (Graham & Perrin, 2006), writing strategy instruction was the most effective writing intervention (average weighted effect size = 0.82), with SRSD being especially potent (average weighted effect size = 1.14).

In the next section, we provide an illustration of how one teacher used the SRSD model to teach second-grade students how to write persuasive text. The six instructional stages of the model are identified as they occur, with the name of the stage in parentheses and italics. This illustration of SRSD is followed by an analysis of how the teacher supported and developed executive functioning via SRSD.

THE SRSD MODEL IN ACTION

Our illustration involves the second-grade class of Ms. Laura Jacobson. She decided to teach a persuasive writing strategy using the SRSD model to her class of 20 students. Included in the class were three students with learning disabilities who struggled with writing and several other students who had difficulty with the writing process. The district's literacy curriculum specified numerous genres to cover at each grade level. To accomplish this, Ms. Jacobson had taught her students a three-step general writing strategy for planning and drafting compositions (POW: Pick my ideas; Organize my notes; Write and say more). She had initially taught students how to use this general strategy when writing stories. Students learned to use a genre-specific planning strategy that helped them complete the second step of POW, organize my notes. With the genre-specific planning strategy, students generated and organized possible ideas for the basic parts of a story (e.g., characters, setting, characters' goals). Ms. Jacobson was now ready to move to a second genre, again using POW as the general approach to planning and drafting but introducing a new genre-specific strategy designed specifically for writing persuasive essays.

Before beginning instruction, Ms. Jacobson had her students write a persuasive essay on whether children should have to go outside for recess. She asked students to plan their essay before writing. After collecting the plans and the essays, Ms. Jacobson reviewed her students' work and noted that many of them had difficulty writing persuasive papers, resulting in incomplete arguments. She also realized, that despite already having been taught a general planning strategy (POW), her students were unable to transfer the strategy to help them write their persuasive essay. Her students with learning disabilities exhibited even greater difficulties and had papers that were short and lacked organization and details. These students failed to plan at all; instead, they started writing immediately. Ms. Jacobson set a goal to teach students how to write a persuasive essay that included a topic sentence, three or more supporting reasons, and a good ending. To do this, she used a genre-specific planning strategy (as the organization step of POW) that we had applied in previous studies (see, e.g., Graham, Harris, & Mason, 2005). The strategy TREE reminded students to Tell what you believe ("State your topic sentence"), give three or more Reasons to support your belief ("Why do I believe this?"), End it ("Wrap it up right"), and Examine your paper ("Do I have all the parts?").

Before starting the persuasive writing instruction, Ms. Jacobson met individually with the students who struggled with writing persuasive essays (*Discuss It*). She discussed each student's previous approach to writing a persuasive essay. Most students said that they wrote down whatever they thought and that they did not engage in any planning. She informed these students that they would learn a new strategy to improve their ability to write a well-organized persuasive essay. This helped prepare them for the upcoming instruction and promote their commitment to learn the strategy. Ms. Jacobson knew that using SRSD to teach narrative writing had helped her students learn to regulate and monitor a writing task effectively, especially her students with learning disabilities. She believed that this strategy would also help her students with this new writing task and excitedly planned for the first lesson.

The first day of instruction started with developing the background knowledge and skills needed to write a good persuasive essay (*Develop Background Knowledge*). Ms. Jacobson first reviewed POW with the class. The class discussed using the POW strategy to write narrative stories. Ms. Jacobson then explained to the students that they would learn how to use POW to write another kind of paper, called persuasive writing. The class discussed the meaning of the words *persuade, fact,* and *opinion*; why and when students might want to persuade another; and the goals of persuasive writing. Ms. Jacobson emphasized that good persuasive writing has a topic sentence that states an opinion, three or more reasons to support the topic sentence, and a strong ending. She then introduced the TREE strategy, integrating it within POW by explaining that TREE was used during the "organize my notes" step. To help the students remember the strategy, the TREE components were compared to a living tree. The topic sentence was compared to the trunk, strong and connected to all other parts; the reasons were like the roots, supporting the trunk; and the ending was like the earth, wrapping around the bottom of the tree. This comparison provided a visual reminder and helped the students understand the reasons for each step. After introducing the strategy, Ms. Jacobson paired each lower-performing student with a higher-performing student to start memorizing the TREE strategy by listing and naming the essential components and describing why each was important (*Memorize It*). The students used cue cards during this introduction to the strategy.

During the next lesson, Ms. Jacobson emphasized the goals of writing better persuasive papers and the necessity of student effort to use and apply the strategy while writing (*Discuss It*). She explained how learning this strategy would enable students to write good persuasive essays. The class then established goals for learning the strategy, and made a commitment to learn it. At the end of the lesson, Ms. Jacobson again paired the students (lower- with higher-performing students) and established writing partners. The writing partner activity was designed to help students transfer the writing strategy to other writing tasks. Ms. Jacobson explained that the writing partners would help each other identify situations when part or all of the strategy could be transferred to other writing tasks, as well as provide help or reminders to use the strategy.

The next day, Ms. Jacobson discussed the parts of a persuasive essay, focusing on the topic sentence and supporting reasons (*Develop Background Knowledge*). She then read aloud an example of a persuasive essay while students followed along on paper. Students raised their hands when they heard one of the TREE components. After identifying the topic sentence, students underlined it on their copy. Ms. Jacobson also included a discussion about transition words, and the students circled the transition words on their copy. The class discussed how transition words help a reader find the reasons in a paper. The students located and labeled each reason with a number, then counted the total number of transition words and reasons in the paper. Finally, the students identified and underlined the end sentence.

Next, Ms. Jacobson introduced the TREE graphic organizer. She demonstrated how to write all of the TREE components from the example essay in note form on the organizer, numbering the reasons as she wrote. Students helped locate the TREE parts in the essay for Ms. Jacobson to write on the graphic organizer. After the topic sentence, reasons, and endings were recorded, Ms. Jacobson then examined the paper to ensure all parts were complete. Students continued to memorize the strategy by working in pairs to practice writing the TREE reminder

(*Memorize It*). This practice activity was continued until each student could name the reminder (TREE) and write the parts on paper from memory. Ms. Jacobson provided additional support and practice for the students with learning disabilities and other struggling writers in the classroom.

During the next lesson, Ms Jacobson introduced self-monitoring and graphing. She asked the students to analyze their previously written persuasive papers on whether children should have to go outside for recess. Ms. Jacobson demonstrated how to read through the paper, using the TREE reminder to look for a topic sentence, three or more reasons, and an ending. She illustrated how to graph each of the parts, which involved coloring in a piece of a rocket for each part in the paper. The students worked on graphing the parts of their papers, while Ms. Jacobson circulated to ensure that everyone was graphing correctly. The students discussed the parts in their papers and which parts to remember to include the next time (*Discuss It*). Ms. Jacobson emphasized that even if a component was included, students could improve it by adding more details or examples to support their reasons or using more sophisticated vocabulary, which she called million-dollar words.

At the end of this lesson, the students met with their writing partners. In a group, the class brainstormed ways to use all or part of the POW or TREE strategy. They discussed how TREE was different from the previously learned narrative writing strategy. They talked about how to transfer the strategies to other writing tasks, such as letters to friends, writing to convince someone, and reports. They also discussed what to do if all or part of the strategy did not work, such as changing parts of TREE or not using TREE if it did not make sense for that writing task. The students made a goal of reporting to their writing partners in the next lesson on how they transferred their strategies. Ms. Jacobson reviewed a chart that helped students record how they transferred their strategy and how they helped their partner transfer the strategy.

In the next lesson, students initially met with their writing partners to complete their "I transferred my strategies/I helped my partner" chart. Ms. Jacobson verbally reinforced each student's effort. The class talked about how they tried to transfer their strategies and the success of their attempts and brainstormed ways to work out problems when transferring strategies, such as asking a writing partner or trying to change some parts of the strategy. Ms. Jacobson established a routine of starting each lesson with the writing partners filling out their charts and a short discussion to guide students through the problems encountered in the transfer task.

During the main part of this lesson, Ms. Jacobson read two more persuasive essays and helped the students verbally identify the parts of the paper (*Develop Background Knowledge*). She showed students how to write their ideas in note form. She then asked the students to add one or two additional reasons to the paper, and she listed these reasons on the graphic organizer. The students were asked to think of transition words for the additional reasons. At the end of the lesson, the group revisited their goal of learning the POW + TREE strategy, including all of the TREE parts and improving all of the parts each time they wrote a persuasive paper.

The following day, Ms. Jacobson posted a copy of POW + TREE, along with the topic "Should students have to give away some of their toys to children who don't have any toys?" Ms. Jacobson modeled how to brainstorm ideas during the "pick my ideas" phase of writing (*Model It*). While modeling, she talked aloud about brainstorming, saying, "I have to let my mind be free. I will take my time, and a good idea will come to me." Ms. Jacobson thought aloud about her ideas on this topic and then decided that her topic sentence would agree that students should have to give toys to children who do not have any. She also modeled brainstorming reasons to support this topic sentence.

During the "organize my notes" phase, Ms. Jacobson modeled how to use the TREE graphic organizer, thinking aloud to develop the essay. Before starting, she set a goal of including all TREE components while writing. During this activity, the students participated by helping Ms. Jacobson plan and make notes for each part. After the "organize my notes" phase was complete, Ms. Jacobson modeled the "write and say more" step using the graphic organizer. She continued to think aloud on how to include the topic sentence, three or more reasons, and an ending. Ms. Jacobson also modeled the recursive nature of writing by making changes to her plan during the writing phase. She remembered to include transition words and used self-statements or questions to help herself organize, stay on task, and address negative self-statements. Ms. Jacobson included self-statements about problem definition ("What do I need to do?"), planning ("First, I need to think of a topic sentence"), self-evaluation ("Does this reason support the topic sentence?"), self-reinforcement ("That is a great reason!"), and coping ("I can do this"). After the first draft was written, the class examined the draft to check if all of the TREE components were present. Ms. Jacobson then verbally reinforced herself for reaching her goal and charted her progress on the graph.

Next, the class discussed the importance of the self-statements people, including Ms. Jacobson, make while writing. Some students offered examples of their own self-statements, and Ms. Jacobson asked the students to identify some self-statements she had made while she was writing. The students then brainstormed a list of positive self-statements.

Ms. Jacobson made sure to address the areas of problem definition, planning, self-evaluation, self-reinforcement, and coping. Each student developed his or her own positive self-statements and recorded them on a card to use while writing. Ms. Jacobson worked with the students in her class who tended to write very little to help them develop positive self-reinforcement and coping statements when discouraged or frustrated with the writing task.

The following day, Ms. Jacobson continued to model the POW + TREE strategy to write a persuasive essay about the topic "Should students have to go to school in the summer?" She followed the modeling procedures in the previous lesson, but in this lesson she encouraged students to take the lead as much as possible. While Ms. Jacobson modeled the process, the students wrote their own notes on a graphic organizer. The class worked through the POW + TREE strategy, focusing on both the process and the self-statements made during the writing process. After the class generated the notes for the paper, they reviewed them to see if they could add more. The students then wrote individual persuasive essays using the class-generated notes (*Support It*). A transition word chart was provided to help students use transition words in the persuasive essay. Ms. Jacobson also encouraged them to use their self-statements as they wrote.

To ensure student success during this phase of instruction (i.e., *Support It*), Ms. Jacobson individualized her support based on student needs. She encouraged more proficient writers to add million-dollar vocabulary words and examples to support their reasons. She conducted a small-group mini-lesson for the students with learning disabilities and the other struggling writers. She had noticed in previous lessons that they continued to require more modeling and support before they could try writing independently. During the mini-lesson, she intentionally forgot a strategy step, and the students discussed the impact and cause of errors. Ms. Jacobson knew these students frequently had difficulty remembering all of the steps of the writing task. She modeled how to remedy the problem and remain focused on the task rather than quitting. Another important lesson for these students was learning to focus on the important attributes of the writing task. Ms. Jacobson modeled how to pay attention to the steps of the POW + TREE writing strategy, rather than attending to the mechanical aspects of writing such as spelling and handwriting. She had seen in the past that many of her struggling writers had difficulty with spelling and handwriting and tended to focus their attention on these skills rather than the higher-level skills of planning and organizing. The small group worked together to generate a paper on the day's topic. At the end of the lesson, all students examined the paper and graphed their progress.

The next week consisted of more collaborative practice with several persuasive writing prompts (*Support It*). Ms. Jacobson continued to monitor individual student progress and provide small-group mini-lessons to children to individualize instruction based on student needs. For the students with learning disabilities, she gradually faded support from modeling the planning phase to reminders to use specific steps. She then faded more support by only providing prompts to pay attention to a specific step. After each paper was completed, students examined their essays and graphed their progress. She allowed students to work at their own pace, as she recognized that her students with learning disabilities required more time to finish a paper. After 2 weeks of practice, most students were proficient in writing a persuasive essay that had a topic sentence, three or more reasons, and a good ending. The students with learning disabilities still required cue cards, transition word charts, and self-statement cards to move through the writing process, but they now required less teacher assistance. At this point, Ms. Jacobson weaned her higher-performing students from the graphic organizers and the graphing process. She taught them how to take notes on blank paper by writing the POW + TREE reminder at the top of the page rather than using the graphic organizer. She also modeled how to make a space for notes on each part of the TREE writing prompt.

Once her students were able to list and describe the POW + TREE components and write a persuasive essay with all of the parts, Ms. Jacobson ended her unit on persuasive writing with two transfer tasks (*Independent Practice*). Before starting the last phase of instruction, she asked the writing partners to share ways they had transferred the POW + TREE writing strategy or some part of it in the last several weeks. Students provided examples of situations in which they were able to transfer the strategy and examples of unsuccessful attempts to transfer the strategy. In the first transfer task, the students read a short story about the Little Red Hen. At the end of the story, Ms. Jacobson asked, "Would you have helped the Little Red Hen? Write a paper telling why or why not." The class discussed whether the POW + TREE writing strategy would work for this paper and the similarities to and differences from previous prompts. At the end of the discussion, the class determined that the POW + TREE strategy would work for this paper. The students worked independently on this writing task, and Ms. Jacobson provided individual support as needed.

The last lesson in the unit focused on individualizing the prompts and self-statements. Ms. Jacobson wanted her students to personalize the strategy in useful ways and to realize that the action plan was flexible and modifiable based on the specifics of the writing task. The class discussed how to improve the strategy and shared with each other the parts that worked best for them. Ms. Jacobson realized that some of her stronger students were able to drop steps of the strategy and still write proficient papers, but some of her struggling writers, especially the students with learning disabilities, continued to require much of the support provided by the graphic organizers. The students were no longer required to use the goal-setting and progress-monitoring pieces but were encouraged to continue using them if necessary to help them meet their goals. As a final writing assignment, the class completed the second transfer task based on a story about the Roman hero Hercules. At the end of the story, Ms. Jacobson asked, "Should Hercules help the old man? Write a paper telling why or why not." After the persuasive essay was finished, the class celebrated their success in learning to write a good persuasive essay and agreed to participate in review sessions to help promote maintenance and generalization.

How SRSD Addressed Problems in Executive Function and Facilitated Its Development

SRSD includes instructional procedures that address problems in executive function, as defined earlier in this chapter. Specifically, SRSD addresses the following aspects of executive function: analysis, decision making and planning, execution and coordination of mental and affective resources, attentional control, and flexible adaptation. The next section provides a representative sample of common instructional procedures included in SRSD (as applied by Ms. Jacobson) that address aspects of executive function involved in the writing process.

Analysis

An important aspect of analysis in writing involves defining the problem and identifying the necessary elements of the task. SRSD incorporates such task analysis by explicitly teaching students how to define the problem and the elements of a writing task. Ms. Jacobson discussed the goals of persuasive writing during the *Develop Background Knowledge* and *Discuss It* stages. The elements of persuasive writing were compared and contrasted to the elements of narrative writing, a previously mastered genre. This discussion helped students identify situations in which writing a persuasive paper using the TREE strategy would be appropriate. Next, Ms. Jacobson modeled how to define the problem and identify the elements of the task specific to persuasive writing (*Model It* stage). Students were then given opportunities to practice these skills during the *Support It* and *Independent Practice* stages of SRSD. Ms. Jacobson had noted that her students with learning disabilities tended to writing immediately begin, before defining the problem and identifying the elements of the writing task, and were thus unable to determine an appropriate approach to the task. Discussing, modeling, and supporting task analysis were critical for these struggling writers to help them differentiate among the elements of different writing tasks.

Generalization and transfer of task analysis were promoted by having students work with writing partners to identify elements of other writing tasks that lent themselves to using all or part of POW + TREE. Each day, the writing partners met to discuss previous opportunities to transfer their strategies to another writing task. During this time, the partners helped each other identify the elements of writing tasks that were appropriate for using all or part of the POW + TREE writing strategy. The writing partners were encouraged to define the problem of a specific writing task and to analyze whether the strategy would work.

Decision Making and Planning

Decision making and planning in writing require goal setting, making a decision to plan, exploring possible approaches and outcomes, and selecting or devising a plan of action. These skills are critical for skilled writing; however, they can be overwhelming to students with learning disabilities who already face a taxing cognitive load. The handwriting and spelling demands for these students are often so demanding that their decision-making and planning abilities are minimized (McCutchen, 1988). SRSD's instructional procedures explicitly model decision-making and planning skills while scaffolding instruction until students are able to perform these tasks independently.

Ms. Jacobson addressed goal setting before starting persuasive writing instruction. She held individual conferences with the students with learning disabilities and her other struggling writers, in which they discussed their previous approaches to persuasive writing and began the process of setting goals to learn the strategy. For the students with learning disabilities, this process highlighted the contrast between their previous ineffective approaches and the new approach, providing an incentive for students to buy into the benefits of the strategy. With the entire class, Ms. Jacobson introduced goal setting throughout the SRSD process. Students set a goal to learn the POW + TREE strategy and engaged in daily practice to learn and describe the strategy components and to include all of the parts in their persuasive essay (*Memorize It*; *Discuss It*). Ms. Jacobson also promoted flexible goal setting by encouraging students to modify their goals as they became more proficient in using the strategy. This process of goal setting helped boost motivation and increase persistence for the struggling writers (Graham & Harris, 1994).

SRSD also includes a series of steps that encourage students to be deliberate in their prewriting phase. Many beginning writers fail to plan or to consider the organization of their essay (Graham & Harris, 1997; Hillocks, 1984). Ms. Jacobson explicitly modeled how to make a decision to plan, explore possible approaches, and then select a plan of action (POW + TREE) to write a persuasive essay. Again, students were given opportunities to master these planning skills during the *Support It* and *Independent Practice* stages of SRSD. This action plan is especially powerful for students with learning disabilities and other struggling writers, who often approach academic tasks in an ineffective or inefficient manner (Harris, 1982), and increases the likelihood that students will incorporate the planning strategy into their existing writing routine (Graham & Harris, 2005b).

Execution and Coordination of Mental and Affective Resources

Writing tasks are inherently complex and require planning, drafting, and revising skills, all of which depend on basic reading, language, spelling, and handwriting skills, as well as knowledge, metacognition, attitudes, motivation, and memory processes (Abbott & Berninger, 1993; Hayes, 1996; Hayes & Flower, 1980; Kellogg, 1987; Scardamalia & Bereiter, 1987). In addition, each written composition is framed by the expected genre, goals, and needs of its audience. SRSD incorporates instructional procedures to support the execution and orchestration of cognitive, metacognitive, and affective resources necessary to carry out multiple demands in writing tasks.

Ms. Jacobson made sure students had the skills and knowledge needed to executive the strategy effectively. (*Develop Background Knowledge*) she introduced the goals and components of a good persuasive essay, as well as important vocabulary words such as *fact, opinion,* and *persuade.* This knowledge of the task was further strengthened during the *Model It, Support It,* and *Independent Practice* stages as students received help writing persuasive essays.

Another way SRSD strengthens execution and orchestration of resources is by incorporating several stages of strategy development. Students memorize the strategy, observe it modeled several times, receive scaffolded support based on individual needs, and engage in independent practice once the strategy has been mastered. This process improves students' knowledge of how to write a good persuasive essay and is designed to support them until they are able to be successful on their own. SRSD is both individualized and criterion-based, meaning that students receive instruction tailored to their needs and do not proceed to the next stage until they have met criteria for doing so. Ms. Jacobson addressed this requirement by allowing students to work at their own pace and conducting mini-lessons with small groups of children who required similar support. For the struggling writers, mini-lessons featured more modeling and support, while mini-lessons for higher-performing students taught more advanced skills.

SRSD also incorporates self-regulation components, which are thought to be important in skilled writing due to the complexity of the writing process (Zimmerman & Riesemberg, 1997). Ms. Jacobson modeled and taught the use of self-statements to monitor and regulate cognitive, metacognitive, and affective resources, addressing the areas of problem definition, planning, self-evaluation, self-reinforcement, and coping. Students were further encouraged to personalize their self-statements to their problem areas. Ms. Jacobson worked with the students with learning disabilities to help them first develop self-statements related to self-reinforcement and coping, since she had seen that these students had negative attitudes about writing and gave up easily. Once these students were able to sustain effort throughout the writing task, they added other self-statements related to the cognitive and metacognitive aspects of the task, such as problem definition and planning.

Attentional Control

Due to the complexity of writing, attentional control is an important component of the composing process. Skilled writers delay responding and put aside typical approaches that may be ineffective. They must also inhibit interfering behaviors and focus on the important attributes of the task. Finally, they must be able to sustain their effort and attention throughout the writing process.

Ms. Jacobson noticed that many of the students with learning disabilities had difficulty sustaining effort and attention while writing. Students with learning disabilities and other struggling writers often have difficulties with transcription skills, such as handwriting and spelling (Graham, Harris, MacArthur, & Schwartz, 1991), which consume a great deal of attention while composing (Berninger, 1999; Graham, 1999; Graham & Harris, 2000). Having to concentrate on the mechanical aspects of writing inhibits students' abilities to focus on the planning and content generation of the paper (Graham, Schwartz, & MacArthur, 1993). This focus on transcription skills leads students to judge writing quality as good handwriting and spelling rather than the organization and substance of the paper (Graham, 1992; Graham et al., 1993).

The instructional procedures in SRSD helped Ms. Jacobson strengthen her students' attentional control. She started by asking students to make a commitment to learn the new strategy. She emphasized that learning a new strategy requires substantial effort. At this time, she also stressed the benefits of learning the strategy to motivate students throughout the process. She provided a supportive environment by expressing her belief that all students would be able to learn the strategy and write good persuasive essays. As students progressed through SRSD stages, they charted their progress, which enabled them to see the benefits of using the strategy. Their motivation to continue using the strategy increased, thereby improving their ability to maintain attentional focus.

The use of specific strategies such as POW + TREE increases student attention to the essential components of the writing task. Using the graphic organizer for TREE taught students to focus on the essential components: the topic sentence, reasons supporting the topic sentence, and a good ending. It also directed students to examine their paper afterward to ensure that all of the parts were present. Ms. Jacobson addressed students' concerns about good handwriting and spelling by incorporating a draft process in which they were able to rewrite their paper to improve the spelling and handwriting. Students were able to maintain their focus on the essential components of the writing task, knowing that they could rewrite their paper later.

While students were learning the persuasive writing strategy, Ms. Jacobson provided visual cues, prompts, and cue cards, along with graphic organizers and graphing sheets to help them maneuver through the writing process. As they became more proficient in their ability to manage this process, Ms. Jacobson slowly removed the visual supports and taught students to make their own cues and prompts.

The use of personalized self-statements also helped students improve their attentional control. Ms. Jacobson first modeled the use of self-statements on problem definition, planning, self-evaluation, self-reinforcement, and coping. She then led a discussion about the benefits of self-statements and had students develop their own to address individual challenges. Ms. Jacobson made sure that the students with learning disabilities and other struggling writers had simple self-statements that addressed sustaining effort and positive reinforcement, as she had noticed that these students tended to have a negative attitude about writing and were therefore prone to giving up quickly. The students reviewed their self-statements each lesson, and the self-statements were always available to them while they were writing. Ms. Jacobson continued to model the use of self-statements during whole-group and small-group mini-lessons to demonstrate how they could help students focus on the writing process.

Flexible Adaptation

The writing process requires flexible adaptation; skilled writers monitor, evaluate, and modify their use of specific writing strategies based on their past and present success (Zimmerman & Riesemberg, 1997). Writing plans and goals may need to be adjusted to meet changing situations or new information. Flexible adaptation is also essential for transfer and generalization of strategy use.

Ms. Jacobson's use of SRSD to teach several different writing strategies addressed flexible adaptation in several ways. First, Ms. Jacobson explicitly taught transfer by linking the general planning strategy (POW) to a new genre-specific strategy (TREE). Students in her class had previously learned to use POW with narrative writing and were able to transfer this strategy to a new genre. Using the same general writing strategy to teach multiple genre styles greatly enhanced her students' ability to monitor, evaluate, and adapt the strategy in several writing situations.

Second, Ms. Jacobson set up writing partners to help focus students on using all or part of POW + TREE in writing situations outside of the persuasive writing instruction. The writing partners dedicated the first part of each day's lesson to brainstorming and discussing ways to transfer their learned strategies to other writing tasks. The partners also made goals of helping each other remember to use the strategies and providing assistance in using the strategies, if necessary. The pairing of higher-performing students with lower-performing students helped ensure that at least one student in the pair would be able to recognize other writing tasks in which to apply the strategy.

Third, students graphed their progress as they continued to master the use of the strategy. Students had set goals to write a good persuasive essay with all of the parts included, and graphing helped them monitor their ability to meet their goals. Students who did not meet their goals could work on adapting the strategy or changing their use of it to be more successful next time. Students who met their goals were encouraged to set new goals to improve their next persuasive essay.

Finally, Ms. Jacobson incorporated transfer tasks within her instruction to promote her students' ability flexibly to adapt the POW + TREE strategy to similar persuasive writing tasks. In addition to the transfer tasks, Ms. Jacobson worked with students to personalize their strategy use by determining the parts of the strategy that worked most effectively for them and to modify the strategy as necessary.

CONCLUSION

In our opinion, a major strength of the SRSD model is that it supports the development of a variety of executive function skills that are essential to becoming a skilled writer. For those who are interested in an additional example of how SRSD addresses executive function issues, we refer you to a previous chapter of ours, which addresses how SRSD addresses problems in executive function, attention, and memory within the context of teaching a sophisticated report-writing strategy (Graham & Harris, 1996). If you are interested in additional information on SRSD or effective writing strategies, please see Graham and Harris (2005b).

REFERENCES

Abbott, R. D., & Berninger, V. W. (1993). Structural equation modeling of relationships among developmental skills and writing skills in primary- and intermediate-grade writers. *Journal of Educational Psychology, 85,* 478–508.

Bereiter, C., & Scardamalia, M. (1987). *The psychology of written composition.* Hillsdale, NJ: Erlbaum.

Berninger, V. W. (1999). Coordinating transcription and text generation in working memory during composing: Automatic and constructive processes. *Learning Disabilities Quarterly, 22,* 99–112.

De La Paz, S., Swanson, P., & Graham, S. (1998). The contribution of executive control to the revising of students with writing and learning difficulties. *Journal of Educational Psychology, 90,* 448–460.

Durst, R., & Newell, G. (1989). The uses of function: James Britton's category system and research on writing. *Review of Educational Research, 59,* 375–394.

Graham, S. (1982). Composition research and practice: A unified approach. *Focus on Exceptional Children, 14,* 1–16.

Graham, S. (1990). The role of production factors in learning disabled students' compositions. *Journal of Educational Psychology, 82,* 781–791.

Graham, S. (1992). Issues in handwriting instruction. *Focus on Exceptional Children, 25,* 1–14.

Graham, S. (1997). Executive control in the revising of students with learning and writing difficulties. *Journal of Educational Psychology, 89,* 223–234.

Graham, S. (1999). Handwriting and spelling instruction for students with learning disabilities: A review. *Learning Disability Quarterly, 22,* 78–98.

Graham, S. (2006a). Writing. In P. Alexander & P. Winne (Eds.), *Handbook of educational psychology* (pp. 457–478). New York: Guilford Press.

Graham, S. (2006b). Strategy instruction and the teaching of writing. In C. MacArthur, S. Graham, & J. Fitzgerald (Eds.), *Handbook of writing research* (pp. 187–207). New York: Guilford Press.

Graham, S., & Harris, K. R. (1994). The role and development of self-regulation in the writing process. In D. Schunk & B. Zimmerman (Eds.), *Self-regulation of learning and performance: Issues and educational application* (pp. 203–328). New York: Erlbaum.

Graham, S., & Harris, K.R. (1996). Addressing problems in attention, memory, and executive functioning: An example from Self-Regulated Strategy Development. In R. Lyon & N. Krasnegor (Eds.), *Attention, memory, and executive function* (pp. 349–365). Baltimore: Brookes.

Graham, S., & Harris, K. R. (1997). Self-regulation and writing: Where do we go from here? *Contemporary Educational Psychology 22*, 102–114.

Graham, S., & Harris, K. R. (2000). The role of self-regulation and transcription skills in writing and writing development. *Educational Psychologist, 35*, 3–12.

Graham. S., & Harris, K. R. (2003). Students with learning disabilities and the process of writing: A meta-analysis of SRSD studies. In L. Swanson, K. R. Harris, & S. Graham (Eds.), *Handbook of research on learning disabilities* (pp. 383–402). New York: Guilford Press.

Graham, S., & Harris, K. R. (2005a). Improving the writing performance of young struggling writers: Theoretical and programmatic research from the center on accelerating student learning. *Journal of Special Education, 39*, 19–33.

Graham, S., & Harris, K. R. (2005b). *Writing better: Teaching writing processes and self-regulation to students with learning problems*. Baltimore: Brookes.

Graham, S., Harris, K. R., MacArthur, C. A., & Schwartz, S. (1991). Writing and writing instruction with students with learning disabilities: A review of a program of research. *Learning Disability Quarterly, 14*, 89–114.

Graham, S., Harris, K. R., & Mason, L. (2005). Improving the writing performance, knowledge, and motivation of struggling young writers: The effects of Self-Regulated Strategy Development. *Contemporary Educational Psychology, 30*, 207–241.

Graham, S., & Perrin, D. (2006). *Writing next: Effective strategies to improve writing of adolescents in middle and high school*. Washington, DC: Alliance for Excellence in Education.

Graham, S., Schwartz, S., & MacArthur, C. (1993). Learning disabled and normally achieving students' knowledge of writing and the composing process, attitude toward writing, and self-efficacy for students with and without learning disabilities. *Journal of Learning Disabilities, 26*, 237–249.

Harris, K. R. (1982). Cognitive-behavioral modification: Application with exceptional students. *Focus on Exceptional Children, 15*, 1–16.

Harris, K. R., & Graham, S. (1996). *Making the writing process work: Strategies for composition and self-regulation*. Cambridge, MA: Brookline.

Hayes, J. R. (1996). A new framework for understanding cognition and affect in writing. In C. M. Levy & S. Ransdell (Eds.), *The science of writing: Theories, methods, individual differences, and applications* (pp. 1–27). Mahway, NJ: Erlbaum.

Hayes, J. R., & Flower, L. S. (1980). Identifying the organization of the writing process. In L. W. Gregg & E. R. Steinberg (Eds.), *Cognitive processes in writing* (pp. 3–30). Hillsdale, NJ: Erlbaum.

Hillocks, G. (1984). What works in teaching composition: A meta-analysis of experimental treatment studies. *American Journal of Education, 93,* 133–170.

Hooper, S., Swartz, C., Wakely, M., de Kruif, R., & Montgomery, J. (2002). Executive functioning in elementary school children with and without problems in written expression. *Journal of Learning Disabilities, 35,* 57–68.

Kellogg, R. T. (1987). Effects of topic knowledge on the allocation of processing time and cognitive effort to writing processes. *Memory and Cognition, 15,* 256–266.

MacArthur, C., Graham, S., & Fitzgerald, J. (Eds.). (2006). *Handbook of writing research.* New York: Guilford Press.

McCutchen, D. (1988). Functional automaticity in children's writing: A problem in metacognitive control. *Written Communication, 5,* 306–324.

National Commission on Writing (2004). *Writing: A ticket to work . . . or a ticket out—A survey of business leaders.* New York: College Board.

National Commission on Writing. (2005). *Writing: A powerful message from state government.* New York: College Board.

Persky, H., Daane, M., & Jin, Y. (2003). *National assessment of educational progress: 2002 report card for the nation and the states.* Washington, DC: U.S. Department of Education.

Scardamalia, M., & Bereiter, C. (1983). The development of evaluative, diagnostic, and remedial capabilities in children's composing. In M. Martlew (Ed.), *The psychology of written language: Development and educational perspectives* (pp. 67–95). New York: Wiley.

Scardamalia, M., & Bereiter, C. (1985). Development of dialectical process in composition. In D. Olson, N. Torrance, & A. Hildyard (Eds.), *Literacy, language, and learning: The nature and consequences of reading and writing* (pp. 307–329). Cambridge, UK: Cambridge University Press).

Scardamalia, M., & Bereiter, C. (1987). Knowledge telling and knowledge transforming in written composition. In S. Rosenberg (Ed.), *Advances in applied psycholinguistics: Reading, writing, and language learning* (Vol. 2, pp. 142–175). New York: Cambridge University Press.

Swedlow, J. (1999). The power of writing. *National Geographic, 196,* 110–132.

Thomas, C., Englert, C., & Gregg, S. (1987). An analysis of errors and strategies in the expository writing of learning disabled students. *Remedial and Special Education, 8,* 21–30.

Zimmerman, B. J., & Riesemberg, R. (1997). Becoming a self-regulated writer: A social cognitive perspective. *Contemporary Educational Psychology, 22,* 73–101.

CHAPTER 11

The Strategic Math Classroom
*Executive Function Processes
and Mathematics Learning*

**BETHANY N. RODITI
JOAN STEINBERG**

Before learning the strategies to become a successful math student, the equations and formulas were scattered in my head and did not have a place to go. Luckily, after learning to use three-column notes and other techniques, I was able to sort them into little "file cabinets" in my head.
—EMILY, NINTH GRADER (cited in Meltzer et al., 2006, p. 95)

EXECUTIVE FUNCTION PROCESSES IN TODAY'S MATH CLASSROOM

In an educational era that emphasizes problem solving and meaningful instruction, there has been a significant increase in the number of tasks that require students to plan, initiate, organize, prioritize, shift, and check their work. These executive function processes are particularly important for effective learning in the math classroom. Students need to come to class prepared, complete and pass in homework, take organized notes, study efficiently, and perform well on tests. These executive function processes generally do not come naturally to many math students, especially students with learning and attention difficulties (Brownell, Mellard, & Deshler, 1993; Bull, Johnston, & Roy, 1999; Bull & Scerif, 2001; Geary, 1990; Mazzocco & Myers, 2003; Meltzer et al., 1996, 2006; Miller & Mercer, 1997; Montague & Marger, 1997; Pressley, 1995). Further, these students often lack math skills and strategies as well as the motivation and confidence needed for success in the mathematics classroom. Providing students with systematic and strategic instruction and teaching them how to utilize accommodations effectively in the classroom are essential to enable them to navigate the math curriculum. In this chapter, we discuss the impact of executive function and dysfunction in the mathematics classroom, with a particular focus on students with learning disabilities and attention problems.

Trends in Math Teaching: From Rote Memory to Meaning

The ongoing theoretical debate between using a rote mathematics instructional model and a meaningful instructional paradigm affects students who struggle with executive function processes. Teaching styles have changed to address the new math curriculum trends, but these new styles do not necessarily accommodate those students who cannot independently generate the structures, templates, and self-regulation strategies they need to learn effectively in the math classroom (Miller & Mercer, 1997; Montague, Warger, & Morgan, 2000). In fact, a number of studies have shown that curricula and methods of instruction can have a significant impact on the math performance of students with learning disabilities and attention problems (Baroody & Hume, 1991; Carnine, 1997; Miller & Mercer, 1997).

Back in the 1960s and 1970s, when math curricula reflected a rote instructional paradigm, teachers provided math rules, algorithms, and step-by-step procedures using direct instruction. They often stood up in front of the class, lecturing and writing the steps for math problem solving on the board. They assigned worksheets for homework and, the following day, reviewed the homework with the class, problem by problem. Then they collected the homework, graded it, and wrote comments on each student's paper. The teachers developed their own tests that mimicked the skills and strategies that they taught directly in class. In these traditional math classrooms, the teachers acted as the executives, providing math instruction in a structured, systematic way within highly organized classroom environments. Therefore, it is not surprising that students were not identified as having executive function difficulties at that time.

In 2000, for the first time, the National Council of Teachers of Mathematics composed new national standards for the mathematics curriculum that embody a blend of rote and meaningful instructional approaches in math (National Council of Teachers of Mathematics, 2000). Currently, students are expected to be "reasonably computationally fluent" (Russell, 2000), and, at the same time, they must learn how to apply these computational skills to solve higher-level mathematical problems. Within a constructivist paradigm, students who have difficulties with executive function processes are more vulnerable than others to experiencing difficulty in discovering their own mathematical conjectures as well as remembering and internalizing all the steps necessary for meaningful problem solving. These students have difficulty organizing knowledge for themselves because they need scaffolds and templates to help them learn how to learn. If they struggle for too long in the math classroom, they begin to develop "learned helplessness" (Diener & Dweck, 1978) and no longer have the motivation to engage in learning mathematics. That is, they no longer have what Moran and Gardner (Chapter 2, this volume) describe as the "will" or "skill" to go up the "hill." Therefore, a major challenge facing math teachers today is how to provide an open structure for meaningful problem solving and, at the same time, the systematic, strategic scaffolds necessary for students with executive function processes who struggle to learn in the math classroom.

Meaningful Problem Solving

Math problem solving involves a four-step approach (Polya, 1957): *understanding* the problem, *organizing a plan*, *operationalizing* the plan, and *reflecting* on the product and the process. Polya's system incorporates multisensory approaches and strategies for math problem solving. The challenge for the teacher is how to make these problem-solving steps explicit for students who have difficulty with the metacognitive processes that are critical for effective problem solving (Meltzer et al., 1996, 2006; Montague et al., 2000). These students need to be taught about the underlying concepts and structures of math problems (Hutchinson, 1993; Xin, Jitendra, & Deatline-Buchman, 2005), and they need explicit "roadmaps" for the process of solving word problems from the initial conceptualization to the solution.

Mathematical *word problems* are particularly difficult for students with executive function weaknesses. When students are presented with word problems to solve, they must first read and understand what the problem is asking. They then have to make a plan and select a strategy, such as a list, table, or chart, to help them organize and solve the problem. They must also translate the words into meaningful numbers and operations, determine the relevant information, hold words and numbers in working memory, control their impulsivity and self-monitor for accuracy and feasibility, and shift to a different strategy if they discover errors. After solving word problems, teachers require them to communicate their answers and the process they have used for problem solving and to reflect on whether or not their solutions make sense.

In general, students with executive function weaknesses, math learning difficulties, and/or attention problems often struggle with both the input and the output of new knowledge and skills. Much of their success in these areas is dependent on *how* the information is presented and how they are asked to show what they know when learning complex quantitative concepts and solving higher-level math problems. They benefit from direct, explicit math instruction on how to solve problems using rules, schemas, and strategies (Fuchs & Fuchs, 2005; Meltzer et al., 1996, 2006; Montague et al., 2000; Xin et al., 2005).

MATH STRATEGIES THAT ADDRESS EXECUTIVE FUNCTION

Though several studies have cited the effectiveness of strategy and schema-based instruction in mathematics (Harris & Graham, 1992; Montague et al., 2000; Xin et al., 2005), teachers face the challenge of how to translate theory into practice in their math classrooms. Math strategies can be taught explicitly as students follow various pathways of math problem solving from beginning to end. Incorporating math strategies and schemas into the problem-solving process utilizes a step-by-step approach and requires systematic documentation. This direct strategy instruction along with documentation helps students with executive weaknesses initially to apply strategies with teacher modeling and assistance, to internalize strategies gradually, and ultimately to use strategies independently. Though teachers can provide a menu of multisensory strategies to the entire math class, they may have to make accommodations for students with executive function weaknesses. These students need individual assistance in choosing the strategies that match their learning styles and that address specific types of math problems. Further, they need direct instruction to learn how to record the strategies in a usable form in their math strategy notebooks (Meltzer et al., 1996, 2006). The executive processes of remembering, organizing, shifting, prioritizing, and checking are all essential to higher-level math success. The following sections discuss specific strategies in each of these areas.

Memory Strategies

Memory strategies are important for automatic math fact recall, memorizing the order of operations, and remembering the overall steps in the problem-solving process. These strategies are especially critical for students with executive function difficulties, who tend to become overwhelmed by numerous details. Several studies have linked math performance with executive function skills, in particular with working memory weaknesses (Bull et al., 1999; Bull & Scerif, 2001; Geary, 1990; Miyake et al., 2000; Swanson, 1993).

Checklists, acronyms, and templates are memory strategies that are particularly helpful for students with executive function weaknesses to bypass their learning and attention problems. Examples of multisensory memory strategies are described below.

Verbal Strategies

Acronyms such as PEMDAS (see Figure 11.1) help students remember the steps in the order of operations in pre-algebra and initiate the process of math problem solving or computation. These types of verbal strategies, while helpful to all students, are essential for students with executive function weaknesses, who often do not know where to begin in terms of solving algebraic operations. Providing students with acronyms or verbal strategies such as PEMDAS helps them remember the important details and steps that can make a major difference in their performance and result in success. When students attempt to solve algebraic equations without a strategy, their answers are often wrong and result in students' confusion because of their inability to remember the order of operations.

Another example of a verbal strategy for overall math problem solving that incorporates remembering key words, operations, and steps

---

PEMDAS Acronym: Memory strategy for remembering the sequence of steps for simplifying algebraic equations

Parentheses

Exponents

Multiplication

Division

Addition

Subtraction

FIGURE 11.1. "Please Excuse My Dear Aunt Sally: PEMDAS."

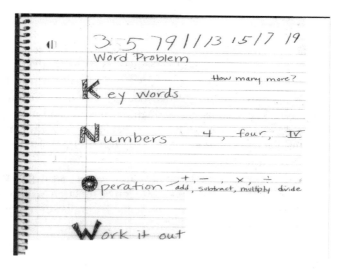

FIGURE 11.2. Example of a math roadmap: KNOW.

in problem solving is KNOW. Figure 11.2 is an example of a student's math strategy notebook page where the KNOW strategy is recorded as a means to remember the important problem-solving steps.

Memory strategies are also particularly helpful for learning math facts. Many students experience math difficulties because they cannot easily store and retrieve arithmetic facts from long-term memory (Garnett & Fleischner, 1983; Geary, Harrison, & Hoard, 2000; Jordan & Montani, 1997; Ostad, 1997). Some benefit from learning a rhyme for a particular fact, and others rely on visual or hands-on strategies. For students with executive function weaknesses, it is important both to practice the strategy and to record it in their math strategy notebooks.

Visual Strategies

Some math performance deficits are associated with deficits in visual–spatial competencies (Geary, 2004; McLean & Hitch, 1999). Combining visual strategies with verbal strategies can enhance conceptual understanding, attention, and memory. Further, when students record a rhyme in a math strategy notebook, the verbal strategy is reinforced visually, can be used for future reference, and helps them bypass long-term-memory problems.

Another example of a visual strategy is a drawing of a group of items, a cartoon, or an array for remembering math concepts and procedures, in the case of Figure 11.3, a problem that is based on multiplication and/or division. The advantage of this strategy is that math students with executive function problems can focus on *one* model, a visual representation that scaffolds across multiple content areas, from multiplication to division, fractions, decimals, percentages, and algebra. By grounding their knowledge in a mathematical array or area model, they can retrieve this one mathematical schema to help them initiate the problem-solving process.

Another visual model for multiplication is the "stoplight strategy" (Schroeder & Washington, 1989). Here, a picture of a stoplight is used for the 3x table. The red light signifies the facts $3 \times 1 = 3$, $3 \times 2 = 6$, $3 \times 3 = 9$. In a variation of the strategy developed at the Institute for Learning and Development, students are told that these facts are for younger children, who are "stopped" from doing particular activities and have more limits than older children. The yellow light facts, $3 \times 4 = 12$, $3 \times 5 = 15$, and $3 \times 6 = 18$, are the "teen facts." Teenagers have more permission than younger children but are still encouraged to slow down. Finally, the "green facts," $3 \times 7 = 21$, $3 \times 8 = 24$, and $3 \times 9 = 27$, are for adults in their 20s who have a green light and rely on their own judgment. In a graphical way, students learn to group the red facts, yellow facts, and green facts and can reduce the burden on their long-term memory by linking the fact to prerequisite knowledge relating to life experience in the form of a story and color.

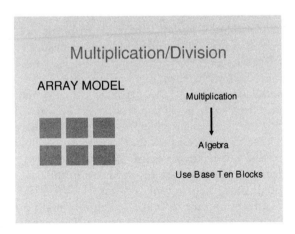

FIGURE 11.3. An array or area model, a visual representation of the multiplication problem, $2 \times 3 = 6$.

Hands-On Strategies

Many students benefit from strategies that are hands on as well as visual
and verbal. One strategy for remembering 7 × 7 is both visual and
hands-on. Students bend pipe cleaners, changing the two 7's into a 4
and a 9, rather than drawing the numbers or arrays in their notebooks
(Schroeder & Washington, 1989). The 2 × 3 array represented in Figure
11.3 can also be taught as a hands-on strategy by having students
manipulate cubes, tiles, or any discrete objects in order to represent multiplication problems in an array format.

In summary, multisensory memory strategies—verbal, visual, and
hands-on—can help students with executive function difficulties and can
be easily incorporated into the math classroom. One critical component
is for students to document the specific strategies that they find useful in
a math strategy notebook. By doing so, they compensate for weaknesses
in working memory, long-term memory, and automatic retrieval, processes that are essential when solving math problems. Over time, they
develop and internalize their own strategies, which become their habits
of problem solving through guided practice, repetition, and consistent
strategy use.

Organizing Strategies

Students with executive function difficulties often become so overwhelmed that they cannot organize the important information necessary
to solve math problems. These students with weak organizational skills,
math learning disabilities, and/or attention problems need roadmaps,
direct strategy instruction, and guided practice to ensure effective strategy use (Miller & Mercer, 1997; Swanson, 2000). They need direct strategy instruction to help them learn how to differentiate relevant and irrelevant information so that they can organize the information enabling
them to initiate the problem-solving process. They often do not know
how to begin to solve a math problem, resulting in impulsive and inaccu-
rate attempts that mislead teachers and parents into thinking that students are lazy and not trying to learn. It is not that they will not pay
attention to learning but that they cannot learn in the way the information is presented; thus, their output is minimal. When they embark on
their problem-solving journey to find a solution to math problems, they
need roadmaps to plan and organize their route. The math strategy notebook becomes a critical tool that assists them with organizing key information and reminds them of usable math strategies that can assist in the
problem-solving process.

Using Lists, Charts, and Tables

Vocabulary lists, charts, and tables recorded in a math strategy notebook assist students with executive function weaknesses to analyze and organize the language of math problems. Verbal cues in the strategy notebook help them understand what a problem is asking (see Table 11.1). Once the information is organized in this way, they can begin to shift from words to numbers, from planning to problem solving.

Roadmaps for Organizing Information for Math Problem Solving

One example of a math strategy that helps compensate for poor organizational skills is RAPS, a road map for math problem solving (Meltzer et al., 1996, 2006; see Figure 11.4).

Once the students have set their goal as solving a math problem (which in itself is a challenge for students with weak executive function) they must read the problem with understanding (R), so they may have to *reread and rephrase* the information. They may draw out the problem in such a way that the pictorial representation helps them in the planning phase of problem solving. Many students need to learn how to depict a problem in an *artistic* way (A), which helps them think about possible strategies for solving it. Some students with executive function weaknesses, learning disabilities, and attention problems, especially those who are not cognitively flexible, tend to be impulsive at this point. Working memory, along with poor attention control and the inability to inhibit irrelevant information, can also affect their math learning and problem solving (Geary, 2004). These students tend to select an approach randomly rather than think of all the possibilities and select the most relevant. They must estimate and then calculate. They have to *pre-*

TABLE 11.1. Translating Words to Mathematical Operations

Addition	Subtraction	Multiplication	Division
All together	Take away	Each has	Share
Total	Less than	The group	Dealing cards
In all	Lost	All together	Each one has?
Got more	How much left?	Getting bigger	Getting smaller
Sum	Difference	Product	Quotient

Name_____
Date _____

R A P S

R ead and **R** ephrase

A rt

P lan and Predict

S olve

FIGURE 11.4. Roadmap for problem solving.

dict the outcome so that they can evaluate their progress in the problem-solving process and the meaningfulness of the answer (*P*). Then they must shift once again in case the answer does not make sense. Finally, they *solve* the problem using the procedural knowledge they have learned, always mindful of the meaning behind the numbers (*S*). Thus, the RAPS roadmap is one example of a directly taught math strategy that is critical for students with executive function difficulties as it helps them focus on salient details and employ an organized approach to solving math problems.

Three-Column Note Taking

The math application of Triple Note Tote (BrainCogs; Research Institute for Learning and Development & FableVision, 2005), three-column note taking, is an extremely helpful organizing strategy. Because students with executive function weaknesses often have difficulty distinguishing relevant from irrelevant information, they feel barraged with massive amounts of detail in which they cannot find usable information (Meltzer & Krishnan, Chapter 5, this volume)

Three-column note taking (see Table 11.2) is a powerful tool if students with executive function problems are taught how to create the template, how to embed their own words into the definitions and rules, and how to use it as a study tool. Students may benefit from recording details about the use of a given strategy in their strategy notebooks (see Figure 11.5).

TABLE 11.2. Example of Three-Column Note Taking or Triple Note Tote, in a Math Strategy Notebook

Term	Definition	Example
Fraction	Part of a whole or a group	2/6, 6 pieces total *** I get 2 pieces out of 6 total or 2/6 ***
Decimal	Another way to write a fraction	2/6 = 2 divided by 6 = .33 = 33/100
Percent	Part of a hundred	33/100 means 33%
LCD (lowest common denominator)	Lowest number both denominators "go into"	LCD of 1/3 and 3/5 is 15

What is a Math Strategy Notebook: Triple Note Tote?

It is a way to keep your math facts, rules, schemas, and steps organized.
It is a way to make studying for math tests easier.

When do I use it?

• In class, when you take notes.
• At homework time, to record important concepts, vocabulary rules, and schemas.
• At study time, when you are preparing for a test or quiz.

How do I use it?

First column: Write down the math term, equation, or concept you want to know.
Second column: Read the meaning of the term but write it in your own words.
Third column: Write or draw a strategy or schema that will help you remember the information in the first two columns.
Study by reviewing all three columns.
Cover up the middle column and test yourself by looking at Column 1 and/or 3.

FIGURE 11.5. The "what, when, and how" for Triple Note Tote.

Shifting Strategies

To solve a math problem, students must shift their thinking from one numerical representation to another and, at the same time, retain the meaning of the numbers as they relate to the specific problem. Thus, students must shift flexibly from words to numbers, specifically from letters, words, and sentences in word problems to numbers, operations, algorithms, and equations. Math students with executive function weaknesses that negatively affect inhibition and working memory find it difficult to shift sets flexibly and to preserve the meaningfulness of the number representations as they problem-solve (Bull & Scerif, 2001; Miyake et al., 2000). Math instruction needs to ensure that students can switch sets while they construct, connect, decipher, and communicate their multiple representations of mathematical ideas (National Council of Teachers of Mathematics, 2000). They need to learn *when* and *how* to shift from one problem-solving strategy to another to find solutions that are accurate and make sense. Shifting strategies can emphasize real-life experiences, math talk, drawing pictures and diagrams, math-based schemas, and other representations. Below are some examples.

Shifting Representations

POSITIVE AND NEGATIVE NUMBERS

Students begin their study of integers by establishing connections with known concepts. Different concepts appeal to different learners. Some students, particularly those living in colder climates, connect to their knowledge of winter temperatures as "below zero." Others use the analogy of money, with earned money represented by positive numbers and spent or lost money represented by negative numbers. Students well versed in sports may envision a football field, where one gains and loses yards. Some students with math learning disabilities and executive function difficulties benefit from thinking about one analogy and using it consistently in order to bypass working memory difficulties and sustain focus on the relevant concept while they engage in the problem-solving process.

In addition to real-life models, many students with math difficulties benefit from the opportunity to use multiple representations to model integers. For example, some may use the traditional number line for adding and subtracting integers, others respond better to a vertical number line, and still others may want to use number chips to calculate with integers. Choosing a model and sticking with it is one way that students with executive function difficulties assume ownership of their learning and begin to approach math problems with a plan and a strategy.

RATIONAL NUMBERS

Understanding rational numbers also involves shifting representations. Students must shift from the numerical fraction or percent (e.g., 8/12, 75%) to a visual and/or conceptual image that makes sense to them. By thinking about how rational numbers relate to their experience, such as sharing brownies or chocolate bars, the concept of rational numbers comes alive. Students with weak executive function need to refer to these real-life models more frequently than their peers, and they also need strategy sheets in their math strategy notebooks that describe the step-by-step processes for computing with fractions and other rational numbers. Mnemonic strategies may help cement the steps into memory. One example of a mnemonic is using the word BIT to remind students that they need to divide the "*Bottom Into the Top*" when changing fractions to decimals or mixed numbers.

Shifting Formats

STUDY GUIDES

In general, students with executive function weaknesses benefit from learning strategies to compensate for their inability to shift easily, and these strategies help students perform well on tests measuring their newly acquired knowledge. A shift in the format of the questions on a test or the overall layout of the test often confuses them. They may not recognize the problem type, which interferes with their ability to use the strategies they learned to solve particular types of math problems. They benefit from study guides that present math problems in the same format as the problems they will encounter on the test. Despite students' knowledge of the mathematical concepts and procedures, even subtle changes in the test format can result in numerous errors and poor grades.

PRIORITIZING STRATEGIES

Many students with math learning disabilities have difficulty prioritizing and selecting the appropriate strategies for problem solving, especially those students who struggle with executive function processes (Miller & Mercer, 1997; Steele, 2004). They become overwhelmed and often do not know where to begin. They are confused by the sequence of steps they need to follow in the problem-solving process and by the symbolism linked to solving the math problem. Since these students are often not systematic, step-by-step approaches that include visual templates and schemas that link to the mathematical concept are very effective and easy to incorporate into the classroom.

Step 1	Slope Intercept Formula	$y = mx + b$
Step 2	m is slope	$m = \boxed{}$
Step 3	b is y intercept	$b = \boxed{}$
Step 4	point of 4 intercept	$(0,b) = (0,\underline{})$
Step 5		Graph

FIGURE 11.6. Template for linear equations.

Students with executive function weaknesses do not know what information is important and where to begin when they are presented with an algebraic equation to graph. Figure 11.6 is a template that helps students, especially those with executive function weaknesses, organize the steps involved in understanding and graphing the algebraic equation for a straight line, that is, $y = mx + b$.

In this schema, $y = mx + b$ represents the linear equation of a straight line. The x and the y represent points on the line, that is, (x,y) coordinates. The m represents the slope of the line, and b represents the y-intercept. $(0,b)$ is the coordinate for the y-intercept point, the point where the line intersects the y-axis. This template helps students prioritize the information and follow the procedural steps necessary to graph the line. The structure gives them a plan and a map to follow. The first step is to identify the type of figure they are graphing. They can then match the presented equation with the line or the $y = mx + b$ template. The second step is to find the m or the slope, the b or the y-intercept, and then the point $(0,b)$, the y-intercept. By using the template, they can successfully graph the line.

Drop an Anchor

Students benefit from math instruction that focuses on one major concept and set of procedures that can be applied to variations of the problem. (Carnine, 1997; Meltzer et al., 2006; Steele, 2004). For example, the linear equation template described above can be applied to any basic linear equation; then, teachers can provide scaffolds to increase the difficulty of problems systematically. Many students with executive function problems need to learn using a strategy called "A Twist at a Time," meaning they need sufficient practice at one difficulty level before the difficulty is increased and that any increase in difficulty needs to be by one step at a time (Meltzer et al., 2006). The key to initiating the task of graphing a linear equation is first to "Drop an Anchor."

Drop an Anchor is a prioritizing strategy that helps students with executive function difficulties to know what to do *first* when faced with complex problems. Students "anchor" themselves by recalling known concepts and schemas that relate to the given problem—in this case, the linear equation template. After the students read the problem, they can anchor themselves first by identifying the type of problem, then select the particular schema that represents its mathematics. Once they diagram the problem, they can take the next step of shifting from the schema to the mathematical equation that represents the problem then, solve it and check. Drop an Anchor applied to linear equations can be schema-based, as described, or formula-based. If students know they are graphing a linear equation, then they anchor themselves by writing down the formula $y = mx + b$. They write down the information that they know, such as points on the line, the slope, and the y-intercept, and figure out the solution using their prerequisite knowledge as the scaffold for problem solving. They may use a table to graph points, the slope and a point to figure out the graph, or the schema. The anchor in this case is the formula $y = mx + b$.

Another example, Distance = rate × time, can be formula-based or schema-based (see Figure 11.7). Problems can be diagrammed differently depending on the problem type (i.e., two equal distances or one distance with varying rates and time). Students who use general strategies to navigate the problem-solving process will solve it using RAPS (see Figure 11.4), but some students will also need to use a math-based schema to solve the problem systematically. Xin and colleagues (2005) offered a good example of a schema used for *proportion* (see Figure 11.8).

The Drop an Anchor strategy is particularly effective when presented with an open-response problem on a math test. Students first read over the problem, then drop an anchor in known information. For example, sup-

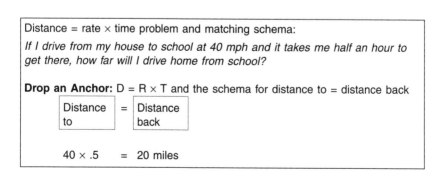

FIGURE 11.7. Schema for Distance = Rate × Time.

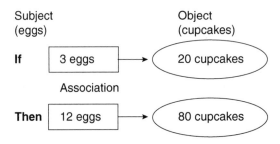

FIGURE 11.8. Schema for proportion.

pose the problem involves determining which of two cell phone plans offers the best deal. Students read over the problem, then remember similar problems that have involved algebraic equations and graphing systems of equations. Similarly, if the problem involves sale prices, students drop an anchor into the realm of percents and easily recall the process of calculating percents and subtracting to find sale prices.

Red-Flag Strategy

This is a strategy for prioritizing on a test to avoid spending too long on a difficult question. Students mark the hard question with a question mark or "red flag" and return to the red-flag questions after they have completed the rest of the test (Research Institute of Learning and Development & FableVision, 2005).

Checking Strategies

In studies that have focused on children's mathematical skills in relation to executive function, students' difficulties with inhibition and working memory often result in problems for them with shifting, monitoring, and evaluating strategies for a given task (Bull & Scerif, 2001; Miyake et al., 2000). In order to learn mathematics and perform well on math tests, students need to attend, self-monitor, self-reflect, and self-regulate, and these actions are often compromised when there is a concomitant math learning disability and/or attention problem (Gross-Tsur, Manor, & Shalev, 1996). Math strategy instruction that focuses on checking is critical for these students.

Although many of these students are eligible for the accommodation of extended time on tests, they often do not know how to make efficient use of that time, and they lack the strategies first to identify and then to self-correct their errors. It is critical to teach checking strategies to help them focus their attention strategically to self-monitor and self-correct their errors. For these students, this level of *reflecting back* does not come easily. They need to check their answer to see if it makes sense, but they also have to reexamine their process in a systematic way. Below are some examples of checking strategies that help students with executive function difficulties. Direct strategy instruction on *how* to check their work can enhance their math performance, resulting in success and increased motivation, which lead to more positive engagement, effort, and persistence.

Error Analysis

In preparation for teaching a checking strategy, teachers must help students search for their individual patterns of test errors. Once the teacher helps students identify their most common errors, they can create a checklist or chart of typical errors together. Students then have to learn how to correct these errors.

Top Three Hits

Once the student and the teacher have identified the student's most common errors, or the teacher has alerted students to the typical errors they tend to make with a particular type of problem, a checklist of the main three error types can be created. Students are advised to write their Top Three Hits, the three errors that they typically make, on the top of their test before they begin taking it (see Figure 11.9).

Top Three Hits

My personal checklist of typical errors (Examples)

- 1.
- 2.
- 3.

Tips to remember:
~ Write these down on top of my test.
~ Change pens to shift mindset.
~ Search for TOP 3 Errors and correct them!

FIGURE 11.9. Example of a checking strategy: Top Three Hits.

This action often helps them catch themselves before they are about to make a typical error.

Test Taker to Test Checker

Math students with executive function weaknesses benefit from differentiating the process of test taking from the process of checking for errors. Students are encouraged initially to take the test with one color of pen or pencil. When they have completed their first attempt at taking the test, they are taught to switch pens or pencils and start the test all over again but, this time, thinking about checking for their typical errors. Some students actually write their Top Three Hits, or typical errors, on the top of the test page before they begin the checking process. They resume reviewing the test, searching for the error types that they typically make. By switching pens, they are symbolically making a cognitive shift from test taker to test checker, often resulting in more accurate solutions and higher grades that better reflect their mathematical knowledge.

THE STRATEGIC MATH CLASSROOM: CASTING A SAFETY NET FOR STUDENTS WITH WEAK EXECUTIVE FUNCTION

Creating a strategic math classroom that incorporates systematic math strategy instruction is beneficial for all students, but it is critical for students with weak executive function, math learning disabilities, and attention problems. These students need teachers who understand how executive function affects their learning and who provide strategy-based schemas, templates, checklists, scaffolds, and accommodations to help them learn *how* to learn math in the classroom. Often students with executive function weaknesses have very strong quantitative abilities that go unrecognized because they may not perform well on tests due to their problems in planning, organizing, shifting, prioritizing, and checking. They do not need a rote approach to math instruction, but they do need step-by-step approaches for meaningful math problem solving. Math strategy notebooks that are set up in an organized way for them can be the centerpiece of math strategy instruction (Meltzer et al., 2006; Roditi, 1996). Their notebooks can include strategy cards, Triple Note Totes, sample strategies and schemas that address various math curriculum areas, and strategy checklists and templates.

Teachers can encourage a strategic mindset in the classroom in several other ways. Modeling how to take notes in a math strategy notebook is an important first step. Giving the students the time needed to record steps is also critical. Structuring time for students to write down particular rules in their math strategy notebooks is essential. Grading their notebooks to make sure they are using specific strategies helps students value the importance of these strategies.

Students who value strategy use tend to improve academically (Meltzer et al., 1996, 2006; Pressley & Woloshyn, 1995; Swanson, 2001). Classroom discourse among students is helpful for encouraging them to value and share strategies that work for them. Strategies they create for themselves generate a "buzz" about strategies in the classroom. When students assimilate strategies into their repertoire, they enthusiastically share them with their peers. *Strategy shares* can be captured by the teacher on *strategy-of-the-week bulletin boards* (see Figure 11.10).

For example, a visually pleasing bulletin board can be created that incorporates multiple strategies for learning a particular math content area (i.e., five various strategies for positive and negative numbers).

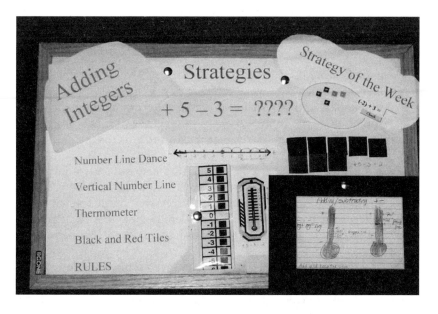

FIGURE 11.10. Math strategy bulletin board—integers.

Strategy labs can be formed in flexible groupings to help students with weak executive function learn a particular set of strategies. Some teachers have set up their own websites where they introduce strategies to help students with homework assignments and conduct strategy chats, or online strategy shares.

Many strategies and accommodations are helpful to all students in the math classroom but critical for those students whose executive function difficulties interfere with math learning and achievement. The familiar accommodations often made for students with attention problems also apply to those students with executive function weaknesses (i.e., preferential seating, extended time, and discrete ways to help them refocus their behavior). In addition, the following accommodations may also promote math learning for all students and help students with weak executive function processes to adopt a can-do attitude to keep them motivated to learn in the math classroom.

Classroom Accommodations for Students with Weak Executive Function

- Provide math-based schemas and strategies when presenting new math concepts and procedures.
- Check in frequently to make sure that students have initiated the problem-solving process and are on the right track.
- *Homework start-ups* help students begin problems and identify strategies or templates to use and ensure that they know how to complete the homework.
- Collect homework every night, grade homework and strategy notebooks, and build similar predictable routines into the classroom.
- Develop a grading system that makes the effective use of strategies count.
- Hold student–teacher conferences that help students understand why success in math is so difficult for them and identify what strategies they need to use to be successful. With teacher assistance, students can set goals and identify strategies to help them achieve these goals, then review them with the teacher at a later date.
- Use the math strategy notebook as a centerpiece for individualized strategy instruction, have notebook checks, and use these notebooks to chart progress and for discussion at parent and student conferences.

Test Accommodations for Students with Weak Executive Function

- Allow all students to reference their math strategy notebooks during test.
- Encourage students to make corrections on test that will ultimately improve their knowledge as well as give them an opportunity to raise their math grades.
- Teach students how to use checking strategies when they take advantage of extended time on tests.
- Provide study guides with math questions that mirror the format and layout of the test.
- Use multiple modes to evaluate students' knowledge, including teacher-made tests; fill-in-the-blank, open-response, and matching questions; projects, board demos, and verbal discussion; notebook checks, homework, strategy use, and test corrections.

CONCLUSION

Teaching strategies directly, utilizing math-based schemas, and providing accommodations in a highly structured but engaging way can provide the scaffolds that students with weak executive function, math learning disabilities, and attention problems desperately need in order to learn mathematics. By doing so, math teachers can change their students' self-perceptions. Math students with executive function difficulties no longer perceive themselves as dumb or incapable of learning math, but are empowered with a can-do attitude. Perhaps a brilliant mathematical mind will be discovered in your strategic math classroom, and that same math student who struggles with EF today will be a leading "business executive" tomorrow.

REFERENCES

Baroody, A. J., & Hume, J. (1991). Meaningful mathematics instruction: The case of fractions. *Remedial and Special Education, 12*(3), 54–68.

Brownell, M. T., Mellard, D. F., & Deshler, D. D. (1993). Differences in the learning and transfer performances between students with learning disabilities and other low achieving students on problem-solving tasks. *Learning Disability Quarterly, 16*, 138–156.

Bull, R., Johnston, R. S., & Roy, J. A. (1999). Exploring the roles of the visual-spatial sketch pad and central executive in children's arithmetic skills:

Views from cognition and developmental neuropsychology. *Developmental Neuropsychology, 15,* 421–442.

Bull, R., & Scerif, G. (2001). Executive functioning as a predictor of children's mathematics ability: Inhibition, switching, and working memory. *Developmental Neuropsychology, 19,* 273–293.

Carnine, D. (1997). Instructional design in math for students with learning disabilities. *Journal of Learning Disabilities, 30,* 142–150.

Diener, C. I., & Dweck, C. S. (1978). An analysis of learned helplessness: Continuous changes in performance, strategy, and achievement cognitions following failure. *Journal of Personality and Social Psychology, 36*(5), 451–462.

Fuchs, L. S., & Fuchs, D. (2005). Enhancing mathematical problem solving for students with disabilities. *Journal of Special Education, 39*(1), 45–57.

Garnett, K., & Fleischner, J. E. (1983). Automatization and basic fact performance of normal and learning disabled children. *Learning Disability Quarterly, 6,* 223–230.

Geary, D. C. (1990). A componential analysis of an early learning deficit in mathematics. *Journal of Experimental Child Psychology, 49,* 363–383.

Geary, D. C. (1993). Mathematical disabilities: Cognitive, neuropsychological, and genetic components. *Psychological Bulletin, 114*(2), 345–362.

Geary, D. C., (2004). Mathematics and learning disabilities. *Journal of Learning Disabilities, 37,* 4–15.

Geary, D. C., Hamson, C. O., & Hoard, M. K. (2000). Numerical and arithmetical cognition: A longitudinal study of process and concept deficits in children with learning disability. *Journal of Experimental Child Psychology, 77,* 236–263.

Gross-Tsur, V., Manor, O., & Shalev, R. S. (1996). Developmental dyscalculia: Prevalence and demographic features. *Developmental Medicine and Child Neurology, 38*(1), 25–33.

Harris, K. R., & Graham, S. (1992). *Helping young writers master the craft: Strategy instruction and self-regulation in the writing process.* Cambridge, MA: Brookline.

Hutchinson, N. L. (1993). Effects of cognitive strategy instruction on algebra problem-solving of adolescents with learning disabilities. *Learning Disability Quarterly, 16,* 34–63.

Jordan, N. C., & Montani, T. O. (1997). Cognitive arithmetic and problem solving. A comparison of children with specific and general mathematics difficulties. *Journal of Learning Disabilities, 30*(6), 624–634.

Mazzoco, M., & Myers, G. (2003). Complexities in identifying and defining mathematics learning disability in the primary school age years. *Annals of Dyslexia, 53,* 218–253.

McLean, J. F., & Hitch, G. J. (1999). Working memory impairments in children with specific arithmetic learning difficulties. *Journal of Experimental Child Psychology, 74,* 240–260.

Meltzer, L., Roditi, B., Haynes, D., Biddle, K. R., Paster, M., & Taber, S. (1996). *Strategies for success: Classroom teaching techniques for students with learning problems.* Austin, TX: Pro-Ed.

Meltzer, L., Roditi, B., Steinberg, J., Biddle, K. R., Taber, S., Caron, K. B., et al. (2006). *Strategies for success: Classroom teaching techniques for students with learning differences* (2nd ed.). Austin, TX: Pro-Ed.

Miller, S. P., & Mercer, C. D. (1997). Educational aspects of mathematical disabilities. *Journal of Learning Disabilities, 30*(1), 47–56. Available at www.ldonline.org/ld_indepth/math_skills/mathld_mercer.html.

Miyake, A., Friedman, N. P., Emerson, M. J., Witzki, A. H., Howerter, A., & Wager, T. D. (2000). The unity and diversity of executive functions and their contributions to complex frontal lobe tasks: A latent variable analysis. *Cognitive Psychology, 41*, 49–100.

Montague, M., & Warger, C. (1997). Helping students with attention deficit hyperactivity disorder succeed in the classroom. *Focus on Special Education, 30*, 1–14.

Montague, M., Warger, C., & Morgan, T. (2000). Solve it! Strategy instruction to improve mathematical problems solving. *Learning Disabilities Research and Practice, 15*(2), 110–116.

National Council of Teachers of Mathematics. (2000). *Principles and standards of mathematics 2000.* Reston, VA: Author.

Ostad, S. A. (1997). Developmental differences in addition strategies: A comparison of mathematically disabled and mathematically normal children. *British Journal of Educational Psychology, 67*, 345–357.

Polya, G. (1957). *How to solve it.* New York: Doubleday.

Pressley, M., & Woloshyn, V. (1995). *Cognitive strategy instruction that really improves children's academic performance* (2nd ed.). Cambridge, MA: Brookline.

Research Institute for Learning and Development & FableVision. (2005). *BrainCogs.* Watertown, MA: Fablevision, Inc.

Roditi, B. (1996). Automaticity and problem solving in mathematics. In L. Meltzer et al. (Eds.), *Strategies for success* (pp. 87–121). Austin, TX: Pro-Ed.

Roditi, B., & Steinberg, J. (2006). Math strategy instruction: Assessment for strategic teaching. In L. Meltzer et al. *Strategies for success* (2nd ed., pp. 95–128). Austin, TX: Pro-Ed, Inc.

Russell, S. J. (2000). Developing computational fluency with whole numbers in the elementary grades. *The New England Math Journal, 32*(2), 40–54.

Sharma, M. (n.d.). *Six levels of knowing, math notebooks.* Framingham, MA: Berkshire Mathematics, Center for Teaching/Learning Mathematics.

Steele, M. (2004). A review of literature on mathematics instruction for elementary students with learning disabilities. *Focus on Learning Problems in Mathematics, 24*, 37–60.

Swanson, H. L. (2001). Searching for the best model of instructing students with learning disabilities. *Focus on Exceptional Children, 34*(2), 1–16.

Swanson, H. L., & Beebe-Frankenberger, M. (2004). The relationship between working memory and mathematical problem solving in children at risk and not at risk for math disabilities. *Journal of Education Psychology, 96*(3), 471–491.

Schroeder, M. A., & Washington, M. (1989). *Math in bloom.* East Moline, IL: Linguisystems. (Individual copies available.)

Xin, Y. P., Jitendra, A. K., & Deatline-Buchman, A. (2005). Effects of mathematical word problem-solving instruction in middle school students with learning problems. *Journal of Special Education, 39*(3), 181–191.

CHAPTER 12

Teaching Metacognitive Strategies That Address Executive Function Processes within a Schoolwide Curriculum

IRENE WEST GASKINS
MICHAEL PRESSLEY

During the 30 years since educators were introduced to John Flavell's (1977) and Ann Brown's (1978) early formulations of metacognition, instruction in how to take charge of and monitor thinking has played an increasingly prominent role in how teachers work with students, especially struggling readers. Over the years, educators' conceptualization of metacognition has continued to evolve through the lenses of contemporary scholars who have applied and expanded notions of metacognition to teaching executive function processes (e.g., setting goals, applying strategies, and initiating behavior) in many aspects of the elementary and middle school curricula (see Israel, Block, Bauserman, & Kinnucan-Welsch, 2005; Zimmerman & Schunk, 2001). In this chapter, we describe the goals and instructional approach we believe should be part of an upper elementary and middle school, across-the-curriculum program to develop metacognitive strategies and enhance executive processes. Although the goals and instruction we describe are good instruction for all students, they are particularly important for at-risk students, who tend not to discover these strategies and processes on their own.

The conception of instruction that we describe in this paper is based on Benchmark School's schoolwide metacognition curriculum (Gaskins, 2005).

At a general level, metacognition involves knowing about thinking and knowing about how to employ executive function processes to regulate thinking (Corno, 2001; McCombs, 2001). Metacognition is also about flexible knowledge of thinking strategies, including the executive function processes of applying strategies to assist in thinking, selecting strategies that match specific situations, and implementing and orchestrating a variety of strategies (Paris, Byrnes, & Paris, 2001). Often not mentioned in discussions of metacognition but a centerpiece in working with struggling readers is that metacognition is also about knowledge of personal attributes (e.g., reflectivity and persistence) and beliefs (e.g., "I'm a poor reader, so I must be dumb") and, most important, the executive function process of taking charge of those attributes that may be maladaptive and capitalizing on those that are more positive (Corno, 2001; Gaskins, 1984, 1998). Critical to metacognition are such executive function processes as setting and protecting goals, applying skills and strategies (e.g., planning, organizing, prioritizing, shifting mindsets flexibly, self-checking), and initiating behavior (intentionality) (Goldberg, 2004; Meltzer & Krishnan, Chapter 5, this volume; Meltzer, Sales Pollica, & Barzilla, Chapter 8, this volume).

METACOGNITIVE GOALS

With respect to metacognitive development and the executive function processes that are the take-charge elements of metacognition, we have a vision of what students should know or be able to do by the time they complete middle school. An awareness of this vision is a place to begin in creating a program that aims to develop students who, when faced with the challenges of learning, thinking, and problem solving, know how to and do take charge of person, situation, task, and text variables (see Gaskins, 2005, for a discussion of these variables).

Students Who Meet Metacognitive Standards

• *Know strategies, including when to use them and why they are helpful, and initiate action based on this knowledge.* By the time students graduate from middle school, they should know effective strategies for recognizing words (i.e., decoding) and for understanding text, as well as effective strategies for writing, problem solving, conducting experiments, studying for tests, and organizing their lives. These students should not only know the strategies, but also actually use them, understanding when and where the strategies should apply and why a particular strategy is appropriate for accomplishing a specific goal. Such metacognitive knowledge is built up over years of practicing the strategies in a schoolwide metacognitive curriculum grade 1–8. The graduates of such a program recognize that the strategies they have learned and now use daily are not intellectual crutches reserved for struggling readers but are the strategies used by skilled thinkers as they read, write, and problem-solve (e.g., Flower & Hayes, 1981; Polya, 1957; Pressley & Afflerbach, 1995). Strategies that we believe these students should use from their first year in elementary school through middle school and on into high school and college include accessing what is known, predicting, questioning, imaging, clarifying, and summarizing.

• *Know academic success is the result of smart effort and put this knowledge to work.* We also envision middle school graduates who independently use the strategies they have learned because, over their years in school, they have developed the important metacognitive understanding that academic success comes not through working hard, but by working smart. That means exerting effort to use the reading, writing, problem-solving, organizational, and study strategies they have learned (e.g., Borkowski, Carr, Rellinger, & Pressley, 1990). The result is that they are intellectually active when reading, writing, and problem solving. They both know how to and do tackle academic tasks.

• *Know how to monitor and use strategies flexibly and take initiative to apply this knowledge.* Once students recognize that they need to use a strategy in a situation (e.g., they are confronted by a word they do not automatically recognize, a text that is challenging to understand, or a math problem that clearly is difficult), they know how to organize themselves to confront the task and use their strategies. They know to stop and make certain they understand the situation as well as possible, perhaps even using self-talk to do so. Once they understand the situation, they might remind themselves to come up with a strategic plan, then carry out the plan and reflect on whether it worked. That is, they are generally planful in the face of difficulties. All of these actions reflect extensive metacognitive knowledge (Meichenbaum & Biemiller, 1998). Good thinkers know that intellectual obstacles require such deliberate action.

Graduates of a grade-1-through-8 metacognitive program also recognize the value of being persistent, realizing that the first sizing up of a problem might not be accurate or complete and are prepared to re-size it up if it becomes clear they do not completely understand it. Moreover, they know that the first strategy attempted is not always the best strategy, with strategies changing as the need for different or additional processing becomes apparent. They have developed the very important metacognitive understanding that intellectual difficulties are signals to apply the strategies they have learned and sometimes are signals to shift gears. This understanding often has replaced a dysfunctional metacognitive belief some students held earlier in their school careers: that intellectual difficulties were a signal to give up.

How do students come to such understandings? It is largely because they are taught consistently to self-monitor their learning (Greeno, Collins, & Resnick, 1996). They are taught to reflect on how they are doing and to recognize that how they are doing depends very much on what they have just done—what strategies they used, what knowledge they accessed as they thought about a situation.

• *Know a lot of important ideas related to content areas and use this knowledge to generate and recall other important ideas.* These middle school graduates know more than strategies. They know a great deal of mathematical content (from basic arithmetic facts to basic geometry), science concepts (e.g., the nature of systems, the adaptation process, conservation, the characteristics of scientific models, scientific classifications), and ideas from social studies (e.g., people's ideas change the way they live; all people have the same basic needs, which are met in different ways; geography affects the way people live; people explore new lands for economic reasons) (Gaskins, 2005). These students have conceptual knowledge, or generalized understandings of the world, more than knowledge of disconnected facts. For example, given years of immersion in American history, these students would certainly know many facts about the colonial, revolutionary, Civil War, and 20th-century periods, but they also would know how those periods relate to one another temporally and conceptually.

A very important metacognitive understanding that emerges from experiencing conceptually based content instruction is that learning content is not about learning isolated facts. Rather, facts are always related to one another, often through general conceptual understandings. For example, the understanding that "all parts of a system are interrelated; thus, a change in one part affects the whole system" permits students to make memorable connections between the facts they are learning when studying body systems (e.g., circulatory, digestive, and nervous) and related health problems (e.g., arteriosclerosis, stroke). This same conceptual understanding about systems also helps students integrate and remember information about the various ecosystems they study (e.g., barrier reefs, deserts, wetlands). The piecemealism that so fragments many elementary and middle school content curricula is replaced with a curriculum connected by essential understandings, with the result that students think about content as a woven fabric, its various threads and strands connecting into larger patterns. They know the overarching themes in science, social studies, and literature and can use this knowledge to guide their processing and understanding of new specific science and social studies content encountered in high school as well as the novels read in English classes.

• *Know how the mind works with respect to thinking and learning and use this knowledge to maximize learning.* Teachers introduce students to principles of understanding and learning that are based on how the brain works. As one example, students might be taught that what people learn is based on what they already know; therefore, it is good practice to call to mind information related to what they are learning and attach new information to the known information. It is also a good strategy to use what is known to figure out what is unknown. Students might also be taught that learning requires active involvement—that they must take charge of and monitor their construction of knowledge, rather than passively hope that their presence in an academic environment will result in understanding. In classes in which students learn about how the mind works, they learn that organized knowledge is easier to recall than random information, that information that is thoughtfully and deeply processed is likely to be understood and used, and that concepts and strategies that are repeatedly practiced and applied are not easily forgotten. Understanding principles of how the brain works provides students with a foundation upon which to base decisions for taking charge of their learning.

• *Know that applying knowledge and strategies is more important than biology and take action to use these knowledge and strategy assets to overcome any perceived deficits.* Just as important as the thinking that currently goes on in the heads of students is the thinking that does *not* go on now, although it may have earlier in these students' school careers. Some students arrive at school believing they cannot do schoolwork and, most saliently, cannot learn how to read. They may believe they are dumb or have a biological difference that prohibits them from learning and performing well in school. In contrast, the graduates we envision know they can do well in school and can learn to read, developing these beliefs over years of success in school. They know that doing schoolwork well depends on learning how to do it, with the lessons taught providing that information and the knowledge honed through years of applying what they have learned to challenging school tasks. By middle school graduation, these students are not thinking about biological differences between them and other children but recognize that the differences that matter are those related to knowledge and using what they know and know they have the knowledge permitting success in future schooling. They know that whether they succeed will depend on whether they apply what they have learned. In short, these students have a very different metacognitive outlook by eighth grade than when they entered school. Many have been transformed from pessimists to optimists and from individuals who believe in biological inevitability as determining their future to individuals who believe they are in charge. Some arrived at school believing they did not have what is required to do well in school (i.e., whatever it was, it was not given to them) and leave knowing they definitely have it (i.e., knowing that intellectual abilities are learned and earned rather than given). For graduates of our envisioned metacognitive program, dysfunctional thinking that may have at one time discouraged and interfered with learning is gone, replaced by functionally healthy thinking.

• *Know the importance of active involvement and reflectivity and put this knowledge to work to set and protect goals and apply strategies.* By eighth grade, students are active thinkers. At one time, some may have been passive thinkers who retreated from academic tasks and active classroom life, but by eight grade the students we envision are intellectually alive. They read and reflect on novels; they try to make sense of math problems and work away, making progress; they surf the Internet for information to connect with science and social studies projects; and they are always drafting, revising, or editing something they have written, keeping at it until the writing accomplishes its purpose and is coherent and mechanically sound. These students are anything but passive, and they will not be academic wallflowers when they begin classes in high school. They no longer retreat from intellectual challenges or habitually give up.

Some other students were not so much passive in their early schooling as they were impulsive and distractible. In contrast, we envision students who do not respond before thinking, but think very deliberately and then respond, after focusing carefully on the task and considering alternative solutions. They do not get upset if the task is not easily doable, but keep their emotions under control, with rapt attention to their task replacing the emotionally driven inattention that resulted when they were challenged as 7- or 8-year-olds.

• *Know themselves as learners and what works for them and initiate actions based on this knowledge.* Although our envisioned middle school graduates have acquired powerful strategic understandings, important and transformative motivational beliefs (e.g., that achievement comes from effort, that difficulties signal the need to try harder), and substantial conceptual understanding of academic content, they also have developed metacognitive understandings of themselves as individual learners (for example, they know that some strategies work better for them than others), and they act on these personal metacognitive understandings. They also realize that not everyone learns in the same way, that one student may remember information from a text by writing notes for each page, while another may find that reading a section of text straight through, then writing a summary works best for him. Still another may remember best by stopping periodically to visualize the content that was just read.

By the time students graduate from middle school, some teachers have them develop a portfolio that describes their learning style and includes their personal plan for learning. In it, they describe what they have found works for them. Some students, for example, know they understand better when they listen to complex text read out loud. Others know they need to restate directions to someone in their own words to be sure they understand assignments. Still others realize that their pace of reading and writing is exceptionally slow and that they need to request extra time when taking tests, reading texts for classroom discussions, or solving math problems.

Summary of Metacognitive Goals

Middle school graduates in an across-the-grades, across-the-curriculum metacognitive program know how to do challenging academic tasks essential for academic success—reading, writing, problem solving, organizing, and studying. They know strategies for each of these processes in the abstract, but they also know the strategies very concretely, having used and adapted them over years of practice in a complete elementary and middle school curriculum. Math, science, and social studies provide many opportunities for students to apply the reading and writing strategies they have learned. The result is that these graduates know how, when, where, and why to use the strategies and knowledge they have acquired, and they take initiative to do so. Moreover, they are motivated to use what they know because of metacognitive beliefs they have developed, including that strategic effort matters and that they can succeed by exerting such effort, consistent with the types of effort that very capable, very smart people make as they go through school. They have also extinguished other metacognitive beliefs they once had that interfered with their learning, including believing they are dumb or biologically disabled and believing that not being able to do a task immediately is a signal to give up.

The result is that graduates of an across-the-grades metacognitive program are intellectually active as they tackle academic tasks. They are self-directed and self-regulated in that they both know how to and do learn and accomplish small and large assignments. The goal is to develop students who so self-manage that they are described by their teachers as persistent and effective learners. They are also reflective students. Rather than spitting out the first thought that comes to mind, they know to gather data and size up a situation and to respond only after carefully thinking about a question and potential solutions. They are flexible in their thinking, recognizing that there are alternative interpretations of texts and problems and alternative ways to go about processing texts and solving problems.

When these graduates get stuck, they know to try to rethink a situation and, if that does not work, to seek help from a teacher, a text, or the Internet. As they make progress in a challenging situation, they reflect on what they are doing and why it is working (or not), and they become better learners and problem solvers because of their self-assessment, perhaps learning new strategies or content knowledge. They are continuously learning and self-modifying because they know to keep at problems, seek assistance when needed, and reflect on their efforts as they try potential solutions to academic problems they face (Costa & Kallick, 2004; Zimmerman, 1998).

How does this metacognitive knowledge develop? It occurs through instruction and school experiences.

THE INSTRUCTIONAL MODEL

There are two basic elements to the instructional model, both very traditional and with a long history. One element is direct teaching, especially direct explanation and modeling of strategies (Duffy, 2003; Duffy, Roehler, & Herrmann, 1988). Teachers explain and model for students strategies for word recognition, comprehension, writing, problem solving, organization, and studying (see Gaskins, 2005, for examples).

The second element is practice. Students practice the strategies they learn in rich contexts, such as reading stories, literature, social studies, science, and math and responding to what is read, often as part of a discussion, but also in writing. Practice permits students to construct a complete understanding of the strategies they are learning, including when the strategies work, how they can be adapted, and the benefits they confer (Pressley, Harris, & Marks, 1992). An important by-product of such practice is that students learn a great deal of content: learning and reflecting on the great life lessons in the Newberry Award–winning novels they read in the upper elementary and middle school years, acquiring and reflecting on important science and social studies understandings, and figuring out how to solve the math problems that elementary and middle school students everywhere must learn how to solve. From day one of first grade, students hear about strategies. They hear direct explanations of how to implement them, see their teachers model them, and then practice the strategies themselves.

In the remainder of the chapter, we discuss five aspects of the instructional model: explaining strategies, discussing how the brain works, modeling self-talk, orchestrating self-assessment, and encouraging students to monitor and control person, situation, task, and text variables. Each aspect is explained by the teacher, followed by scaffolded practice.

Explaining Strategies

To make strategy instruction more concrete and to elaborate on some of the critical elements of such instruction, consider what reading comprehension strategies instruction might look like in the primary grades of a school with an across-the-grades metacognitive program. From the very first day, teachers emphasize that people read to get meaning from text, with this point made often in the small reading group, where much of reading and reading strategies instruction occurs. Reading the words is important, but a major message is that reading is all about getting meaning. Even the youngest readers know that reading must make sense. Of course, this metacognitive message clashes with the metacognition that some of these readers bring to class. Some may be so upset by not being able to read the words that they begin to believe reading is about pronouncing the words correctly. To counter this, meaning is emphasized right from the start as is the message that meaning can be acquired by being active while reading in the ways that good readers are active, by using strategies in combination with prior knowledge that can be related to ideas in the text.

Basic Strategies

Early in that first year, students begin to learn that good readers make predictions about what might be in a story or informational text by paying attention to clues in the title and pictures and by using their prior knowledge. This is their introduction to comprehension strategies. The teacher leads students on picture walks through stories as a first step in getting students to understand that they should habitually preview a text and make predictions about it based on the title and pictures and what they already know. Then, as students read the story, the teacher nudges them to notice whether their predictions were on target.

Lessons on making predictions will be salient for much of the first year and continue in subsequent years, although the teacher will have to do less and less nudging as students begin to internalize the strategy. Students will also use their prior knowledge more and more flexibly, using it to make predictions but also to make connections as they read and hear stories, at first in response to teacher modeling and nudges to look for connections. More and more, however, conversations in small reading groups start to include comments by students about how something in the story is like something they already know or like something that happened in another story. More and more, students make such connections on their own, and as they do so, the teacher backs off, letting students take control of their own thinking as they read. Such nudging and backing off is at the heart of scaffolded strategies use (Wood, Bruner, & Ross, 1976). Once students have begun to learn a strategy, teachers provide reminders and other assistance to encourage the use of the strategy when students are not using it on their own. As the students begin to take charge of their reading and learning, the teacher lets them do so. The nudges were scaffolds, analogous to the scaffolds that hold up a building under construction; they are removed as the structure is able to stand on its own (Wood et al., 1976).

Of course, these students use more than just prediction and prior knowledge activation. Teachers explain and model mental imagery for the students, talking about pictures that emerge in their heads of what is occurring in the text. They urge their students to form such images when they read, and, at first, teachers even suggest portions of the text that would benefit from students forming images. Eventually, students begin to report images they are getting on their own and learn to formulate questions as they read, look for answers, notice when they are confused, seek clarification (e.g., by rereading), and summarize.

Metacognitive Strategies for the Executive Function Processes to Monitor and Control

Sense making is further emphasized by encouraging students to monitor whether reading is making sense and that, if it is not, that is a signal to take control and do something about it. Such monitoring and control of sense making can play out at the word level: if the word just read does not make sense in context, students learn that that is a cue to analyze the sound–letter matches in the word until it is recognized as one that does make sense in its sentence, paragraph, and story context.

Sense making is also encouraged above the word level. Thus, as students continue reading, they are encouraged to stop and summarize along the way; if they cannot summarize, they are taught to interpret that as a cue to change reading tactics, perhaps to reread or to slow down with subsequent reading. Similarly, as students attempt to construct mental images, they learn that not being able to do so is a signal to reread and to read more carefully, in order to get the meaning of the text, which is essential if an effective mental image is to be constructed. In short, as strategies are taught, teachers also teach students to monitor whether they are understanding text. Such encouragement of monitoring goes well beyond word recognition and strategies instruction, with students encouraged to monitor themselves constantly. For example, when students are discussing text, they learn that if they cannot remember enough of what was read to discuss it, that is a signal that they need to reread and to read more carefully in the future. In general, students are taught to interpret failures to be able to do something as signals to become more actively involved or to use a different tactic, as illustrated by this example:

> In a reading group of four 8- and 9-year-olds, a teacher asks students to read silently for a purpose the group has agreed upon. One student finishes quickly, and the teacher passes him a pencil and an index card suggesting that he jot down a few ideas he would like to share with the group regarding the purpose question. The student sits with the pencil poised above the index card for 10 seconds or so, then tells the teacher he needs to reread the page because he does not have any ideas to share.

Through her simple request to jot down ideas, the teacher scaffolded metacognition. As a result, the student reflected, monitored, and took control of the situation. Later, the teacher will find an opportunity to point out to the student that taking time to think (reflection) proved to be a great strategy for him and allowed him to make valuable contributions to the discussion. Instances of scaffolded metacognition such as this occur in classrooms every day in schools where metacognition is emphasized across the curriculum, with these instances part of a larger message that students should continually self-assess.

In addition to monitoring and taking charge of sense making, as students progress through the grades they monitor and control other mental processes such as completing tasks, controlling emotions, being motivated, and thinking positively, to name just a few. Control is the executive process that directs successful learning, thinking, and problem solving. One important component of control is planfulness, which starts with students being taught a very explicit set of strategies for analyzing a challenging task. Students are taught to ask themselves the following questions and come up with answers to each before moving on to the next: "What do I need to do?" (i.e., sizing up the situation). "How will I do it?" (i.e., formulating a plan). "What characteristics do I have that could get in the way and what strengths do I have that could assist me? What situation, text, or task variables could get in the way or help me to succeed?" (i.e., more sizing up of the situation, in terms of personal strengths and weaknesses and other variables that could affect success). Then, after understanding the situation well and formulating a plan to deal with it, students attempt to carry out the plan, monitoring progress along the way by consistently asking and answering another question: "How am I doing?" Students know that if the answer to that is "not very well," they need to revise their strategic plan of attack in light of their continuing to develop understanding of the task and variables that affect performance in the situation. After they do so, they also know to continue by trying the new plan and asking, the same question.

Reading Comprehension Strategies Instruction Spirals

Although all of these reading comprehension strategies can be introduced and practiced in some form with simple first-grade texts, they are re-introduced and practiced additionally in subsequent grades. In fact, practicing the application of the comprehension strategies with increasingly complex texts is a major focus of small-group reading throughout the elementary years. The comprehension strategies curriculum spirals as Bruner (1960) conceived of a spiraling curriculum. At first, the strategies are applied only with a great deal of urging by the teacher and with simple texts. With practice, students increasingly use the strategies on their own and do so with increasing flexibility and more complex texts.

As an example of how the use of a strategy spirals, consider the case of the story grammar strategy. In the early grades, students learn to figure out in the first page or two of a story who the characters are and what the setting is. Then, they look for the problem or two experienced by these characters and their attempts at problem solution until a solution is found. By the end of the elementary grades, students are using a form of the story grammar strategy to acquire much more information about the multiple characters that often appear in a novel and to understand the more complex settings that occur in novels. They watch for problems and solutions over chapters and learn to recognize that the climactic problem and solution probably will occur near the end of the book. They also understand that the characters may be transformed from what they were in the beginning of the book through the adventures they encountered and lessons they learned.

Instruction Is Long Term

Comprehension strategies instruction and practice is a constant from a student's first day of school until he or she graduates from middle school. It is decidedly long-term instruction, as is all other strategies instruction in grades 1 through 8. Writing, organizational, problem-solving, and study strategies are all first taught in the youngest class, with expansions and refinements learned and practiced over the entire elementary and middle school curriculum. Students practice using the strategies over years and over every type of content—reading, writing, problem solving, organization, and studying occur in math, social studies, and science. The sum of so much application and practice is many opportunities to learn how to adjust strategies and stretch them, as well as many opportunities to learn when and where to use the strategies being learned and to figure out which strategies work for the particular student.

In short, a simple strategy once used only when cued by the teacher develops into a more complex strategy that students increasingly use on their own in this spiraling comprehension strategies instructional curriculum. Such development does not occur with respect to just one strategy but with respect to all of the comprehension strategies, with the most impressive reflection of this in the small reading groups. By the end of the elementary years, the small reading groups are filled with student predictions, reports of images and connections being made, questions, comments about being confused and rereading for clarification, and attempts at interpretive summaries. In short, as the students read silently and discuss together, they report their active thinking, or strategy use, with the result being great conversations about the texts (Gaskins, Anderson, Pressley, Cunicelli, & Satlow, 1993), conversations consistent with the instructional conversations that typify language arts instruction producing the greatest language arts achievement (Applebee, Langer, Nystrand, & Gamoran, 2003).

Discussing How the Brain Works

Lessons about the Nature of Mind

Instruction as described above provides many opportunities for students to learn lessons about their minds, but teachers go many steps further to ensure that students know why they are learning strategies and how to use them. There is a great deal of explicit teaching about the nature of mind, some of it in the context of lessons within content-area classes and some of it in the middle school mentor period. These lessons involve providing explicit instruction to students about the healthy functioning of the mind. Good thinking involves being in control of one's thinking, using the strategic processes used by good learners, and monitoring when thinking is working well and when it is not. Students learn that high-ability people have well-developed prior

knowledge and that they use the knowledge they possess to understand new content, which often proves connectable to what the learner
already knows. They learn about the importance of self-efficacy (e.g.,
Bandura, 1997)—that is, believing that one can read, write, problem-
solve, learn, and perform well academically. As part of this, they assess
their own self-efficacy with respect to these important processes. Students also learn about the importance of goals, including that one's
goals go far in determining what one is willing to do (e.g., having a
goal of learning a lot is more likely to result in learning than having a
goal of getting a high grade or doing better than classmates; Ames,
1984). They assess their own goals and how these goals might be
adjusted to improve their learning. Students learn that it is much more
motivating to attribute one's successes to effort, which is controllable,
than to high ability, good luck, or an easy task, none of which is controllable. They also learn that it is more motivating to attribute failure
to lack of effort or use of the wrong strategies, which can be reme-
died, than to low ability, bad luck, or a too difficult task, none of
which is under one's control. Goals of this instruction are to increase
students' understanding of why they are learning strategies and acquiring content knowledge, to make clearer why their teachers continuously point out their successes following their efforts, and to increase
their awareness that trying to learn and improve pays off much more
than wanting to do better than classmates. The rich instructional focus
on strategies and content learning provides many specific opportunities
for experiences that have metacognitive implications.

Principles of Learning

At the center of metacognition is understanding the nature of knowing
and learning. Therefore, in teaching heuristics and strategies, teachers
have learned that an important motivational factor is sharing with students the rationale for the strategy they are about to teach (Paris,
Lipson, & Wixson, 1983). For example, when teachers introduce a new
concept in social studies or science, they often initially assign books on
an easy reading level about the topic. The metacognitive understanding
they want students to grasp is that what people learn is based on what
they already know. They want students to understand that subsequent
learning will be easier if they take steps to develop background knowledge on a topic that is new to them. Reading books on an easy reading
level is a heuristic for developing background knowledge, a heuristic students will be able to implement on their own in any learning situation.
This point is emphasized before the students read the easier books and
again, when the students tackle the target concepts, which can be under-

stood more easily by relating the background knowledge developed through reading the easier books. The students acquire a strategy, and they understand why it works, an understanding that should motivate its continued use according to metacognitive theory and research (e.g., Pressley, Borkowski, & O'Sullivan, 1984, 1985).

When students learn a memory strategy, teachers try to make certain students understand why the strategy works and why it makes sense based on what is known about brain functioning. For example, in the middle school social studies program, students might be taught to remember the specific details of life among Native American tribes by using the strategy of attaching what they are learning to what they already know. What they know in this case is the geographic characteristics of various parts of the United States. These were taught in earlier grades and reviewed earlier in the year in this class. What they want to learn is how early Native American tribes in various parts of the United States met their needs for food, shelter, clothing, and safety. Students are taught to attach what they are learning about how the Native American tribes met their needs to what they already know about the geography of the areas in which the tribes lived. For example, in heavily wooded areas of the Northeast, Native Americans lived in lodges made from trees and traveled in canoes also made from trees. In the Southwest, where there were few trees but ample claylike soil, homes were adobe pueblos and travel was on foot. Teachers explain that it is the nature of learning that new information will be easier to understand, remember, and use if it is attached to prior knowledge (Gaskins, 2005) and if it is rendered sensible by that prior knowledge. That is, the students are using a variety of elaboration—they are thinking about why the tribe's lifestyle made sense in the environment where its members lived. Connecting new information to prior knowledge by thinking about why the new information makes sense is a very powerful learning strategy, one that produces huge positive effects on learning (for a review, see Pressley, Wood, et al., 1992).

In a similar manner, teachers introduce students to other principles about understanding and learning that are based on how the brain works. Students learn that organized knowledge is easier to recall than random information because we have limited slots in short-term memory (Miller, 1956). Thus, it makes sense to take notes and summarize information. They learn that information that is thoughtfully and deeply processed is likely to be understood and used (Craik & Lockhart, 1972). Therefore, it is beneficial to take part in discussions where participants are expected to elaborate on, relate to, and put in their own words important information that has been presented. Teachers also guide students in coming to grips with a very basic premise of understanding and learning: that concepts and strategies that are repeatedly practiced and applied are not easily forgotten (Marzano, 2003). Psychologists have understood for more than a century that if practice does not produce perfect learning, it definitely produces better learning (Thorndike, 1913–1914), a lesson worth impressing on students.

Modeling Self-Talk

Teachers explain to students that talking to oneself (usually not aloud, except for the youngest students who subvocalize) is a metacognitive skill that can help them become engaged in tasks and self-monitor how well they are doing (Meichenbaum, 1977). Students are encouraged to talk their way through implementing strategies and to elaborate and construct explanations in their heads. They are also encouraged to self-reinforce (Meichenbaum, 1977), to tell themselves when they are doing a good job. Teachers model the talk-to-yourself strategy almost daily (Duffy et al., 1988). For example, a teacher might say:

> "If I were you, I might be saying to myself: 'Does the response I just wrote make sense when I think about the other information I have already learned about the main character?' "

On another occasion, the teacher might say:

> "I know I tend to rush through reading story problems in math class. This time I'm going to write notes to myself as I read the problem. That should slow me down and help me be more reflective."

Orchestrating Self-Assessment

In the early elementary years, self-assessment begins with teacher guidance during weekly goal-setting conferences. There are also daily mini-conferences about goals. During these conferences, students are asked to assess their strengths and the roadblocks that seem to be getting in the way of their making the progress they would like to make. Prior to the weekly goal-setting conference, and to create awareness among students of their strengths, teachers try to catch students demonstrating executive control. It is not unusual to hear a teacher make such comments as in this example:

> "Wow! I can't believe you knew how to revise your story to make it so interesting. You reflected on your piece, decided you didn't like your word choices in several places, and came up with wonderful,

juicy words. I think you have just become the class expert on juicy words."

When asked about a roadblock, a student often needs a teacher's reminder of some specific instance when the student was not as successful as he or she would have liked to be. For example, the following scenario might occur.

TEACHER: What seemed to get in the way of your successfully completing your written responses to reading the last several days?

STUDENT: I wasn't paying attention and the directions changed. I wasn't sure about the directions, but I just went ahead and completed my responses the *old* way.

TEACHER: What might your goal be for this week?

STUDENT: To take time to listen to directions and ask questions when I'm not sure how to do something.

The goal is written on a card that is taped to the student's desk. Each time the student listens to directions and proceeds based on those directions or asks a question for clarification when unsure, he or she makes a check on the card, creating concrete feedback for him- or herself with respect to the target behavior. With self-assessment being such an integral part of each school day over the primary years, students become aware of their strengths and constraints and learn how to take charge of them or to adapt as necessary to particular situations even during their early years in school.

Self-assessment with older students usually takes a variety of forms. A self-assessment in a social studies class might be a few questions at the beginning of the class to which students write responses about last night's homework. After answering the questions, students are asked to write how they prepared for today's class, how successful they thought their preparation was, and how and if they will prepare differently when completing tonight's homework. On another occasion, students in a discussion group may be asked to evaluate the group's discussion on a scale of 1 to 5 and to provide a rationale for their rating, telling what they will do the same and differently tomorrow. On other occasions, students may be asked to share what they learned about themselves as learners.

Self-assessment of the presence or absence of characteristics usually exhibited by successful learners is a frequent topic of discussion between students and teachers. Teachers spend much effort talking to students about personal-style characteristics of successful learners— characteristics that are often found missing in struggling readers. These include attentiveness, active involvement, reflectivity, persistence, adaptability, and organization (Gaskins, 2005). Individual students reflect with teachers about which of these characteristics they need to develop. Then teachers challenge students to make plans to take charge of themselves and improve with respect to the characteristics, with the plan including students' self-assessment about when and whether they are making progress in improving with respect to the characteristic.

Encouraging Students to Monitor and Control Person Variables

Personal Style

As discussed above, some students demonstrate maladaptive personal styles. Sometimes as a result of difficulty in meeting classroom expectations, students tend to be inattentive and/or passive. From the perspective of a struggling reader, it may seem less damaging to one's self-image to fail as a result of not paying attention (or not being involved) than to attend (or be actively involved) and fail. Teachers employ every-pupil-response activities to keep usually inattentive, uninvolved students engaged and to help students discover that, when they are paying attention and actively involved, they are successful. Other personal-style issues that teachers address are impulsivity (e.g., by orchestrating reflectivity, then pointing out to students the benefits they reaped when they were reflective), giving up easily (e.g., by scaffolding success that resulted from persistence), inflexibility (e.g., by mediating willingness to improve work by considering alternative approaches that lead to success), and disorganization (e.g., by helping students construct checklists or making sure that homework is written down correctly in an assignment book).

Beliefs, Attitudes, and Attributions

Teachers make students aware of the impact beliefs, attitudes, and attributions have on motivation and of the need for students to take charge of those that are dysfunctional. They guide students to assess their beliefs, attitudes, and attributions regarding learning tasks and explicitly explain to students how they can take charge of them. To increase student understanding of how beliefs, attitudes, and attributions affect motivation and the achievement of goals and to promote more functional ones, teachers may initiate mini-experiments as described below.

Some students believe that they will never be able to spell words correctly because they have inherited a disability from one of their parents. We hear students say: "Dad can't spell well and neither can my granddad, so I will never be able to spell well." Students are asked how sure they are that nothing will change their inability to spell well, with the teacher making certain students remember their predictions. Then, students enter a program in which they chart their spelling improvement score each week, after being guided through a specific routine for learning words (Gaskins, 2002). Their spelling does improve, and over time they begin to believe that they can control how well they spell. When asked what they have learned about their belief that they will always be poor spellers, their responses often include such comments as the following: "When I study a word by looking at every letter and matching letter patterns to the sounds, I usually am able to remember how to spell the word"; "I believe I can be a good speller if I use the Word Detectives study strategy for spelling" (i.e., the strategy they have been taught)"; "I am in charge of how well I spell."

Other students believe that smart people do not have to work hard to learn. Thus, they believe some students, including themselves, must be dumb because learning is hard work for them. Others believe that working hard means putting in time at their desk or looking at a book. In both cases, students need to be guided to understand that being actively involved applying smart, strategic effort is what counts. Teachers often deal with these situations by having students track what they did in preparing work that received satisfactory teacher feedback and what they did differently when they received less satisfactory teacher feedback. When these findings are shared in small-group discussions about attributions, students usually learn that those who consistently receive the most positive teacher feedback are those who work hard by applying strategic effort, and these are the students others regard as smart.

Beliefs, attitudes, and attributions are not the only person variables that students need to be aware of and for which control strategies need to be taught. For example, students need to be aware of the impact of affect, both temperament and emotion, on learning and develop personal strategies with teacher guidance (e.g., such as those discussed by Meichenbaum, 1977) to take control of affect. In addition, teachers can discuss with students the control each has over interest and how interest affects motivation to learn.

One technique is for a teacher to share how he or she handled a lack of interest in something that had to be learned. As one example, listen to what one teacher had to say who was about to teach a unit on the period of reconstruction that followed the Civil War.

"When I was your age, I was passionate about everything related to medieval times, especially novels set in that period. History in general, however, didn't interest me, especially when it was about wars, which seemed mostly what history was about. Early in the school year, due to my lack of interest and inactive reading and discussion of assignments, I did poorly on a test covering the Civil War. Thinking I had studied hard, I asked the teacher what the secret was to learning history. She said I had to find a way to be interested—to attach what was being presented in class to something I was interested in and knew a lot about. Not wanting to look like the poor student I had been in the Civil War unit, I forced myself to try her suggestion. I did my best to relate what was being taught about reconstruction to what I knew about medieval times. I thought about how each happening during reconstruction was similar to or different from medieval times. Much to my surprise, I found myself interested in what I was studying, and I learned much more about history than I had in previous years. Finding a reason to be interested really helped."

Interest also stirs the fire of motivation.

Motivation and Volition

Motivation is viewed by many as the emotional energy behind behavior that affects persistence in learning goals (Bransford, Brown, & Cocking, 2000). Others focus on motivation as wishes, wants, needs, and goals (Snow, Corno, & Jackson, 1996) and describe volition as the process that mediates the enactment of goals and intentions, the will to take action that involves the self-regulation of effort (Cronbach, 2002). Setting realistic learning goals and self-regulating their accomplishment are executive function processes that are taught and scaffolded in a program that puts students in charge of their motivation and volition.

Most students have lots of wishes, wants, needs, and goals when it comes to becoming better readers and students. What often is missing is the willful self-regulation of effort. How can teachers guide students to fulfill the goals they set? One way is to teach students to set incremental goals that lead to the accomplishment of the major goal and to self-reinforce the accomplishment of these incremental goals. Even students who faithfully hand in daily assignments can appear totally unmotivated when it comes to completing long-term projects, even ones in which they seem interested. When explicitly taught to break a long-term assignment into doable daily assignments for which they hold themselves accountable by checking off each daily increment in accomplishing the goal, a more motivated student appears. Students discover they can control their motivation and volition.

Encouraging Students to Control and Monitor Situation, Task, and Text Variables

There are also important metacognitive understandings about situation, task, and text variables that teachers can share with students. Situation variables, for instance, include understanding the appropriateness of one's study environment for promoting or interfering with learning, the availability of study tools that can promote achievement, opportunities for collaboration that can increase learning, and the impact of a student's schedule of extracurricular activities on achievement. Students also need to understand that task variables matter in how one prepares. For example, students need to learn that studying should be different if the test is going to cover factual information than if it covers more general understanding. They need to learn about text variables as well, including learning to size up the difficulty of a text and, if it is too difficult for them, to consider the possibility of looking for an easier text to read that covers much of the same content or listening to a recording of it. They also need to learn to size up whether the texts they have read provided enough information for their current needs and, if not, to seek other texts that might be able to fill in gaps (e.g., if they are writing a report on a topic). Being metacognitive means taking charge of situation, task, and text variables in whatever way appropriate, monitoring whether progress toward an academic goal is occurring, and, if it is not, making changes to improve the situation, deal better with the task, or locate a text more likely to be readable or more equal to the task at hand.

SUMMARY

In this chapter, we described the goals and instructional approach of a grades-1-through-8, across-the-curriculum program to develop metacognitive strategies and enhance executive function processes. These goals include knowing a lot about five categories of information and taking executive control of this information to become successful learners, thinkers, and problem solvers. The five categories of information are (1) strategies, (2) motivation and volition, (3) essential content-area understandings, (4) person, situation, task, and text variables, and (5) principles of how the brain works and how learning develops (see Table 12.1).

The characteristics of the instructional approach we recommend are: explaining strategies, discussing how the brain works, modeling self-talk, orchestrating self-assessment, and encouraging students to monitor and control person, situation, task, and text variables. Teachers explicitly explain each aspect of this instructional model, with each explanation followed by scaffolded practice.

TABLE 12.1. Metacognitive Strategies and Executive Processes for Grades 1–8

Know and implement strategies for monitoring and taking charge of learning and problem solving.
1. Know strategies, how to implement them, and when and why to use each for reading, writing, problem solving, organization, studying, and learning.
2. Know themselves as learners and what works for them.
3. Understand that progress toward achieving academic goals should be monitored using some form of self-assessment and that a different strategy needs to be selected if things are not going well.
4. Understand that academic achievement depends on active involvement and effort to use strategies that are well matched to specific academic tasks.
5. Know how to use strategies flexibly and in combination to accomplish complex tasks.

Know a lot about factors that affect motivation and volition and take charge of those factors to enhance learning, thinking, and problem solving.
1. Understand that explaining successes and failures in terms of strategic effort goes far in motivating academic efforts and promoting achievement.
2. Understand that explaining successes and failures in terms of ability (especially biologically determined ability), luck, or the difficulty or lack of difficulty of tasks undermines motivation.
3. Know the value of reflective persistence and that academic difficulty is a signal to try harder, size up a situation more completely, perhaps formulate a new plan of attack, and continue to monitor as additional attempts at the task are made.
4. Know that explicitly talking oneself through a situation often helps in planning and carrying out actions that lead to achieving one's goal.

Know a lot of important concepts and use these concepts to generate and remember
1. Understand that important content knowledge is conceptual, rather than a bundle of facts.
2. Understand that known concepts can be used to understand and learn new information.

Know that person, situation, task, and text variables interact to determine what one learns and take charge of these variables.
1. Understand that one can affect the outcome of learning by taking charge of person variables that may interfere with learning and by capitalizing on those that may enhance learning.
2. Understand that one can often change a learning situation to make learning more likely and to accomplish a task more efficiently by such tactics as analyzing the task into component parts and using texts other than the given one if it is too difficult, dense, or otherwise inappropriate.

Know and apply the basics of how the brain works and how learning develops.
1. Understand how the brain works and principles of learning and use this knowledge to guide the selection of strategies for accomplishing learning tasks.
2. Understand that intellectual development takes time and is not given, but rather earned as a result of instruction, practice, and reflective refinement and elaboration.
3. Understand that the intellectual tools learned in elementary and middle school will continue to serve one and with elaboration become even more powerful.

Although the metacognitive and executive function process goals and instructional approach described above are good instruction for all students, they are especially important for struggling readers. Prototypical struggling readers have many metacognitive beliefs that reflect their previous academic failures and that contribute to future academic failure if permitted to persist. Most struggling readers do not believe they can learn to read or be good students, based on their school failures to date. They often think they lack the ability required to be readers or good students and can see no reason to try. Should they try an academic task and experience difficulty, they take the difficulty as an indication they should give up. They become passive students who shrink from the action in the classroom, students who become inattentive or attentive to anything except what is to be learned.

Our recommended response is to teach the student strategies and important conceptual understandings: reading, writing, problem-solving, organizational, and study strategies with much direct explanation, teacher modeling of the strategies, and practice, often in the context of small groups of peers, always under the watchful eye of teachers who scaffold students, providing just enough help so that each can make progress without doing the task for them. In addition, teachers reflect with students about their learning (e.g., helping them see when they do well and when they do not and the covariation between doing well and using the strategies and knowledge being taught in the school) to convince students of the power of the skills and knowledge they are acquiring. Teachers encourage students to do such reflection on their own as well, since good students and thinkers of all sorts habitually reflect on their behaviors, noting when they are effective and ineffective and changing behaviors to be more effective. Instruction and scaffolded practice of the strategies goes on for years, with the complexity of the strategies increasing gradually, as does the breadth of their application to new situations, more challenging tasks, and an increasing array of texts.

The result of such an education is that what the student knows about learning and thinking is very different when he or she leaves the type of school described here than is usually found in other students entering high school.

REFERENCES

Ames, C. (1984). Competitive, cooperative, and individualistic goal structures: A motivational analysis. In R. Ames & C. Ames (Eds.), *Research on motivation in education* (Vol. 1, pp. 117–207). New York: Academic Press.

Applebee, A. N., Langer, J. A., Nystrand, M., & Gamoran, A. (2003). Discussion-based approaches to developing understanding: Instruction and achievement in middle and high school English. *American Educational Research Journal, 40*, 685–730.

Bandura, A. (1997). *Self-efficacy: The exercise of control*. New York: Freeman.

Borkowski, J. G., Carr, M., Rellinger, E. A., & Pressley, M. (1990). Self-regulated strategy use: Interdependence of metacognition, attributions, and self-esteem. In B. F. Jones (Ed.), *Dimensions of thinking: Review of research* (pp. 53–92). Hillsdale, NJ: Erlbaum.

Bransford, J., Brown, A., & Cocking, R. (Eds.). (2000). *How people learn: Brain, mind, experience, and school* (Expanded ed.). Washington, DC: National Academy Press.

Brown, A. L. (1978). Knowing when, where, and how to remember: A problem of metacognition. In R. Glaser (Ed.), *Advances in instructional psychology* (Vol. 1, pp. 77–165). Hillsdale, NJ: Erlbaum.

Bruner, J. (1960). *The process of education*. Cambridge, MA.: Harvard University Press.

Corno, L. (2001). Volitional aspects of self-regulated learning. In B. Zimmerman & D. Schunk, *Self-regulated learning and academic achievement: Theoretical perspectives* (2nd ed., pp. 191–225). Mahwah, NJ: Erlbaum.

Costa, A. L., & Kallick, B. (2004). Launching self-directed learners. *Educational Leadership, 62*, 51–55.

Craik, F. I. M., & Lockhart, R. S. (1972). Levels of processing: A framework for memory research. *Journal of Verbal Learning and Verbal Behavior, 11*, 671–684.

Cronbach, L. (Ed.). (2002). *Remaking the concept of aptitude: Extending the legacy of Richard E. Snow*. Mahwah, NJ: Erlbaum.

Duffy, G. G. (2003). *Explaining reading: A resource for teaching concepts, skills, and strategies*. New York: Guilford Press.

Duffy, G. G., Roehler, L. R., & Hermann, B. A. (1988). Modeling mental processes helps poor readers become strategic readers. *The Reading Teacher, 41*, 762–767.

Flavell, J. H. (1977). *Cognitive development*. Englewood Cliffs, NJ: Prentice-Hall.

Flower, L. S., & Hayes, J. R. (1981). A cognitive process theory of writing. *College Composition and Communication, 32*, 365–387.

Gaskins, I. W. (1984). There's more to a reading problem than poor reading. *Journal of Learning Disabilities, 17*, 467–471.

Gaskins, I. W. (1998). There's more to teaching at-risk and delayed readers than good reading instruction. *The Reading Teacher, 51*, 534–547.

Gaskins, I. W. (2002). *Word Detectives intermediate program (B)*. Media, PA: Benchmark Press.

Gaskins, I. W. (2005). *Success with struggling readers: The Benchmark School approach*. New York: Guilford Press.

Gaskins, I. W., Anderson, R. C., Pressley, M., Cunicelli, E. A., & Satlow, E. (1993). Six teachers' dialogue during cognitive process instruction. *Elementary School Journal, 93*, 277–304.

Goldberg, E. (2004). *The executive brain: Frontal lobes and the civilized mind*. New York: Oxford University Press.

Greeno, J. G., Collins, A. M., & Resnick, L. (1996). Cognition and learning. In D. Berliner & R. Calfee (Eds.), *Handbook of educational psychology* (pp. 63–84). New York: Macmillan.

Israel, S. E., Block, C. C., Bauserman, K. L., & Kinnucan-Welsch, K. (2005). *Metacognition in literacy learning*. Mahwah, NJ: Erlbaum.

Marzano, R. J. (2003). *What works in schools: Translating research into action.* Alexandria, VA: Association for Supervision and Curriculum Development.

McCombs, B. L. (2001). Self-regulated learning and academic achievement: A phenomenological view. In B. Zimmerman & D. Schunk, *Self-regulated learning and academic achievement: Theoretical perspectives* (2nd ed., pp. 67–123). Mahwah, NJ: Erlbaum.

Meichenbaum, D. (1977). *Cognitive-behavior modification: An integrative approach.* New York: Plenum Press.

Meichenbaum, D., & Biemiller, A. (1998). *Nurturing independent learners: Helping students take charge of their learning.* Cambridge, MA: Brookline.

Meltzer, L. (2005, November). *Executive function in the classroom: Metacognitive strategies for fostering academic success and resilience.* Paper presented at the 20th Annual Learning Differences Conference, Boston, MA.

Miller, G. A. (1956). The magical number seven, plus-or-minus two: Some limits on our capacity for processing information. *Psychological Review, 63,* 81–97.

Paris, S. G., Byrnes, J. P., & Paris, A. H. (2001). Constructing theories, identities, and actions of self-regulated learners. In B. Zimmerman & D. Schunk, *Self-regulated learning and academic achievement: Theoretical perspectives* (2nd ed., pp.253–287). Mahwah, NJ: Erlbaum.

Paris, S. G., Lipson, M. Y., & Wixson, K. K. (1983). Becoming a strategic reader. *Contemporary Educational Psychology, 8,* 293–316).

Polya, G. (1957). *How to solve it.* New York: Doubleday.

Pressley, M., Borkowski, J. G., & O'Sullivan, J. T. (1984). Memory strategy instruction is made of this: Metamemory and durable strategy use. *Educational Psychologist, 19,* 94–107.

Pressley, M., & Afflerbach, P. (1995). *Verbal protocols of reading.* Mahwah, NJ: Erlbaum.

Pressley, M., Borkowski, J. G., & O'Sullivan, J. T. (1985). Children's metamemory and the teaching of strategies. In D. L. Forest-Pressley, G. E. MacKinnon, & T .G. Waller (Eds.), *Metacognition, cognition, and human performance* (pp. 111–153). Orlando, FL: Academic Press.

Pressley, M., Harris, K. R., & Marks, M. B. (1992). But good strategy instructors are constructivists!! *Educational Psychology Review, 4,* 1–32.

Pressley, M., Wood, E., Woloshyn, V. E., Martin, V., King, A., & Menke, D. (1992). Encouraging mindful use of prior knowledge: Attempting to construct explanatory answers facilitates learning. *Educational Psychologist, 27,* 91–110.

Snow, R. E., Corno, L., & Jackson, D. (1996). Individual differences in affective and conative functions. In D. Berliner & R. Calfee (Eds.), *Handbook of educational psychology* (pp. 243–310). New York: Simon & Schuster Macmillan.

Thorndike, E. L. (1913–1914). *Educational psychology.* New York: Teachers College, Columbia University.

Wood, S. S., Bruner, J. S., & Ross, G. (1976). The role of tutoring in problem solving. *Journal of Child Psychology and Psychiatry, 7,* 89–100.

Zimmerman, B. J. (1998). Developing self-fulfilling cycles of academic regulation: An analysis of exemplary instructional models. In D. Schunk & B. Zimmerman, *Self-regulated learning: From teaching to self-reflective practice* (pp. 1–19). New York: Guilford Press.

Zimmerman, B. J., & Schunk, E. H. (2001). *Self-regulated learning and academic achievement: Theoretical perspectives* (2nd ed.). Mahwah, NJ: Erlbaum.

CHAPTER 13

Deficits in Executive Function Processes

A Curriculum-Based Intervention

DAVID ROSE
KATHERINE ROSE

Executive function manages top-down or conceptually driven processing in which goals, expectations, and context drive the learning process. Executive function processes allow us to pick out information relevant to our goal while ignoring the sea of irrelevant stimuli. Students with deficits in executive function processes face many barriers to achievement in typical classrooms. In this chapter, we argue that typical interventions—those that focus on rehabilitating or remediating students so that they can overcome those barriers—are not robust enough. Instead, we argue that the curriculum itself needs rehabilitation and remediation and that the tools and techniques to do so are now available.

While our ultimate aim is to find solutions to the problem of students with deficits in executive function processes, our immediate approach is to focus on the disabilities in the curriculum rather than in the student. Our intent is to avoid looking for solutions in the old places and, powered by modern technologies and universal designs, to begin to look in some new places.

THE IDEA OF CURRICULUM-BASED DISABILITIES

A school's general education curriculum is a plan for instruction, a framework for teaching and learning. A curriculum usually identifies the goals (or standards) for instruction and the means for achieving those goals—the materials and methods that can be used, the sequence of instruction, and the ways progress can be measured.

Recent policies and practices in education (e.g., Individuals with Disabilities Education Improvement Act, 2004; No Child Left Behind Act, 2002) have increasingly mandated that the general education curriculum apply to all students. All students, including those with disabilities, are to be educated, evaluated, and held accountable within the same general education curriculum, including students with deficits in executive function processes.

Unfortunately, few general education curricula were designed or validated for students with disabilities. Instead, most curricula are designed by regular education teachers and content specialists. Their materials and methods have been designed and validated only for "regular" students, and the means of evaluation are often standardized in ways that exclude students with a wide range of disabilities.

The general education curriculum, the only curriculum in which students with executive function deficits are educated and held accountable, has not been designed for them. Consider an analogous situation from the field of architecture. In older buildings, the needs of individuals in wheelchairs were not considered as part of the design. As a consequence, these buildings pose serious obstacles to these individuals, such as stairs. For most people, stairs work well—they facilitate access to interior spaces—but for individuals in wheelchairs, the stairs are a barrier. While in some environments these individuals may be completely capable, the building creates or exaggerates their disability. It is sometimes said that such individuals have a building-based disability.

Do curriculum designs disable some students? Yes. For instance, it is now common to refer to some students as having print-based disabilities. That is, they have difficulties in learning that are created or exaggerated by the fact that their schools are overly dependent on print-based learning technologies. Students with dyslexia and students who are blind are among those who are increasingly considered as print-disabled (CPB/WGBH National Center for Accessible Media, 2006). Under most conditions, they may not demonstrate a learning disability at all, but under the restricted learning conditions of the classroom, learning difficulties may be marked. They have a curriculum-based disability.

What about students with deficits in executive function processes? Is the traditional curriculum effective for them, or might it inadvertently erect barriers to them? Let us consider this question briefly.

Most schooling, across cultures, begins during the developmental period immortalized by Sheldon White as the "five-to-seven" shift (Sameroff & Haith, 1996). Most cultures recognize that, prior to that period, most children do not have the maturity—many would say they do not have the executive capacity—for formal schooling. Subsequent to that period, cultures recognize that typically developing children are ready for formal schooling and its demands. Specifically they are increasingly ready to delay immediate gratification, to sustain attention and focus, to adopt plans and strategies for classroom activities, and to execute, monitor, and adapt those plans as needed—what are commonly called the executive processes.

From about age 5 to 7, executive processes are increasingly assumed, an implicit challenge in the curriculum. For most students, the increasing executive demands of the curriculum parallel their increased executive capacities. For others, such as those with executive function deficits, the executive demands of the curriculum increasingly outstrip their capabilities and begin to intrude on the explicit curriculum. By the later grades, the executive demands create potential barriers that extend throughout the curriculum: visually complex and textually inconsiderate textbooks require high-level metacognitive strategies to extract useable knowledge; science and history projects extend over long stretches of time and require extensive planning, time, and progress monitoring; classroom activities are increasingly collaborative and require careful social goal setting and constant negotiation, and so forth. Faced with these potential barriers to achievement, students with executive function deficits have limited options.

In contrast, consider the two kinds of options available to students with print-based disabilities. The first option, common in learning, is assistive technology. For students with print-based disabilities, there is an abundance of assistive technology to help them overcome the barriers they typically face. Most districts, some on a statewide basis, have provided digital versions of textbooks along with software applications that automatically translate text into speech. With this assistive technology, many of the barriers inherent in printed books evaporate for students who are blind or have learning disabilities. It has been much less clear what kind of assistive technology is ideal for students with deficits in executive function processes, and even those that are commonly used with adults are not typically considered part of the school's responsibility.

A second option, also common in schools, is to provide remedial instruction for students who need help. Students who have dyslexia, for example, are provided with a panoply of individual and group services directed at teaching them the remedial or compensatory skills that they need to overcome the typical barriers in school (not always successfully). Much research has suggested that students with executive function deficits can benefit from analogous training in remedial and compensatory skills. Indeed, the benefits of strategy instruction are clear for students with a wide range of learning disabilities and abilities (Deshler & Schumaker, 1999), but such teaching is infrequently implemented in practice. The kinds of executive strategies that students with executive function deficits find difficult to apply are just the kinds of strategies that teachers find most difficult to teach. Most teachers in the upper grades are focused on content, not process—the executive skills are implicit in the curriculum rather than explicit. As a result, the kinds of skills that students with executive function deficits need to learn are often taught implicitly rather than explicitly through incremental trial-and-error learning rather than through organized and consistent pedagogy. Some students build executive function skills adequately in this way, but many do not. The classroom environment is not an optimal place to learn those skills for any student, but particularly for students who have demonstrable weaknesses in this area.

There are three prominent barriers to successful instruction in executive function skills and strategies. First, teachers are usually ill-trained in effective teaching of such strategies, and the curriculum provides little guidance or support. Recent research suggests that it takes teachers several years to learn how to provide reading strategy instruction since it requires a shift from teacher-directed instruction with a focus on asking and answering questions to teaching focused on thinking processes, problem solving, and interactive learning with students (Duffy, 1993). In general, many teachers find this approach very difficult to implement (Duffy, 1993). As a result, teachers are ill-prepared to deliver the direct, systematic instruction that strategic development requires and that students with executive function deficits need.

Second, effective strategy instruction requires an abundance of opportunities for supported practice because good results depend upon frequent and sustained practice with plentiful, individualized feedback. With 8–15 students in a resource room or 20–30 in a regular classroom, the typical teacher lacks the time and resources to achieve intensive strategy interventions or to provide the accumulated opportunities for supported practice that students with deficits in executive function processes need.

A third barrier to the implementation of strategy instruction is the increasing diversity of today's classrooms. In the wake of the Individuals with Disabilities Education Improvement Act amendments, classrooms host more varied student populations, presenting a broad spectrum of strengths and weaknesses. To meet students' varied needs and preferences, teachers are finding that they need additional training, time, and resources in order to individualize instruction. With regard to students with deficits in executive function processes in particular, teachers are rarely able to provide the ongoing support or adaptations within the curriculum that would allow individual students to overcome their difficulties and make progress. The kinds of instruction and support that a student with a decoding-based learning disability like dyslexia needs are very different from those required for students with deficits in executive function processes. Teachers simply do not have the skills or resources to individualize instruction for the range of students that they now encounter.

ONE SOLUTION: UNIVERSAL DESIGN FOR LEARNING

A fundamentally different kind of solution emerged in the field of architecture about 20 years ago. That solution, now a widespread movement, is called universal design. In universal design, the approach is to plan and construct buildings that, from the outset, are as barrier-free and accessible as possible. The success of universal design derives primarily from the fact that alternatives—both stairs and a ramp or stairs and an elevator—are built into the original design. Such alternatives increase access for everyone; people with disabilities are a minority of those who use ramps or elevators every day. Universal design has grown considerably because proper design is much less expensive than retrofitting poorly designed and inaccessible buildings and because the benefits, unlike those of assistive technologies, are available for individuals with and without disabilities.

Within the field of education, an analogous movement has recently taken hold. That movement, called universal design for learning (UDL), focuses on the learning process (Rose & Meyer, 2002). Just as universally designed buildings provide options to accommodate a broad spectrum of users, universally designed curricula offer a range of options for accessing, using, and engaging with learning materials in order to accommodate a broader spectrum of learners. Begun at the Center for Applied Special Technology (CAST) more than a dozen years ago (Rose & Meyer, 2002), UDL theory and practice is now the focus of research in many areas and of policy and practice in many states and districts. At the heart of UDL is the recognition that individual differences are substantial, and new kinds of curricula are essential to optimize and differentiate learning in the face of these differences. "Universal" does not mean one size fits all; rather, it means that learning is conceived and designed to accommodate the widest possible range of learner needs and preferences, usually by providing alternatives.

The UDL framework consists of three principles that guide the processes of considering learner differences, anticipating curriculum barriers, and designing a curriculum that offers the alternatives necessary to minimize barriers and maximize learning. The framework is structured according to three essential learning elements proposed by Vygotsky, Hanfmann, and Vakar (1962): recognition of the information to be learned, application of strategies to process that information, and engagement with the learning task. These three learning elements correspond to three broad learning components of the nervous system (Cytowic, 1996): recognition networks in the posterior areas of cortex, strategic networks in the anterior regions of cortex, and affective networks in the central and interior regions.

Successful learning requires all three learning elements and components. A widely circulated report of the National Reading Panel (Snow, Burns, & Griffin, 1998) summarized "three potential stumbling blocks" in learning to read:

> The first obstacle, which arises at the outset of reading acquisition, is difficulty understanding and using the alphabetic principle—the idea that written spellings systematically represent spoken words. It is hard to comprehend connected text if word recognition is inaccurate or laborious. The second obstacle is a failure to transfer the comprehension skills of spoken language to reading and to acquire new strategies that may be specifically needed for reading. The third obstacle to reading will magnify the first two: the absence or loss of an initial motivation to read or failure to develop a mature appreciation of the rewards of reading. (pp. 4–5)

Consequently, the three principles of UDL call for flexibility with regard to each learning component—that is, providing multiple flexible methods of presentation, options for expression and apprenticeship, and options for engagement (Rose & Meyer, 2002).

The Power of New Media for Universal Designs

Until recently, it was not practical to think about developing curricula that had such alternatives because of the labor intensiveness and high cost, due in large part to the predominance of print technology in our classrooms. While an excellent medium for instruction, and even a preferable medium for most proficient readers, printed books are inadequate platforms for universal design because they provide little flexibility. Existing print technologies deliver the same book, the same challenge, to each student—one size fits all. With prominent individual differences in students, this creates enormous barriers to learning. With printed books, the entire burden of individualizing instruction and support is left to the teacher. Few teachers have the knowledge to individualize instruction without help, and almost none have the time to do so on a consistent basis with their students. As a result, most students receive instruction and support that is inappropriate for them and continually face reading material that is not in their zone of proximal development.

Additionally, printed books provide little support for the emergent or struggling reader who is trying to practice new skills of comprehension. On the one hand, many students are still investing much of their cognition in decoding words rather than in striving for meaning. For those students, there is little payoff in trying to focus on learning new comprehension strategies at the same time. Even for students who are able to decode fluently, the early trials of new strategies often need considerable modeling, scaffolding, and monitoring. Such supports can be made available with a teacher in a tutorial role or with elaborate classroom preparation for such interventions as the reciprocal teaching method (Palincsar & Brown, 1984). The vast majority of time, the student reading alone using a printed book has no supports whatsoever for his or her apprenticeship in learning to use reading strategies.

Fortunately, advances in technology and the availability of digital text have made it possible seriously to pursue the development of UDL-based books and curricula. With these new kinds of learning technologies, it is considerably easier to provide alternatives. Reading in a digital medium can be very different from reading in a print medium. Unlike printed text, digital text is highly flexible. Because of word processors, most people are aware of the rudiments of this flexibility. Once a document is opened, its appearance can be subtly or radically altered with a keystroke or two. The user can change from one font, size, or color to another with ease. These alterations in display are not particularly interesting to most readers, but for individuals with visual, attentional or learning disabilities they are critical.

This flexibility of visual representation on the screen is only the tip of the iceberg. The real power and flexibility of digital content stems from the separation of content and display. Unlike printed text, where content and display are fused, digital content can be presented in countless ways. For example, digital text can be automatically converted to spoken words (through text-to-speech technology), and the words can be highlighted on screen as they are spoken, making the connection between written and spoken forms more evident. The same words can also be converted into tactile words through a refreshable Braille device. Thus, students who cannot see or decode printed text at all can read digital text and construct meaning. For students who face barriers in the language itself, a simple click on a word can bring up a contextually appropriate definition in multiple languages. In these and many other ways, this new kind of text can reduce barriers for students with disabilities, struggling readers, English language learners and so forth.

Another beneficial aspect of digital content's flexibility is its ability to be variably and reversibly marked. With hypertext markup language (HTML), the same content can be displayed on many different computers and devices in unique ways for different users without losing the integrity of the original content. A concrete example is the way that a single webpage can be displayed on a large desktop, a small laptop, and even a handheld device all because the webpage is marked up in HTML. HTML works by tagging different pieces of content. Structural tags, for example, can indicate that one line of text is a header, another set of lines is the body of a paragraph, and another piece of text is a sidebar or title. Once tagged, the different components can be assigned different display characteristics by the user. Headers can be large or small, purple or blue; content can be displayed or hidden, depending on the user's needs and preferences.

With the newer extensible markup language (XML), the tags are not only structural, but also semantic, enabling elements to be identified based on their meaning and not just their structure or syntax. For example, a body of text can be labeled as a summary, explanation, narrative, or query and, at a later time, selectively manipulated (gathered, hidden, or displayed). With semantic tagging, it is possible to begin to create digital texts that are strongly pedagogical rather than simply informational. For example, one can create documents with highly individualized supports for learning within a common content. Supplemental background knowledge can be inserted, accessed, and formatted on a person-by-person basis. Individuals who do not need it need not display the information at all. Others, particularly those for whom a lack of background knowledge would create a barrier, might display and even highlight the information. For still other individuals, barriers in syntax, vocabulary, structure, and logic can be reduced by embedding alternatives that make content more readable.

With pedagogical tags, it is possible to embed scaffolds or supports for learning in text documents. These supports can help students construct meaning or learn new reading skills. For example, CAST is conducting studies that embed research-based techniques like reciprocal teaching directly into students' core reading materials. In these digital "Universal Learning Editions," middle school students find prompts and supports built into their books, guiding and scaffolding them as they learn to summarize, ask questions, predict, or visualize meanings. An example of a supported reading environment is shown in Figure 13.1.

With these new digital editions every student reads the same content, but supports for learning and the level of scaffolding that the content provides are selected and displayed individually for each student because pedagogical supports and scaffolds are embedded with tags and can be selectively displayed depending on students' needs (Rose & Meyer, 2002). Using this approach to individualizing, smart, flexible learning materials can support students in their zone of proximal development, much the way a skilled human tutor does (Wood, Bruner, & Ross, 1976).

Meeting the Needs of Students with Executive Function Deficits with Universal Designs

Realizing the promise of UDL for students with deficits in executive function processes requires two understandings. First, it will take under-

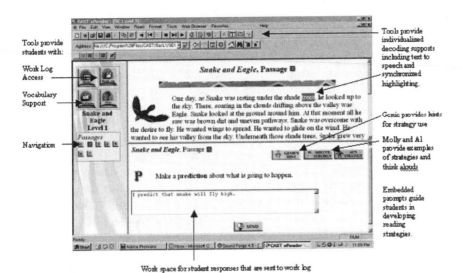

Work space for student responses that are sent to work log

FIGURE 13.1. Screen shot of a Universal Learning Edition, a scaffolded reading environment developed by CAST (a prototype for Thinking Reader).

standing these deficits. What kind of problem are we trying to solve? In what significant ways do students with such deficits differ from "regular" students? What are the sources of the difficulties that we need to design solutions for? Second, it will take a similarly sharp understanding of curriculum design, especially curriculum design in the world of new and flexible media. How can new media increase the options in curricula? With answers to those questions, we begin to answer the real question: What should be included in a UDL curriculum to accommodate the learner with deficits in executive function processes?

First, consider deficits in executive function processes—what needs to be addressed? To do that, we will adopt the framework of UDL. In what ways do students with deficits in executive function processes differ from other students? What kinds of factors are likely to lead to disabilities that can be characterized as executive function deficits?

Executive Function and the Frontal Lobes: Strategic Cortex

Most neurological discussions of executive function deficits begin (and often end) with the frontal lobes, particularly with prefrontal cortex. The anterior part of the brain (the frontal lobes) comprises the networks responsible for knowing *how* to do things—holding a pencil, riding a bicycle, speaking, planning a trip. Actions, skills, and plans are highly patterned activities, requiring the frontal brain systems to generate such patterns. Frontal strategic systems are critical for all tasks that involve learning how to act effectively in the world. Frontal systems allow us to learn to read, compute, write, solve problems, plan and execute compositions, and complete projects (see Fuster, 2003; Goldberg, 2001; Stuss & Knight, 2002). In many respects, Phineas Gage is the poster child for deficits in executive function. A responsible and personable railroad worker, Gage was involved in an accident that permanently altered his life and gave us a glimpse of the role of the frontal lobes. While blasting for a new railroad, Gage was struck by a tamping rod that entered through his cheek and exited the top of his skull, damaging his prefrontal cortex. He made a full physical recovery, but the damage to his frontal lobes left him irresponsible, unable to keep a job, and socially inappropriate. Since then, lesion and neuropsychological studies have confirmed the frontal lobes' participation in executive function (Duncan, Burgess, & Emslie, 1995; Stuss & Benson, 1984). The advent of functional magnetic resonance imaging (fMRI) has further elucidated the role of the frontal lobes in behavior and planning (Elliott, 2003).

The inability to engage in top-down, goal-directed processing has marked effects on culling information from many sources, including text, pictures, and aural sources. Similar frontal systems are critical in any kind of information processing and any act of cognition. In reading, for example, competency is not simply in recognizing patterns in visual text, but in knowing how to look for patterns—knowing how to look at the critical features of the letters, how to sound out an unfamiliar word, how to look for the antecedent of a pronoun and an author's point of view. Not surprisingly, the frontal cortex is active in skilled readers (e.g., Sandak, Mencl, Frost, & Pugh, 2004; Shaywitz & Shaywitz, 2004).

Executive Function and the Posterior Lobes: Recognition Cortex

What appears to be a problem in executive function may be the result of difficulty in one of the many systems that work in concert with the frontal cortex. Most of the posterior half of the brain's cortex is devoted to recognizing patterns (Farah, 2000; Mountcastle, 1998). Pattern recognition makes it possible to identify objects on the basis of the visual, auditory, tactile, and olfactory stimuli that reach our receptors. Through recognition systems we learn to know that a particular stimulus pattern is a book, a dog's bark, or the smell of burning leaves. In the reading domain, pattern recognition systems identify basic patterns in orthography, phonology, and semantics, as well as the many higher-level patterns of written syntax, paragraph structure, story grammar, and style.

When recognition systems in the posterior cortex are damaged or undeveloped, the brain's capacity to know what things are—to recognize objects, symbols, or signs by their perceptible properties—is compromised. From a neurological perspective, there are many names for both general and specific types of recognition problems: the receptive aphasias (difficulty recognizing spoken words), the visual agnosias (difficulty recognizing objects that are seen), dyslexias (difficulty recognizing written words), amusia (difficulty recognizing the patterns in music), and so forth. Imaging studies on many types of recognition problems reveal atypical patterns of posterior brain activation; the work on dyslexia is a notable example (Shaywitz & Shaywitz, 2004).

The dyslexic reader who has difficulty recognizing words via the posterior cortex may also show deficits in executive function. Because of the abnormalities in the recognition cortex, the frontal cortex is relied upon more heavily for word reading putting stress on a limited-capacity system (Shaywitz & Shaywitz, 2004). As a result, the struggling reader seems less strategic in comprehending. Consider the analogy of a singer with perfect pitch. This person is able to be quite strategic in his or her musical performance and perception because pitch does not require executive attention or effort. For the rest of us, much of our concentration is focused on getting the right note, which lessens our ability to think about phrasing, dynamics, and tone quality. This is not to say that people without perfect pitch will never be good musicians; with practice and experience, one gets better at recognizing the right note while concentrating on the overall structure of the piece. It is very likely that weaknesses in posterior recognition cortex also can contribute, at least under some circumstances, to excessive cognitive load in the frontal cortex and, therefore, to executive function deficits.

Executive Function and the Limbic System: Affective Cortex

At the core of the brain (the extended limbic system) lie the networks responsible for emotion and affect. Neither recognizing nor generating patterns, these networks determine whether the patterns we perceive matter to us and help us decide which actions and strategies to pursue (Damasio, 1994; Lane & Nadel, 2000; LeDoux, 2003; Ochsner, Bunge, Gross, & Gabrieli, 2002; Panksepp, 1998).

The affective systems, like the strategic and recognition systems, are distinctive parts of a distributed system for learning and knowing (Lane & Nadel, 2000; LeDoux, 2003). Clinicians have shown, for example, that amnesiacs may be totally unable to recognize an object or person and yet able to react appropriately to its affective significance. A patient may be fearful of a doctor who has given him or her a shot, for example, even without conscious recollection of ever having seen the doctor before. As a result of the effective operation of affective systems, we are able to prioritize goals, develop preferences, build confidence, persist in the face of difficulty, and care about learning. Damage to the limbic system can impair these abilities. It is impossible for any individual to act in a strategic, attentive, and goal-oriented fashion if he or she does not care about the goal at all. Rather, that person would appear to be disorganized, inattentive, and unfocused; in other words, he or she would exhibit executive function deficits.

UNIVERSALLY DESIGNED LEARNING ENVIRONMENTS

From a neurological standpoint, disorders in executive function are tightly linked to frontal-lobe functionality. Damage, immaturity, atypical organization, or comparative weaknesses in frontal-lobe systems are all sources of deficits in executive function processes. Students with completely typical frontal-lobe systems can also present under certain circumstances with apparent deficits in executive function—for example, in a novel complex environment where insufficient knowledge is available, in an environment where recognition is difficult, or in a stressful environment where there are predominating affective demands for attention and effort. Differences in the strategic cortex, recognition cortex, or affective cortex may all affect executive function.

Regardless of the cause of deficits in executive function processes or associated behavioral manifestations, what can be done to create more effective instructional environments for learners with executive function deficits? In what follows, we will consider that question in the context of CAST's research and development of UDL environments. These learning environments, or digital books, are highly customizable along the lines suggested by the three brain networks and the UDL principles discussed earlier. Next, we examine how these next-generation books can help students with deficits in executive function processes in ways that are more supportive and instructional than their printed predecessors.

Providing Apprenticeships in Strategy Development

There are two primary priorities in a universal design for students with deficits in executive function processes. The first is to reduce or eliminate the barriers that such students typically face in an instructional environment. The second is to provide the instructional supports that they will need to develop fully the executive functions that are important to their future success.

We will begin with the second priority, providing the instruction and supports that students with deficits in executive function processes need to develop executive strategies and abilities. The key distinction is that executive function processes are skills and strategies—they are ways of acting on the world, not merely information about the world. In Bruner's (1973) terms, executive function processes are about "knowing how," not "knowing that." Both practice and research provide a guide for teaching so that students know how.

For many centuries, cultures have adopted apprenticeship systems in order to inculcate their core skills and strategies. These traditional apprentice practices continue in most challenging fields, from piloting to medicine to construction. In recent years, cognitive scientists have examined the essential elements of apprenticeships and begun to apply them to "cognitive apprenticeships" more in keeping with the demands of learning in the information age (Collins, Brown, & Newman, 1989). Congruently, cognitive neuroscientists (Fuster, 2003; Goldberg, 2001; Jeanerrod, 1997) have examined the underlying mechanisms of apprenticeship forms of learning. These literatures highlight several critical features:

1. Apprenticeships take place in the presence of mentors or experts who can model both the outcomes and the processes of the skills being developed.
2. Apprenticeships typically include an extended period of practice with high levels of support and scaffolding for beginners and a gradual release as independent skills are mastered.
3. Apprentices practice in an environment where feedback is plentiful, relevant, and timely.

How can students, especially those with deficits in executive function processes, find such apprenticeships in their classrooms? We have already noted that their teachers are unlikely sources of some or all of the key elements in such an apprenticeship. Few teachers know how or have the time to mentor strategy development effectively for their students; they teach primarily by telling, providing information about strategies but not the sustained modeling, scaffolding, and feedback that strategy development will require. They have even less time to individualize their mentoring so that it will be effective, especially for students who are in the margins. Students, on the other hand, have little time to practice these new skills with proper graduated support, get feedback that is far too tardy to be of use and is primarily focused on outcome rather than process, and rarely find that the mentor is available at the point when modeling and instruction would be most useful.

We believe that both students and their teachers can only get the supports they need for proper apprenticeships when those supports are built into the curriculum itself. Consider the ways that such supports are built into the *Thinking Reader* program (TR; Tom Snyder Productions/ Scholastic, 2005), based on CAST's research prototypes called universal learning editions. TR presents universally designed versions of core literature that use digital power to provide the kinds of supports that students with many kinds of disabilities need.

Among those supports are the core elements of apprenticeships. Unlike printed texts, students find supports and scaffolds embedded in the digital learning environment. When they are learning a new strategy—predicting, summarizing, or visualizing, for example—they will find a virtual agent available, a highly skilled mentor who can demonstrate how to apply the strategy right at that point in the text. That mentor, unlike a real teacher, is always available with the click of a mouse and is tireless. When students begin to practice the skill themselves, they find scaffolds available that can be withdrawn gradually as fluency builds. They might find, for example, that the text is highlighted to help draw attention to information relevant to predicting or that key points have been presented along with distractors to help them understand how to select the most important information in building a summary. Finally, as students make early choices to construct predictions or select items to include in a summary, they get immediate feedback that is timely and relevant. To help students and their teachers monitor progress, all students' work—and their levels of support—are saved in a worklog for later inspection and further feedback. To summarize, the following elements of apprenticeship are embedded directly within the texts:

- *Mentors and models.* Whenever students are asked to think or act strategically, there is a "just-in-time" virtual model or mentor (often both) that can easily be called up as a guide. The embedded strategy support system of prompts, hints, and feedback scaffolds students' comprehension and acquisition of strategies and is highly individualized to provide the right level of challenge and support.
- *Scaffolded practice.* When learning to apply strategies within the text, students benefit from supports that can be gradually decreased as they become more skillful and independent.
- *Relevant feedback and reflection.* Every time a student is asked to read or respond strategically, to act on the text, or to find support, his or her actions (spoken, written, or chosen) are collected as data within the electronic worklog. Embedded supports may offer him or her some feedback automatically and immediately; other feedback follows reflection on the saved data by both student and teacher.

One final point about the embedding of apprenticeships: while it may help build long-term skills, does it really make the immediate task more accessible to students or does it interfere with the short-term objective? First, prompts are built in to guide a student toward the use of the supports while he or she works. For many students, particularly students with deficits in executive function processes, the long-term objective of building skills is not particularly salient or urgent when compared to the immediate task. For that reason, explicit prompts are necessary to engage students in a timely fashion in the kinds of learning that will have long-term payoffs. Those prompts are strategically placed and chosen to help students in the immediate task, understanding what they are reading. In the early stages of learning, the prompts are primarily assistive, providing interruptions or signals that some kind of mental processing is needed, then guiding students toward ones that are effective. Over time, the prompts become reminders, increasingly internalized as a part of normal learning. The main thing is that students consistently report that these prompts and scaffolds are helpful in their reading, providing structure and guidance that they often find lacking when they read independently. Qualitative findings confirm their impression.

Second, all of the prompts and supports are individualized—they may be at very different levels for each student according to his or her needs. This is a critical feature because it helps avoid the dual-ended problem that is typical in educational settings: students who are bored because the task is too easy, and students who are terrified or reluctant because the task is too hard.

The embedding of apprentice supports within the learning environment is a key factor for students with deficits in executive function processes, but it will be of little use if students' attention and effort are devoted elsewhere. The following section highlights some of the ways that the learning environment can support students in focusing their attention and effort on what is a priority.

Providing Supports for Recognition

At a gym, customers usually find an array of expensive and highly engineered bodybuilding machines designed to focus the workout, allowing individuals to concentrate their exercise on very specific muscle groups. The majority of the expense in creating these machines is for the supports they provide, not the resistance. Those supports position the individual to take advantage of the exercise, to avoid expending energy in nonproductive ways, and to avoid injury. To be effective and safe, these supports are highly adjustable, with many settings that allow them to be configured closely to the size, weight, and experience of the user.

In educational environments, providing such support and scaffolding during learning is equally important. Good teachers succeed not merely by challenging their students, but by supporting them in optimal ways so that they are positioned well for learning. As in physical exercise, customization of supports is critical to their usefulness.

In TR, there are several ways that students who have executive function deficits can find the customized supports that will position them well for learning. We wish to draw attention to the kinds of recognition supports that are provided and the ways in which they can be customized to help students concentrate on the priority skills they need to develop.

For the student who is weak in executive function processes or who is focused on developing those skills, there are many possible distractions in typical learning environments. In books, for example, the individual words need to be decoded before higher-level comprehension skills can be applied. Students who are devoting considerable attention to decoding words are not devoting the requisite attention to higher-level strategies.

One of the advantages of the customizability of a program such as TR is that weak readers, and students with executive function deficits can be positioned better, getting the supported practice that they need to develop more effective strategies. The TR books can provide supports for skills that are not a focus, such as recognition skills, so that students can concentrate their learning on developing new executive capacities that *are* a focus, such as learning to predict, summarize, and question.

For some students, as noted, decoding words is an executive task—they must laboriously sound out the words and actively decode them before any strategies can be applied for making meaning. Unfortunately, the lower-level task competes with the development of higher-level strategies. In TR, there are a number of alternatives—the whole text can read itself aloud, or a student may click on a word in order quickly to confirm or ascertain its sounds. Such alternatives scaffold the struggling reader, providing just enough help so that he or she can continue to read and focus on developing new higher-level strategies.

For other students, the vocabulary may provide an impediment. While looking up an unfamiliar word in a dictionary may seem useful for some students, for most struggling readers or students with executive function deficits, such a task is formidable; by the time they have found a definition, the overall meaning of the text has long been lost. In TR, key vocabulary words, especially ones that may be difficult for the student, are highlighted and clickable. Students can get help that is correct and immediate. The meanings are displayed in pictures and words, even in Spanish if that is the student's first language.

There are two advantages to having such technology-enabled supports built into the text. The obvious one is that they ensure that more children will have sensory, perceptual, linguistic, and cognitive access to the text (e.g., students who are blind, deaf, dyslexic, ELLs, etc. will be able to recognize the words and their meaning). The second advantage, one particularly important for students with deficits in executive function processes, is that the flexibility in available reading supports allows teachers to tailor the text to the individual child and his or her learning needs. Through that support, the texts are considerate of the primary goals for each student, allowing him or her to focus learning more optimally on the high-priority strategies.

Providing Supports for Engagement and Motivation

Without motivation, no student is likely to engage in learning, let alone develop executive capabilities. The first task is to create a learning environment in which students with a wide variety of backgrounds and preferences will be motivated to read and to learn to apply executive skills to their reading.

All students, including those with deficits in executive function processes, display considerable variation (both intra- and interindividual) in the ways in which they can be motivated and engaged in learning. Whether *any* student is successful in learning depends to a large extent on whether he or she is motivated to do so; engaged by the content, the goals, or the teacher; or distracted by competing demands or attractions in the classroom (Koskinen, Palmer, Codling, & Gambrel, 1994).

Students with executive function deficits are likely to be more vulnerable to competing attractors in the learning environment. They seem "stimulus-bound" rather than goal-directed, attracted to stimuli with immediate emotional valence (safety, satisfying hunger, being accepted by peers) rather than longer-term goals and objectives (Goldberg, 2001). The goal is to help students adopt longer-term objectives and stick to them. Any intervention needs to foster this development. Here are some ways in which students with deficits in executive function processes can find a supportive environment in which to begin at the right level for them.

The issue of recruiting initial interest is important. With many competing demands for attention, it is essential that the *content* of books (their stories and characters) be appealing and engaging enough to attract attention from students, including those with deficits in executive function processes. For most students, there are intrinsic rewards from the narrative itself, but there is more to reward than completion of the narrative. Are there any aspects of universal design that reward the development of executive skills? TR, for example, combines instructional supports with the use of an interactive worklog to support students in setting, monitoring, and achieving learning goals and in understanding themselves as learners. As they progress through content, students are prompted periodically through self-reflection and goal-setting sessions, which require them to use their worklogs. Teachers have access to the worklogs and can include comments as well. Flexible worklog viewing tools engage and facilitate students' use and provide automatically generated suggestions about appropriate scaffold levels.

The advantage of electronic worklogs is that they can help to make progress explicit and valued. The worklogs keep track of everything that students produce. In some cases, feedback is immediate feedback. In other cases, particularly in long-term development of strategies, it is not. Instead, rewards can only come from reflection, guided by the teacher. What the worklogs do is make progress explicit—it can be viewed and reflected on by student and teacher alike. Worklogs are part of helping students recognize the progress they are making. The role of the teacher is to guide students' reflection on that progress, emphasizing the value of gains and the significance of results, and eventually to transfer that function to students, building their ability to reflect on their work and to congratulate themselves. This shift to intrinsic, rather than extrinsic motivation, is an important change. Again, a key is that, for each student, the goals, kinds of strategies, and benchmarks be individualizable (see case below).

> Jose, a sixth-grade student with deficits in executive function processes who reads on a third-grade level, is seated at the computer with headphones on, reading a TR version of *The Giver*, an award-winning novel that is required by his school district. He clicks on a read-aloud button to have the text read to him. He encounters an unknown word, *wilderness*, and clicks on it to obtain a definition and a photograph of a forest wilderness, similar to the setting of the novel. As he continues reading, the text occasionally prompts him to stop and think about the story and to use one of the strategies he has learned, such as predicting, questioning, clarifying, and summarizing. Summary writing is somewhat difficult for Jose, so he clicks on his personal coach to get a hint. He writes his summary in the response box and sends it to be posted in his interactive worklog. Before logging off, Jose goes to the online bulletin board and posts a message about his reactions to the novel. He also reads a few messages from other students and looks at a multimedia story map that the class is building. The following week, Jose and his teacher review his worklog and decide he is ready to move to another level of scaffolding, one that provides less structure and will help move him toward more independent use of strategies while he is reading.

Does Universally Designed Curriculum Work?: Preliminary Empirical Results

Beginning in 2000, CAST has conducted research comparing the TR computer-supported condition to traditional strategy instruction using print materials only. The original study was conducted with 102 middle school students, all performing at the 25th percentile or lower on the Gates–MacGinitie Reading Achievement Test, administered prior to the intervention (Dalton, Pisha, Eagleton, Coyne, & Deysher, 2002). Two striking findings emerged. First, results on student reading outcomes demonstrated that these universally designed versions can meaningfully support struggling learners so that they are able to read for understanding, to monitor their understanding and apply a variety of reading strategies, and to build their confidence as readers. Most important, students working with the supported text showed statistically significant gains on standardized reading comprehension assessments when compared to the control group not using the digital texts but receiving the same strategy

instruction. The latter results show that the supports were not only helpful in ensuring that students understood the texts they were presently
reading, but that students also were developing new capacities that
might ultimately transfer to reading any text, including the texts on
statewide reading assessments.

Second, while research was focused primarily on student outcomes,
there was an additional observational finding: the teachers using TR
altered their teaching and became more strategic in their practice. They
focused more on reading strategies in their teaching, taught students to
develop them, and even adopted aspects of the models of mentoring
present in the digital books. These new kinds of books were not only
modeling strategic reading for the students; they were also modeling
strategic teaching for their teachers (Rose & Dalton, 2002).

As a result of these findings, this work has been through a variety of
extended research and development projects to include additional student populations: such as students with cognitive disabilities; deaf students; and English Language Learners. But what about students with
specific deficits in executive function processes? None of our studies has
specifically concentrated on this subgroup but future research will need
to. We believe, on the basis of our observations, anecdotal evidence from
teachers, and the logic of universal design, that these kinds of effects will
be especially helpful for students with deficits in executive function processes.

CONCLUSION

Such customizable books are rapidly becoming available in schools.
While there is much to be learned, especially for students with executive
function deficits, on the basis of the research results publishers have recognized the market value of these new kinds of supported reading environments. While TR is the first to be commercially released, other publishers are following suit, preparing to distribute core textbooks with
flexible supports. Moreover, the U.S. Department of Education has
recently endorsed a National Instructional Materials Accessibility Standard for the publication of textbooks in digital formats so that they are
more accessible to students of all kinds (Hitchcock, Meyer, Rose, &
Jackson, 2005; NIMAS Development & Technical Assistance Centers,
2006).

With these new kinds of universally designed curricula on the horizon for students with deficits in executive function processes, it is essential to conduct the targeted research that will maximize their effectiveness. That they will be more effective than print editions is highly
probable. That they will be as effective as needed remains to be seen.

REFERENCES

Bruner, J. S. (1973). *Beyond the information given: Studies in the psychology of knowing.* Oxford, UK: Norton.

Collins, A., Brown, J. S., & Newman, S. E. (1989). *Cognitive apprenticeship: Teaching the crafts of reading, writing, and mathematics.* Hillsdale, NJ: Erlbaum.

CPB/WGBH National Center for Accessible Media. *NCAM/Print Access Project.* Retrieved June 7, 2006, from ncam.wgbh.org/projects/printaccess.html

Cytowic, R. E. (1996). *The neurological side of neuropsychology.* Cambridge, MA: MIT Press.

Dalton, B., Pisha, B., Eagleton, M., Coyne, P., & Deysher, S. (2002). *Engaging the text: Final report to the U.S. Department of education.* Peabody: CAST.

Damasio, A. D. (1994). *Descartes' error: Emotion, reason, and the human brain.* New York: Putnam.

Deshler, D., & Schumaker, J. (1999). Best practices in intervention research for students with learning disabilities: Introduction. *Learning Disability Quarterly, 22*(4), 239.

Duffy, G. G. (1993). Teachers' progress toward becoming expert strategy teachers. *Elementary School Journal, 94*(2), 109–120.

Duncan, J., Burgess, P., & Emslie, H. (1995). Fluid intelligence after frontal lobe lesions. *Neuropsychologia, 33*(3), 261–268.

Elliott, R. (2003). Executive functions and their disorders. *British Medical Bulletin, 65*, 49–59.

Farah, M. J. (2000). *The cognitive neuroscience of vision.* Malden, MA: Blackwell.

Fuster, J. M. (2003). *Cortex and mind: Unifying cognition.* New York: Oxford University Press.

Goldberg, E. (2001). *The executive brain: Frontal lobes and the civilized mind.* New York: Oxford University Press.

Hitchcock, C., Meyer, A., Rose, D. H., & Jackson, R. (2005). Equal access, participation, and progress in the general education curriculum. In D. H. Rose, A. Meyer, & C. Hitchcock (Eds.), *The universally designed classroom: Accessible curriculum and digital technologies* (pp. 52–96). Cambridge, MA: Harvard Education Press.

Individuals with Disabilities Education Improvement Act of 2004, Public Law No. 108-446, 118 Stat. 2647 (2004) (amending 20 U.S.C. §§ 1400 *et seq.*)

Koskinen, P., Palmer, B., Codling, R. M., & Gambrell, L. (1994). In their own words: What elementary students have to say about motivation to read. *The Reading Teacher, 48*(2), 176–178.

Lane, R. D., & Nadel, L. (Eds.). (2000). *Cognitive neuroscience of emotion.* New York: Oxford University Press.

LeDoux, J. (2003). *Synaptic self: How our brains become who we are.* New York: Penguin.

Mountcastle, V. B. (1998). *Perceptual neuroscience.* Cambridge, MA: Harvard University Press.

NIMAS Development and Technical Assistance Centers. Retrieved April 8, 2006, from nimas.cast.org/

No Child Left Behind Act, 20 U.S.C. §§ 6301 *et seq.* (2002); 34 C.F.R. §§ 200.1 *et seq.* (2003).

Ochsner, K. N., Bunge, S. A., Gross, J. J., & Gabrieli, J. D. (2002). Rethinking feelings: An fMRI study of the cognitive regulation of emotion. *Journal of Cognitive Neuroscience, 14*(8), 1215–1229.

Palinscar, A. S., & Brown, A. L. (1984). Reciprocal teaching of comprehension-fostering and comprehension-monitoring activities. *Cognition and Instruction, 1*(2), 117.

Panksepp, J. (1998). *Affective neuroscience: The foundations of human and animal emotions.* New York: Oxford University Press.

Rose, D. H., & Dalton, B. (2002). Using technology to individualize reading instruction. In C. C. Block, L. B. Gambrell, & M. Pressley (Eds.), *Improving comprehension instruction: Rethinking research, theory, and classroom practice* (pp. 257–274). San Francisco, CA: Jossey Bass.

Rose, D. H., & Meyer, A. (2002). *Teaching every student in the digital age: Universal design for learning.* Alexandria, VA: Association for Supervision and Curriculum Development (ASCD).

Sameroff, A. J., & Haith, M. M. (Eds.). (1996). *The five to seven year shift: The age of reason and responsibility.* Chicago: University of Chicago Press.

Sandak, R., Mencl, W. E., Frost, S. J., & Pugh, K. R. (2004). The neurobiological basis of skilled and impaired reading: Recent findings and new directions. *Scientific Studies of Reading, 8*(3), 273–292.

Shaywitz, S. E., & Shaywitz, B. A. (2004). Reading disability and the brain. *Educational Leadership, 61*(6), 7.

Snow, C. E., Burns, M. S., & Griffin, P. (1998). *Preventing reading difficulties in young children.* Washington, DC: National Academy of Sciences, National Research Council.

Stuss, D. T., & Benson, D. F. (1984). Neuropsychological studies of the frontal lobes. *Psychological Bulletin, 95*(1), 3–28.

Stuss, D. T., & Knight, R. T. (Eds.). (2002). *Principles of frontal lobe function.* New York: Oxford University Press.

Thinking Reader. (2005). Watertown, MA: Tom Snyder Productions/Scholastic.

Vygotsky, L. S., Hanfmann, E., & Vakar, G. (1962). *Thought and language.* New York: MIT Press and Wiley.

Wood, D., Bruner, J. S., & Ross, G. (1976). The role of tutoring in problem solving. *Journal of Child Psychology and Psychiatry, 17*(2), 89–100.

Index

Academic domains, learning disabilities and, 81–83, 81*f*
Academic performance
  learning disabilities and, 88–89, 89*f*
  Metacognitive Awareness System (MetaCOG), 94–96, 95*t*
  nonverbal learning disabilities and, 107
  planning and goal setting, 171
  strategy instruction and, 97–99, 100*f*, 185–186
Academic skill instruction, 122–126. *See also* Strategy instruction
Accommodations in instruction/testing
  assistive technology and, 289
  autism spectrum disorders and, 141, 142*t*–143*t*
  mathematics learning and, 253, 255–257
Achenbach Behavioral Checklist, 115
Achievement, master stage and, 31
Acquisition of executive skills, 152–155, 154*f*
Adaptive coping model, 42
Adult neuropsychology model, 43–45
Analysis in writing, 228–229
ANOW strategy, 211
Anxiety
  executive dysfunction and, 11
  learning disabilities and, 88
  productive role of, 33

Apprentice stage
  educational intervention and, 32–34
  overview, 23–24, 24–28, 31–32, 35
Apprenticeship, cognitive, 119–120
Apprenticeship systems, 299–302
Asperger disorder, 134. *See also* Autism spectrum disorders
Assertiveness, Children's Assertive Behavior Scale: Self-Report, 115
Assessment
  autism spectrum disorders and, 136–139
  developmental perspective and, 50–51
  executive function measures, 90–96, 95*t*
  learning disabilities and, 84–89, 89*f*, 101, 108, 111–115
Attention
  assessment of executive function processes and, 85
  autism spectrum disorders and, 140*t*
  educational perspectives and, 7
  self-regulated strategy development model and, 231–233
Attention-deficit/hyperactivity disorder (ADHD)
  cognitive remediation and, 146
  diagnosis of, 10–13, 85
  educational intervention and, 13–16
  historical overview of, 5–6

Attention-deficit/hyperactivity disorder
(cont.)
  learning disabilities and, 8–10
  multiple aspects of executive
    functioning and, 69
  overview, 2
Attention problems, 79–81, 80f, 81f
Attention Process Training, 146
Attention Training Program, 146
Attentional control, 231–233
Attitudes, metacognitive strategy
    instruction and, 278–280
Attributions, metacognitive strategy
    instruction and, 278–280
Autism spectrum disorders
  assessment of executive function
    processes and, 136–139
  executive function processes and, 135–
    136
  intervention and, 139–141, 140t, 142t–
    143t, 144–149, 145t, 147f, 148f,
    149f, 150f, 151–155, 151f, 152f,
    154f
  intrapersonal intelligence and, 21
  overview, 133–134, 155
Autobiographical memory, 22

Background knowledge
  declarative knowledge and, 207–208
  learning disabilities and, 82, 83, 124
  metacognitive strategy instruction and,
    274–275
  nonverbal learning disabilities and, 124
  reading comprehension in elementary
    school and, 199–201
  self-regulated strategy development
    model and, 222–223, 228–229
Behavior, patterns of, 26
Behavior Rating Inventory of Executive
    Function (BRIEF)
  autism spectrum disorders and, 138–139
  nonverbal learning disabilities and, 111
  overview, 94
Behavior rating scales, 93–96, 95t
Behavioral Assessment System for
    Children, 115
Behavioral problems, 139–140
Behavioral regulation
  autism spectrum disorders and, 148f
  Children's Assertive Behavior Scale:
    Self-Report, 115
  nonverbal learning disabilities and,
    110–111

Beliefs, metacognitive strategy instruction
    and, 278–280
Brain development, 64–67, 65f. See also
    Neurological perspective
Brain functioning. See also Neurological
    perspective
  metacognitive strategy instruction and,
    273–274
  universal design for learning model
    and, 296–298
Brain injury
  attention-deficit/hyperactivity disorder
    and, 10
  cognitive remediation and, 146
  executive dysfunction and, 6
  universal design for learning model
    and, 296–298
BrainCogs
  overview, 99
  test preparation and, 179

Category Shift task, 112–113
Checking strategies, 252–254, 253f
Children's Assertive Behavior Scale: Self-
    Report, 115
Clarity seeking, 145f
Classroom-based strategy instruction. See
    also Strategy instruction
  cognitive flexibility and, 179–182
  creating classrooms that support, 184–
    185, 185f
  Drive to Thrive program, 185–186
  mathematics learning and, 254–257,
    256f
  organizing and prioritizing, 172–174,
    175f–176f, 177, 178f, 179
  overview, 168, 170–174, 172f, 175f–
    176f, 177, 178f, 179–186, 179f,
    180f, 183f, 184f, 185f
  planning and goal setting, 171–172, 172f
  self-monitoring and self-checking, 182–
    183, 183f, 184f
  universal design for learning model
    and, 298–306
Classroom environment, 170–174, 172f,
    175f–176f, 177, 178f, 179–186,
    179f, 180f, 183f, 184f, 185f
Coaching, 152–153
Cognition
  educational perspectives and, 7
  intrapersonal intelligence and, 21
  self-regulated strategy development
    model and, 230–231

Cognitive apprenticeship, 119–120
Cognitive development
  brain development and, 64
  overview, 60–64, 61*f*, 62*f*, 63*f*
Cognitive flexibility
  classroom-based strategy instruction
    and, 179–182
  executive function processes and, 82
  learning disabilities and, 80–81, 81*f*
  mathematics learning and, 247–252,
    250*f*, 251*f*
  reading comprehension in elementary
    school and, 195–196, 202
  self-regulated strategy development
    model and, 233
Cognitive functioning, 49
Cognitive remediation, 146
Communication deficits, 134, 140*t*
Comorbidity, 8–10, 12
Compensatory skills, autism spectrum
  disorders and, 144–149, 145*t*, 147*f*,
  148*f*, 149*f*, 150*f*, 151, 152–153, 152*f*
"Compensatory ways", 15
Comprehension, reading. *See also*
  Metacognitive strategy instruction
  instruction and, 122–126
  learning disabilities and, 82
  overview, 194–196, 212–213
  principles underlying, 196–203, 213
  strategy instruction and, 166
  variables that affect, 203–212, 213
Conditional knowledge, 208–209
Confusion, productive role of, 33
Consequences, natural, 154, 154*f*
Controlling of tasks, 118
Criterion-referenced, process measures, 92–93
Cultural norms
  apprentice stage and, 25
  master stage and, 29
Cultural psychology, 22
Curriculum-based intervention. *See also*
  Intervention, educational; Strategy
  instruction
  overview, 287–291
  universal design for learning model
    and, 291–298, 295*f*, 298–306
Curriculum demands, 85–86

Decision making
  autism spectrum disorders and, 151, 152*f*
  executive function and, 22
  self-regulated strategy development
    model and, 229–230

Decision matrix, 151, 152*f*
Declarative knowledge, 207–208
Decoding skills, 303
Delay of gratification
  developmental perspective and, 47
  master stage and, 31
Delis–Kaplan Executive Function System
  (D-KEFS)
  autism spectrum disorders and, 138
  nonverbal learning disabilities and,
    112–113
  overview, 90–91
  Trail Making Test, 85
Design Fluency task, 112–113
Developmental coordination disorder
  (DCD), 12
Developmental disabilities, 69–70
Developmental Neuropsychological
  Assessment (NEPSY)
  autism spectrum disorders and, 137–
    138
  overview, 90–91
Developmental perspective
  versus adult models, 43–45
  developmental psychology, 22
  modularity of executive functions and,
    40–42
  overview, 39–40, 49–52
  reciprocal partnership with other fields,
    56–58
Developmental processes
  ADHD and, 9–10, 12–13
  apprentice stage and, 24–28
  assessment of executive function
    processes and, 85–86
  brain development, 64–67, 65*f*
  cognitive development, 60–64, 61*f*, 62*f*,
    63*f*
  curriculum-based intervention and, 289
  diagnosis of ADHD and LDs and, 12–
    13
  executive function and, 11, 23–24
  extrinsic and intrinsic influences and,
    46–49
  learning disabilities and, 12–13, 13–15
  master stage and, 28–31
  multiple aspects of executive
    functioning and, 67–69
  overview, 57
Diagnosis
  of ADHD and LDs, 12–13
  confusion regarding, 85
  high-stakes testing and, 86

Diagnostic fuzziness, 85
Differentiation, 51
Digital text options, 291–298, 295f
Direct instruction. *See also* Instruction
  metacognitive strategy instruction and, 268
  nonverbal learning disabilities and, 120–121
Drill, providing, 121
Drive to Thrive program
  overview, 185–186
  writing process and, 176f
Drop an Anchor strategy, 250–252, 250f
Dyslexia. *See also* Learning disabilities
  curriculum-based intervention and, 290
  "dyslexia-plus" conceptualization, 10–11
  multiple aspects of executive functioning and, 69–70

Education reform, 34
Educational interventions. *See also* Instruction
  ADHD and LDs and, 13–16
  autism spectrum disorders and, 139–141, 140t, 142t–143t, 144–149, 145t, 147f, 148f, 149f, 150f, 151–155, 151f, 152f, 154f
  developmental perspective and, 48
  multiple-intelligences perspective and, 32–34
  nonverbal learning disabilities and, 116–122
  social skills and, 126–128
Educational perspectives
  connecting to medical perspectives, 6–8
  multiple aspects of executive functioning and, 69–70
  multiple-intelligences perspective and, 32–34
  overview, 57
  reciprocal partnership with other fields, 56–58
Effort
  assessment of executive function processes and, 85
  learning disabilities and, 87–89, 88, 89f
  Metacognitive Awareness System (MetaCOG), 94–96, 95t
  metacognitive strategy instruction and, 263, 280
  reading comprehension in elementary school and, 199, 205–206

self-regulated strategy development model and, 231–233
  strategy instruction and, 169–170, 263, 280
Effortful control, 47
Emotion
  metacognitive strategy instruction and, 279
  reading comprehension in elementary school and, 204–205
  regulation of, 110–111
Enculturation, 26
Engagement, 303–305
Environment, classroom, 170–174, 172f, 175f–176f, 177, 178f, 179–186, 179f, 180f, 183f, 184f, 185f
Environmental factors
  autism spectrum disorders and, 142t–143t, 145f
  classroom-based strategy instruction and, 184–185, 185f
  developmental perspective and, 47–49
  intervention and, 97
  nonverbal learning disabilities and, 116
  reading comprehension in elementary school and, 209–210
  role of, 88
  social skills and, 127–128
  universal design for learning model and, 298–306
Episodic memory, 22
Error excesses, 13
Evolutionary perspective, 46
"Excessive variability", 8
Executive dysfunction. *See also* Executive function disorders
  ADHD and LDs and, 8–10, 10–13, 13–16
  curriculum-based intervention for, 287–291
  educational intervention and, 13–16
  educational perspectives and, 6–8
  historical overview of, 5–6
  learning disabilities and, 79–81, 80f, 81f, 108–111
  overview, 2, 73
  universal design for learning model and, 295–298, 295f
Executive function disorders. *See also* Executive dysfunction
  historical overview of, 5–6
  overview, 73, 77–78

Executive function overview. *See also*
    Executive dysfunction; Executive
    function processes
    diversity in, 67–69
    modularity of executive functions and,
        40–42
    multiple-intelligences perspective of,
        31–34
    overview, 22–23
Executive function processes
    assessment of, 84–89, 89*f*
    impact of on specific academic
        domains, 81–83, 81*f*
    multidimensionality of, 86–87
    overview, 78–79
Expectations, 25–26
Explicit instruction. *See also* Instruction
    classroom-based strategy instruction
        and, 184
    mathematics teaching and, 240–254,
        241*f*, 242*f*, 243*f*, 245*t*, 246*f*, 247*t*,
        250*f*, 251*f*, 252*f*, 253*f*, 255*f*
    metacognitive strategy instruction and, 281
    nonverbal learning disabilities and,
        120–121, 128
    strategy instruction and, 168–169
Extrinsic influences on executive
    functioning, 46–49

504 Plan, 15
Flexibility, 135
Flexibility, cognitive
    classroom-based strategy instruction
        and, 181–182
    executive function processes and, 82
    learning disabilities and, 80–81, 80*f*
    mathematics learning and, 248–252,
        250*f*, 251*f*, 252*f*
    reading comprehension in elementary
        school and, 195–196, 202
    self-regulated strategy development
        model and, 233
Freedom, master stage and, 34
Frontal lobe functioning
    developmental perspective and, 40, 44–45
    executive dysfunction and, 296–297
    intrapersonal intelligence and, 21
Frontal lobe injury, 6
"Frontal metaphor", 40
Frustration
    learning disabilities and, 88
    productive role of, 33

Functioning, independent
    nonverbal learning disabilities and, 113
    strategy instruction and, 170
Funnel model of executive function, 80–
    81, 80*f*

Generalization, 140*t*, 146, 152–155, 154*f*
Gestalt, establishing, 117–118, 128
Goal achievement, 201–202
Goal-directed behavior
    apprentice stage and, 24–28
    executive function and, 22–23
    learning disabilities and, 87–89, 89*f*
    master stage and, 28–31
    multiple-intelligences perspective of,
        31–34
    reading comprehension in elementary
        school and, 205–206
    regulation of via executive functioning, 19
Goal setting
    classroom-based strategy instruction
        and, 171–172, 172*f*
    learning disabilities and, 89
    metacognitive, 262–268
Goals, metacognitive, 262–268
"Goodness of fit", 49
Grading
    autism spectrum disorders and, 142*t*
    classroom-based strategy instruction
        and, 184
    mathematics learning and, 256
    strategy instruction and, 99
Graphic organizers
    autism spectrum disorders and, 147–
        148, 147*f*, 148*f*, 149*f*, 150*f*, 154*f*
    note taking and, 177, 178*f*
    self-regulated strategy development
        model and, 223–224, 225, 232, 233
    writing process and, 174, 175*f*–176*f*
Gratification delay
    developmental perspective and, 47
    master stage and, 31

Help-seeking
    autism spectrum disorders and, 145*f*
    reading comprehension in elementary
        school and, 210
Helplessness, learned
    learning disabilities and, 89
    mathematics learning and, 239
High-functioning autism, 134. *See also*
        Autism spectrum disorders

Homework assignments
assessment of executive function
processes and, 86
learning disabilities and, 11, 83
mathematics learning and, 256
nonverbal learning disabilities and, 113
planning and goal setting, 171–172,
172f
strategy instruction and, 166

"Ideal self" model, apprentice stage and,
23–24
Ideas, organization of, 173. See also
Organization
Independent functioning
nonverbal learning disabilities and, 113
strategy instruction and, 170
Individuality
developmental processes and, 60
intervention and, 97–98
master stage and, 31
metacognitive strategy instruction and,
278–280
Individualized education plan (IEP)
ADHD and LDs and, 14
autism spectrum disorders and, 141
Individuals with Disabilities Education
Act (IDEA)
autism spectrum disorders and, 144
curriculum-based intervention and,
288, 291
Information, organization of, 173
Information processing, 21
Inhibitory control, 8, 12–13
Insight, 21
Instruction. See also Curriculum-based
intervention; Metacognitive strategy
instruction; Strategy instruction
autism spectrum disorders and, 139–
141, 140t, 142t–143t, 144–149,
145t, 147f, 148f, 149f, 150f, 151–
155, 151f, 152f, 154f
multiple-intelligences perspective and,
33
nonverbal learning disabilities and,
116–122, 122–126, 129
strategy instruction, 97–99, 100f
Instruction, accommodations in
assistive technology and, 289
autism spectrum disorders and, 141,
142t–143t
mathematics learning and, 253, 255–257

Instructional aids, 152–153
Integration, developmental perspective
and, 51
Intelligence, according to multiple-
intelligences theory, 20–21
Intelligence, intrapersonal. See also
Multiple-intelligences theory
executive function and, 22–23
overview, 20–22, 35
Intelligent behavior, 206
Interpolation, master stage and, 30
Intervention, educational. See also
Instruction
ADHD and LDs and, 13–16
autism spectrum disorders and, 139–
141, 140t, 142t–143t, 144–149,
145t, 147f, 148f, 149f, 150f, 151–
155, 151f, 152f, 154f
developmental perspective and, 48
multiple-intelligences perspective and,
32–34
nonverbal learning disabilities and,
116–122
social skills and, 126–128
Intervention, learning disabilities and, 97–
99, 100f, 101
Intrapersonal intelligence. See also
Multiple-intelligences theory
executive function and, 22–23
overview, 20–22, 35
Intrinsic influences on executive
functioning, 46–49

Knowledge. See also Prior knowledge
metacognitive strategy instruction
and, 263, 265–266, 274–276,
282t
reading comprehension in elementary
school and, 206–209
Knowledge-telling model of writing, 218–
219

Language-based learning disabilities
attention-deficit/hyperactivity disorder
and, 10–11
executive dysfunction and, 13–14, 15–
16
Language development, 134
Language skills, 107, 124–125, 140t
Learned helplessness
learning disabilities and, 89
mathematics teaching and, 239

Learning disabilities. *See also* Nonverbal
    learning disabilities
  assessment and, 84–89, 89*f*, 90–96, 95*t*
  attention-deficit/hyperactivity disorder
    and, 8–10
  diagnosis of, 10–13, 85
  educational perspectives and, 7
  executive function processes and, 69,
    69–70, 78–79, 79–81, 80*f*, 81*f*
  impact of on specific academic
    domains, 81–83, 81*f*
  intervention and, 13–16, 97–99, 100*f*,
    101
  language-based, 10–11, 13–14, 15–16
  neuropsychological perspective, 2
  overview, 101
Learning, principles of, 274–276
Learning profiles, 140, 140*t*
Limbic system, 298

Maintenance of executive skills, 152–155,
    154*f*
Master stage
  educational intervention and, 32–34
  overview, 24, 28–31, 32, 35
Mastery, 99
Materials, organization of, 173
Mathematics learning
  autism spectrum disorders and, 140*t*
  classroom-based strategy instruction
    and, 254–257, 255*f*
  cognitive flexibility and, 248–252,
    250*f*, 251*f*, 252*f*
  organization and, 244–246, 245*t*, 246*f*
  overview, 237–240
  problem-solving skills and, 239–240,
    245–246, 246*f*
  strategy instruction and, 162, 240–254,
    240–254, 241*f*, 242*f*, 243*f*, 245*t*,
    246*f*, 247*t*, 247*f*, 250*f*, 251*f*, 252*f*
  visuospatial capacity and, 242–244, 243*f*
Mathematics teaching, 241–244, 241*f*,
    242*f*, 243*f*
Medical perspectives
  connecting to educational perspectives,
    6–8
  overview, 55–56
Memorization, 13
Memory
  ADHD and LDs and, 11, 13, 15–16
  assessment of executive function
    processes and, 85

autism spectrum disorders and, 140*t*
educational perspectives and, 7
frontal lobe functioning and, 44–45
intrapersonal intelligence and, 22
knowledge-telling model of writing,
    218–219
mathematics teaching and, 238–239,
    241–244, 241*f*, 242*f*, 243*f*
metacognitive strategy instruction and,
    275
Mentorships, 300–302
Metacognition. *See also* Metacognitive
    strategy instruction
  classroom-based strategy instruction
    and, 170–171
  educational perspectives and, 7
  intrapersonal intelligence and, 22
  strategy instruction and, 166–169
Metacognitive Awareness System
    (MetaCOG), 94–96, 95*t*
Metacognitive goals, 262–268
Metacognitive strategy instruction. *See
    also* Instruction; Strategy instruction
  discussing how the brain works, 273–
    276
  encouraging students to monitor and
    control variables, 278–281
  explaining strategies, 269–273
  goals and, 262–268
  modeling self-talk, 276
  overview, 261–262, 268–281, 282*t*, 283
  self-assessment, 276–278
Mirror movements. *See* Overflow
    movements
Modeling
  apprenticeship systems and, 300–302
  classroom-based strategy instruction
    and, 184
  metacognitive strategy instruction and,
    276
  multiple-intelligences perspective and, 33
  nonverbal learning disabilities and,
    119–120
  self-regulated strategy development
    model and, 225, 226, 227
  strategy instruction and, 168
Modification in instruction/testing. *See
    also* Accommodations in instruction/
    testing
  assistive technology and, 289
  autism spectrum disorders and, 141,
    142*t*–143*t*

Modularity of executive functions
    developmental perspective and, 50
    overview, 40–42
Moral perspective, 21
Motivation
    apprentice stage and, 27
    assessment of executive function
        processes and, 85
    autism spectrum disorders and, 140t
    classroom-based strategy instruction
        and, 184–185
    learning disabilities and, 87–89, 89f
    master stage and, 30–31
    Metacognitive Awareness System
        (MetaCOG), 94–96, 95t
    metacognitive strategy instruction and,
        280
    multiple-intelligences perspective and,
        33
    planning and goal setting, 171
    reading comprehension in elementary
        school and, 205–206
    strategy instruction and, 98, 169–170
    universal design for learning model
        and, 303–305
Motor control, 12
Motor systems
    autism spectrum disorders and, 140t
    nonverbal learning disabilities and,
        107, 129
    overview, 59
Multiple-intelligences theory
    apprentice stage and, 26
    executive function and, 22–23
    intrapersonal intelligence and, 20–22
    master stage and, 28–31
    overview, 31–34, 35

NEPSY. See Developmental
    Neuropsychological Assessment
    (NEPSY)
NEPSY Visual Attention tasks, 85
Neurological perspective
    ADHD and, 5–6, 10, 12–13
    brain development, 64–67, 65f
    developmental perspective and, 40, 43–
        45, 46
    diagnosis of ADHD and LDs and, 12–
        13
    intrapersonal intelligence and, 21
    learning disabilities and, 12–13, 101,
        107–108

    modularity of executive functions and,
        41–42
    overview, 2, 57
    reciprocal partnership with other fields,
        56–58
    universal design for learning model
        and, 296–298
Neuropsychological testing, 90
No Child Left Behind Act, 288
Nonverbal behaviors, 134
Nonverbal learning disabilities. See also
        Learning disabilities
    assessment and, 111–115
    common executive function deficits
        among, 108–111
    complex academic skill instruction and,
        122–126
    intervention and instruction and, 116–
        122, 122–126
    overview, 106–108, 128–129
    social skills and, 113–115, 126–128
Norm-referenced tests, 90–92
Norms, cultural
    apprentice stage and, 25
    master stage and, 29
Note taking
    classroom-based strategy instruction
        and, 174, 177, 178f
    conditional knowledge and, 209
    mathematics learning and, 246–247,
        246f, 247f
    planning and goal setting, 171–172
    self-regulated strategy development
        model and, 225
    strategy instruction and, 166

Organization
    classroom-based strategy instruction
        and, 172–174, 175f–176f, 177, 178f,
        179
    mathematics learning and, 244–246,
        245t, 246f
    reading comprehension in elementary
        school and, 195–196, 209–211
    self-regulated strategy development
        model and, 222–223
    strategy instruction and, 97–99, 100f
Overflow movements, 12–13

Parent–child interactions, 47
Parent training, 154–155
Parents, role of, 154–155

PEMDAS acronym, 241, 241*f*
Perceptual skills, autism spectrum
    disorders and, 140*t*
Persistence
    assessment of executive function
        processes and, 85
    learning disabilities and, 88
    metacognitive strategy instruction and,
        263–264
Personality, frontal lobe damage and, 21
Personality psychology, 22
Peterson–Quay Behavior Problem
    Checklist, 115
Phonological loop, 11
Planning skills
    autism spectrum disorders and, 151
    classroom-based strategy instruction
        and, 171–172, 172*f*
    reading comprehension in elementary
        school and, 198–199, 209–210
    self-regulated strategy development
        model and, 222, 227, 229–230
Positive psychology, 22
Posterior lobes, 297–298
POW writing strategy
    attentional control and, 232
    decision-making and planning and,
        229–230
    flexible adaptation and, 233
    overview, 221–222
    TREE writing strategy and, 225–228
Practice, providing
    metacognitive strategy instruction and,
        268–269
    nonverbal learning disabilities and, 121
    strategy instruction and, 168
Predictions, metacognitive strategy
    instruction and, 269–270
Prefrontal regions
    assessment and, 91
    developmental perspective and, 44–45
    modularity of executive functions and,
        41–42
Print-based disabilities
    assistive technology and, 289
    curriculum-based intervention and,
        288
Prior knowledge
    declarative knowledge and, 207–208
    learning disabilities and, 82, 83, 124
    metacognitive strategy instruction and,
        274–275

nonverbal learning disabilities and, 124
reading comprehension in elementary
    school and, 199–201
self-regulated strategy development
    model and, 222–223, 228–229
Prioritization
    autism spectrum disorders and, 151,
        152*f*
    classroom-based strategy instruction
        and, 172–174, 175*f*–176*f*, 177, 178*f*,
        179
    mathematics learning and, 249–252
    reading comprehension in elementary
        school and, 195–196, 199
Problem-solving skills
    learning disabilities and, 79–80
    mathematics learning and, 239–240,
        245–246, 246*f*
    modeling, 119–120
    nonverbal learning disabilities and,
        107, 109
    Survey of Problem-Solving and
        Educational Skills (SPES), 92–93
Problematic situation, 124
Procedural knowledge, 208
Process measures, 92–93
Projects, long-term
    learning disabilities and, 83
    strategy instruction and, 166
"Prosthetic frontal lobe", 33
Psychoanalysis, 22

Reading, autism spectrum disorders and,
    140*t*
Reading comprehension. *See also*
    Metacognitive strategy instruction
    instruction and, 122–126
    learning disabilities and, 82
    overview, 194–196, 212–213
    principles underlying, 196–203, 213
    strategy instruction and, 166
    variables that affect, 203–212, 213
Reading comprehension instruction,
    nonverbal learning disabilities and,
    122–126
Reasoning skills, 22
Recall skills, 13
Recess play, social skills and, 127–128
Reciprocal teaching methods, 120
Red-Flag strategy, 252
Reform, educational, 34
Resiliency, 88

Response inhibition
  diagnosis of ADHD and LDs and, 12–13
  multiple-intelligences perspective and, 33
Responsibility, student, 32–34
Rey Complex Figure Test, 91–92
Role play, Social Skills Role-Play Test,
  114–115
Routines, needs for, 125–126

Scaffolding
  apprenticeship systems and, 300–302
  metacognitive strategy instruction and,
    281
  strategy instruction and, 168
Schema theory, 123
Schemata
  declarative knowledge and, 207
  nonverbal learning disabilities and, 123
Schizophrenia, cognitive remediation and,
  146
Segmenting of tasks, 118, 119
Selective attention, 7
Self-advocacy skills, 145f
Self-assessment
  metacognitive strategy instruction and,
    276–278
  reading comprehension in elementary
    school and, 195–196, 202–203
Self-awareness
  autism spectrum disorders and, 145f
  intrapersonal intelligence and, 21
  master stage and, 30
  motivation and, 170
Self-checking
  classroom-based strategy instruction
    and, 182–183, 183f, 184f
  mathematics learning and, 252–254,
    253f
  reading comprehension in elementary
    school and, 195–196, 201–202
Self, development of, 30
Self-efficacy
  learning disabilities and, 88
  metacognitive strategy instruction and,
    274
  planning and goal setting, 171
Self-esteem, 21
Self-management, 153–154
Self-monitoring
  autism spectrum disorders and, 153–154
  classroom-based strategy instruction
    and, 182–183, 183f, 184f

reading comprehension in elementary
    school and, 205–206
  self-regulated strategy development
    model and, 224
  strategy instruction and, 98
Self-reflection, 21
Self-regulated strategy development model
  executive function processes and, 228–233
  illustration of, 221–233
  overview, 162, 220–221, 234
Self-regulation
  developmental perspective and, 51
  executive function processes and, 78
  frontal lobe damage and, 21
  learning disabilities and, 79–80
  planning and goal setting, 171–172
  reading comprehension in elementary
    school and, 205–206
  resiliency and, 88
Self-talk, 276
Semantic clustering, 13
Sensory-motor development, 140t
Sequential learning, 119
Sequential thinking, 147–148
Situational variables
  metacognitive strategy instruction and,
    281
  reading comprehension in elementary
    school and, 209–211
Skill development
  apprentice stage and, 23–24, 26–27
  executive function and, 22–23
  learning disabilities and, 87–89, 89f
  master stage and, 29–30
  multiple-intelligences perspective of,
    31–34
Social psychology, 22
Social skills
  assessment and, 113–115
  autism spectrum disorders and, 133–134
  nonverbal learning disabilities and,
    110–111, 126–128
Social Skills Observation Checklist, 114
Social Skills Role-Play Test, 114–115
Socialization, multiple-intelligences
  perspective and, 35
Spatial problem solving, 109
Spatial working memory, 45
Special education. See also Learning
  disabilities
  ADHD and LDs and, 15
  educational perspectives and, 7

Standardized tests, 90. *See also* Testing, high-stakes
STAR strategy, 99, 100*f*
Strategy instruction. *See also* Classroom-based strategy instruction; Curriculum-based intervention; Metacognitive strategy instruction; Systematic strategy instruction
autism spectrum disorders and, 146
creating classrooms that support, 170–174, 172*f*, 175*f*–176*f*, 177, 179*f*, 179–186, 180*f*, 183*f*, 184*f*, 185*f*
learning disabilities and, 97–99, 100*f*, 121–122
mathematics learning and, 240–254, 241*f*, 242*f*, 243*f*, 245*t*, 246*f*, 247*t*, 247*f*, 250*f*, 251*f*, 252*f*
overview, 166–170, 167*f*, 186–187
Strategy spirals, 272
Strategy use, 94–96, 95*t*
Stroop Color Word Test
autism spectrum disorders and, 138
nonverbal learning disabilities and, 111–112
Structure, needs for, 125–126
Study skills
classroom-based strategy instruction and, 179, 179*f*, 180*f*
learning disabilities and, 83
Support-seeking, 210
Survey of Problem-Solving and Educational Skills (SPES), 92–93
Systematic strategy instruction. *See also* Strategy instruction
autism spectrum disorders and, 146
importance of, 162
nonverbal learning disabilities and, 121–122
overview, 165–166, 169

Tactile perception, 107
Task analysis, 148–149
Task demands
metacognitive strategy instruction and, 281
reading comprehension in elementary school and, 211
TEACCH program, 141, 144
Teaching. *See* Instruction
Technology
autism spectrum disorders and, 142*t*, 146
BrainCogs, 99

curriculum-based intervention and, 289
nonverbal learning disabilities and, 129
universal design for learning model and, 291–298, 295*f*
Temperament
metacognitive strategy instruction and, 279
reading comprehension in elementary school and, 204–205
Test preparation, 179, 179*f*, 180*f*
Test taking ability
checking strategies and, 252–254, 254*f*
classroom-based strategy instruction and, 179, 179*f*, 180*f*
learning disabilities and, 83
mathematics learning and, 255–257
planning and goal setting, 171–172
Testing, accommodations in
assistive technology and, 289
autism spectrum disorders and, 141, 142*t*–143*t*
mathematics learning and, 253, 255–257
Testing adaptations, 142*t*
Testing, high-stakes
assessment of executive function processes and, 86
learning disabilities and, 11, 101
Text structures, 125
Text variables
metacognitive strategy instruction and, 281
reading comprehension in elementary school and, 211–212
Thalamus, 10
Theory of mind, 22
Thinking Reader program, 298–306
Three-column note taking strategy
mathematics learning and, 246–247, 247*t*, 247*f*
overview, 179, 180*f*
Time management
autism spectrum disorders and, 151
learning disabilities and, 83
planning and goal setting, 171–172, 172*f*
reading comprehension in elementary school and, 199, 209–210
Tower Test
autism spectrum disorders and, 137, 138
nonverbal learning disabilities and, 111–112
overview, 91